# Cognitive Predictive M
# Tools for Brain D



This book involves the design, analysis, and application of various cognitive predictive maintenance tests with the help of tools like vibration analysis, ultrasonic analysis, infrared analysis, oil analysis, laser-shaft alignment, and motor circuit analysis in the prediction of various cognitive diseases such as epilepsy, Parkinson's disease, Alzheimer's disease, and depression. These are needed since there are no proper medical tests available to predict these diseases in remote areas at an early stage. Various emerging technologies are analyzed for the design of tests.

Key features:

- Incorporates innovative processes for treating cognitive diseases.
- Early and exact identification and treatment strategies are incorporated.
- Future technologies like artificial intelligence, machine learning, the IoT, and data science are used to find solutions.
- Analysis with existing cognitive disease solutions is incorporated and simulations provided.
- The novelty of the book lies in the accurate prediction of cognitive diseases.

Encompassing future technologies and various communication protocols or devices available for cognitive diseases for the design of new equipment are an outcome of the book. Various parameters like power consumption, productivity, and safety should be taken into account during the analysis, design, and application of a product. The book could well be added to the curriculum of medical colleges and biomedical engineering students. Possible vendors include biomedical research centers like Biotechnika and the Indian Council of Medical Research (ICMR). It would be a breakthrough for biomedical companies to launch their new products.

## Chapman & Hall/CRC Internet of Things: Data-Centric Intelligent Computing, Informatics, and Communication

The role of adaptation, machine learning, computational Intelligence, and data analytics in the field of IoT systems is becoming increasingly essential and intertwined. The capabilities of intelligent systems are growing, depending on various self-decision-making algorithms in IoT devices. IoT-based smart systems generate a large amount of data that cannot be processed by traditional data processing algorithms and applications. Hence, this book series involves different computational methods incorporated within the system with the help of analytics reasoning, learning methods, artificial intelligence, and sense-making in big data, which are effected in an IoT-enabled environment.

This series focuses on attracting researchers and practitioners who work in information technology and computer science within the field of the intelligent computing paradigm, big data, machine learning, sensor data, the IoT, and the data sciences. The main aim of the series is to make available a range of books on all aspects of learning, analytics, and advanced intelligent systems and related technologies. The series covers the theory, research, development, and applications of learning, computational analytics, data processing, and machine learning algorithms, as embedded in the fields of engineering, computer science, and information technology.

***Series Editors*:**
**Souvik Pal**
Sister Nivedita University, (Techno India Group), Kolkata, India

**Dac-Nhuong Le**
Haiphong University, Vietnam

*Security of Internet of Things Nodes: Challenges, Attacks, and Countermeasures*
Chinmay Chakraborty, Sree Ranjani Rajendran and Muhammad Habib Ur Rehman

*Cancer Prediction for Industrial IoT 4.0: A Machine Learning Perspective*
Meenu Gupta, Rachna Jain, Arun Solanki and Fadi Al-Turjman

*Cloud IoT Systems for Smart Agricultural Engineering*
Saravanan Krishnan, J Bruce Ralphin Rose, NR Rajalakshmi, N Narayanan Prasanth

*Data Science for Effective Healthcare Systems*
Hari Singh, Ravindara Bhatt, Prateek Thakral and Dinesh Chander Verma

*Internet of Things and Data Mining for Modern Engineering and Healthcare Applications*
Ankan Bhattacharya, Bappadittya Roy, Samarendra Nath Sur, Saurav Mallik and Subhasis Dasgupta

*Energy Harvesting: Enabling IoT Transformations*
Deepti Agarwal, Kimmi Verma and Shabana Urooj

*SDN-Supported Edge-Cloud Interplay for Next Generation Internet of Things*
Kshira Sagar Sahoo, Arun Solanki, Sambit Kumar Mishra, Bibhudatta Sahoo and Anand Nayyar

*Internet of Things: Applications for Sustainable Development*
Niranjan Lal, Shamimul Qamar, Sanyam Agarwal, Ambuj Kumar Agarwal and Sourabh Singh Verma

*Artificial Intelligence for Cognitive Modeling: Theory and Practice*
Pijush Dutta, Souvik Pal, Asok Kumar and Korhan Cengiz

*Cognitive Predictive Maintenance Tools for Brain Diseases: Design and Analysis*
Shweta Gupta

# Cognitive Predictive Maintenance Tools for Brain Diseases

## Design and Analysis

Edited by
Shweta Gupta

CRC Press
Taylor & Francis Group
Boca Raton London New York

CRC Press is an imprint of the
Taylor & Francis Group, an **informa** business
A CHAPMAN & HALL BOOK

**Chapter 10** Prediction and Maintenance of Alzheimer's Disease using Ultrasound and Infrared Spectroscopy Sensors/Augmented Reality Techniques.............................. 158

*Sasi Smitha and B. V. Srividya*

**Chapter 11** Deep Learning in Mental Illnesses: Understanding Networks................................ 174

*Priya Dev and Abhishek Pathak*

**Index**........................................................................................................................................ 187

# Note on the Editor

**Shweta Gupta** is an all-India topper in her 12th standard and has been awarded Senior Scientist by the Science and Engineering Research Board, Department of Science and Technology, Government of India. She received her doctorate from Dr. K. N. Modi University, Newai, Rajasthan, and also has a degree in Executive Global Business Management from I.I.M. Lucknow, Noida Campus. Her main area of research incorporates cognitive diseases and their treatment. She has published books with international publishers like IGI Global. She was chosen at a very young age to be Section Editor for the journal *Chip Design and Manufacturing*." She is a senior member of the Hong Kong Group of Conferences and has been invited as a speaker at the International Conference on Bioinformatics and Biomedical Technology (ICBBT) 2023, Xi'an China Conference for her work as Session Chair. She is part of the Elsevier Advisory Panel, Amsterdam, the Netherlands. She was Second Runner-up in the TechGig NTT Data Hackathon with a cash prize of Rs. 75,000 in which she demonstrated early prediction of epilepsy. She is a research consultant providing medical solutions for medical and health sciences in Malaysian organizations.

# Contributors

**N. Amuthan**
AMC Engineering College
Bengaluru, India

**K. Anusha**
Jain University
Bengaluru, India

**Meenakshi Bannerjee**
O.P. Jindal Global University
Sonepat, Haryana, India

**Priya Dev**
Banaras Hindu University
Varanasi, India

**B. Gopal Samy**
V.S.B. Engineering College
Karur, Tamil Nadu, India

**Shweta Gupta**
Woxsen University
Telangana, India

**Mohamed Jebran P.**
Jain University
Bengaluru, India

**M. S. Jyothi**
AMC Engineering College
Bengaluru, India

**Sanjay Kumar**
Amity University
Rajasthan, India

**Abhishek Pathak**
Banaras Hindu University
Varanasi, India

**M. S. Rohokale**
SKN Sinhgad Institutes of Technology and Science
Pune, India

**Sasi Smitha**
Dayanand Sagar College of Engineering
Bengaluru, India

**B. V. Srividya**
Dayanand Sagar College of Engineering
Bengaluru, India

**Sangeeta Avinash Tripathi**
SKN Sinhgad Institutes of Technology and Science
Pune, India

# 1 The Brain
## *Its Structure and Functions*

*K. Anusha*
Jain University, Bengaluru, India

*Shweta Gupta*
Woxsen University, Telangana, India

## 1.1 INTRODUCTION

The brain is the mass of nerve tissue that forms a major portion of the central nervous system and is located in the anterior portion of the skull. In appearance the brain can be compared to a walnut that is deeply folded. It is made up of billions of brain cells called neurons (Jorfi et al. 2018). The structure of a neuron is composed of an axon, dendrites, and soma. Axons are the neuron projections that transmit electrical and chemical signals from the brain to other parts of the body. Dendrites are the root-like structures of the neuron that receive signals from other nerve cells. Soma is the core of a neuron that contains genetic information (Birey et al. 2017).

The brain is composed of 60% fat and 40% a combination of water, protein, carbohydrates, and salts (Pistell et al. 2010). The brain itself is a not a muscle. It contains blood vessels and nerves, including neurons and glial cells.

It functions as a primary receiver, organizer, and distributor of information for the body. The transfer of information between the brain cells is due to the transmission of electrical and chemical signals throughout the nervous system in the body. Different signals control different processes, and your brain interprets each one. The brain integrates sensory information and directs motor responses throughout the body (Risso & Valle 2022).

An adult brain on average weighs 1.4 kg (3 lb) and its weight is known to decrease with age (Schwartz et al. 2022). The male brain's weight is 9.8% greater than that of the female brain. This decrease in weight starts at about 50–60 years of age and this progressive decline reach its maximum at the age of 85–90 years, by which time the average weight is reduced by 11% in comparison to the maximum weight in young adults (Brion et al. 2021).

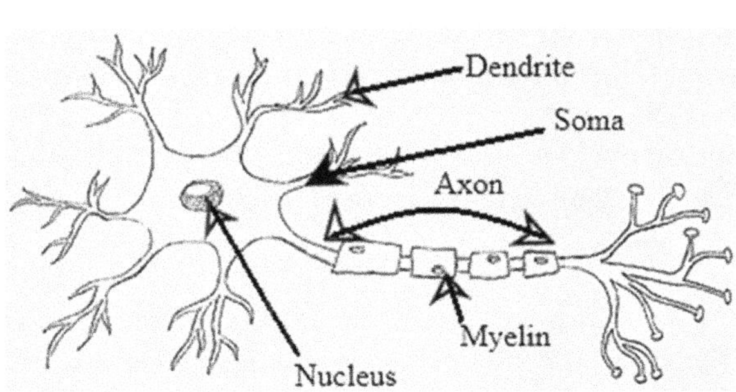


**FIGURE 1.1** Structure of a neuron.

DOI: 10.1201/9781003245346-1

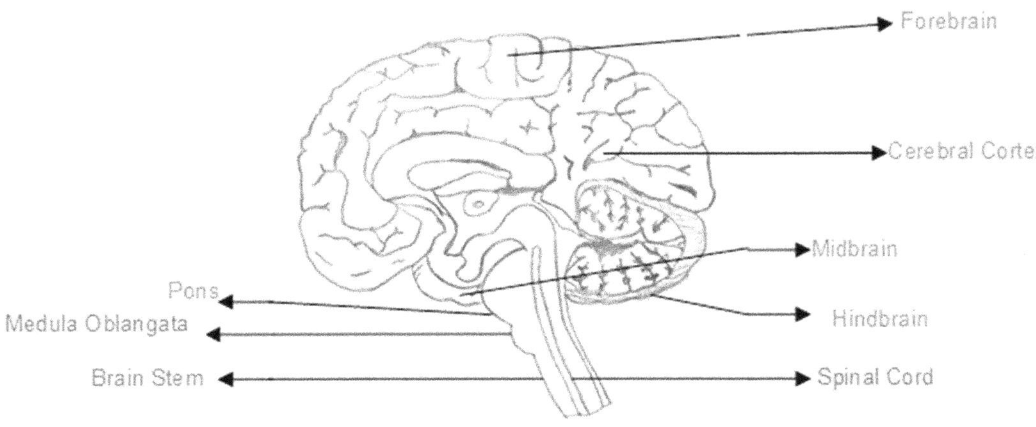


**FIGURE 1.2** Structure of the brain.

## 1.2 STRUCTURE OF THE BRAIN

The brain structure is divided into three main sections:

1. Forebrain;
2. Midbrain;
3. Hindbrain.

### 1.2.1 FOREBRAIN

The cerebrum and cerebral cortex constitute the forebrain. The cerebrum is the largest area of the brain and the cerebral cortex is the outer layer that covers the cerebrum. The cerebral cortex is made up of grey matter that comprises cell bodies and dendrites and it covers the internal white matter (Bit et al. 2021). The cerebrum is made up of both grey and white matter and comprises both cell bodies and nerve fibres. The cerebral cortex contains only grey matter as this section of the nerve lacks the fatty covering material called myelin (white matter). The cerebrum contains both grey and white matter (Hoppstädter et al. 2022).

#### 1.2.1.1 The Cerebrum

The cerebrum defines an individual's personality. It is also responsible for intelligence, memory, personality, emotion, speech, and the ability to feel and move, that is, voluntary muscular movements.

The cerebrum is divided into a right and a left half, called right and left hemispheres. Both halves are connected by a set of nerve fibres called the corpus callosum, which facilitates communication between the two hemispheres. Both hemispheres carry different functions and control different parts of the body (Grant et al. 2021).

The left side is considered the logical, analytical, and objective side. The right side is thought to be more intuitive, creative, and subjective (Assaneo et al. 2019).

#### 1.2.1.2 The Cortex

The cerebral cortex is the outermost covering of the brain's surface. It consists of between 14 and 16 billion nerve cells. The cerebral cortex is responsible for higher-order thinking, consciousness, imagination, language, memory, perception, learning, reasoning, sensation, and problem-solving (Budson et al. 2022).

The sensory information of the sense organs are first transmitted to the cells in the cortex of the brain. This information is then directed to other parts of the nervous system through nerves and neurons in the form of chemical and electrical signals.

The cortex is further divided into four functional sections called lobes. These lobes are named after the overlying cranial bones, namely the frontal, parietal, temporal, and occipital lobes (Bazira 2021).

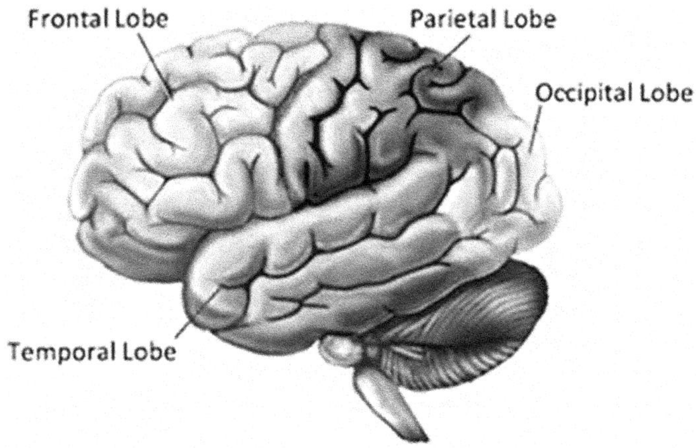


**FIGURE 1.3** The four lobes of the forebrain.

- **The frontal lobe** lies just beneath the forehead. The functions of the frontal lobe regulate attention, concentration, self-monitoring, organization, facial expression, speaking, spontaneity, personality, flexibility, problem-solving behaviour, and the emotions (Tucker & Luu 2023).
- **The parietal lobe** is located at the upper rear portion of brain, and controls complex behaviours, including: vision; touch; body awareness and spatial perception; the ability to identify different sizes, shapes, and colours; judgement; emotions; body positioning and movement; organization; and problem solving (Crowe-Riddell & Lillywhite 2023).
- **The occipital lobe** is located at the back of the brain and is mainly associated with visual processing, such as visual recognition, visual attention, and visual perception of body language, such as posture, expression, and gesture (Arioli et al. 2021).
- **The temporal lobe** is located near the ears and controls visual perception, memory, language comprehension including spoken language, verbal memory, visual memory, language fluency and word-finding, general knowledge, hearing, and sequencing (Chandregowda et al. 2021).

The inner part of the forebrain consists of:

- The thalamus, which coordinates movement and transmits sensory information from other parts of the body to the cortex.
- The hypothalamus, which is a collection of nuclei present along the base of the brain near the pituitary gland. It is responsible for controlling many body functions like hunger, thirst, emotion, body temperature regulation, and circadian movements. It also controls the pituitary gland and hormones that regulate stress, sexual maturity, growth, metabolism, and also balance the water and mineral contents of the body (Timothy & Forlano 2020).
- The pituitary gland is the size of a pea. It is the connecting bridge between the endocrine and nervous system. It is responsible for regulating thyroid-stimulating hormones, adrenocorticotropic hormones, prolactin, sex hormones, follicle-stimulating hormones, luteinizing hormones, growth hormones, melanocyte-stimulating hormones, and dopamine. It also responds to signals from the hypothalamus (Bhushan et al. 2022).
- The pineal gland produces melatonin, the hormone that controls skin pigmentation. The gland has been called a "third eye" because it is controlled by neurons sensitive to light.

### 1.2.2 The Midbrain

The midbrain is the smallest part of the brainstem at a length of 2 cm. It is a connecting bridge between the hindbrain and forebrain. It is located between the thalamus and pons. The midbrain is also known as the mesencephalon as it develops from the mesencephalon of the neural tube and connects the pons to the forebrain (Rahimi-Balaei et al. 2022). It contains relay nuclei for two of the cranial nerves, namely the oculomotor and trochlear nerves that are responsible for processing auditory and visual information. It regulates eye and eyelid movement.

The midbrain is composed of the (Sciacca et al. 2019):

- Tectum – the dorsal part of the midbrain that has four rounded lobes or colliculi that are called the corpora quadrigemina. The superior colliculi are involved in processing visual signals. The inferior colliculi are involved in processing auditory signals.
- Cerebral aqueduct – the canal that passes through the midbrain, which connects the third and fourth cerebral ventricles.
- Cerebral peduncle – which consists of thick nerve tracts connecting the forebrain to the hindbrain.
- Tegmentum – located anterior to the tectum. It contains various nerve tracts, the reticular formation, and cranial nerve nuclei. The two main regions are the red nucleus and the peri-aqueductal gray. It is involved in motor coordination.

The main functions of the midbrain are:

- A centre for visual and auditory reflexes.
- Involved in the processing of visual and auditory information.
- Regulates eye movement and pupil dilation. It is involved in regulating muscle movement and motor control. Together with the other parts of the brainstem, it controls vital autonomic functions. It is involved in regulating pain, mood, breathing, alertness, amongst others (Mesman & Smidt 2020).

#### 1.2.2.1 The Pons

The primary role of the pons is to serve as a bridge between various parts of the nervous system, including the cerebellum and cerebrum. Many important nerves originate in the pons, such as the trigeminal nerve, responsible for feeling in the face, as well as controlling the muscles that are responsible for biting, chewing, and swallowing. It also contains the abducens nerve, which allows us to look from side to side, and the vestibular cochlear nerve, which allows us to hear. As part of the brainstem, a section of the lower pons stimulates and controls the intensity of breathing, while a section of the upper pons decreases the depth and frequency of breaths (Zuperku et al. 2019). The pons is also associated with the control of sleep cycles, and controls respiration and reflexes. It is located above the medulla, below the midbrain, and just in front of the cerebellum. The pons participates in many sensory and autonomic processes such as motor control, arousal, maintaining equilibrium, respiratory functions, muscle tone, and the circadian cycle (Joseph et al. 2021).

#### 1.2.2.2 The Medulla

The primary role of the medulla is regulating our involuntary life-sustaining functions such as breathing, swallowing, and heart rate. As part of the brain stem, it also helps transfer neural messages to and from the brain and spinal cord. It is located at the junction of the spinal cord and brain.

### 1.2.3 The Hindbrain

The cerebellum or hindbrain got its name by its location, as it is present at the back of the head and looks partly tucked under the two cerebral hemispheres. In Latin "cerebellum" means "little brain" and it carries out the processing and sorting of signals necessary to maintain posture and balance, and to coordinate body movements. The cerebellum is considered the second largest part of the brain, its large surface area being accommodated within the skull by elaborate folding, which gives it an irregular, pleated look (Gur et al. 2021).

In humans, the cerebellum relays impulses for movement from the motor area of the cerebral cortex to the spinal cord; from there, they pass to their designated muscle groups. At the same time, the cerebellum receives impulses from the muscles and joints that are being activated and in some sense compares them with the instructions issued from the motor cortex, so that adjustments can be made. The cerebellum thus is neither the sole initiator of movement nor a simple link in the chain of nerve impulses, but a site for the rerouting and in some cases refining of instructions for movement. The right and left hemispheres of the cerebellum each connect with the nerve tracts from the spinal cord on the same side of the body, and with the opposite cerebral hemisphere. For example, nerve impulses concerned with movement of the left arm originate in the right cerebral hemisphere, and information about the orientation, speed, and force of the movement is fed back to the right cerebral hemisphere, through the left half of the cerebellum. The nerves responsible for movement at the ends of the arms and legs tend to have their origin near the outer edges of the cerebellum (Zhang 2019, Hou & Qi 2022).

## 1.3 BRAIN DISEASES

The brain is the control centre of the body. It regulates growth, development, and bodily functions. All of our thoughts, feelings, and actions begin there. A network of nerves carries signals to the spinal cord and brain from the body and the outside world. The brain processes the signals and sends responses back out through the spinal cord and nerves. A wide range of diseases and disorders affect the brain. They can alter a person's behaviour, personality, and their ability to process information and function. Many brain diseases impact a person's capacity to carry out daily activities (Jensen et al. 2020).

### 1.3.1 Types of Brain Diseases

There are many types of brain diseases, ranging from injuries and infections to brain tumours and dementia. They can impact on the ability to function and carry out daily activities. Outcomes vary widely depending on the type of disease, location, and severity of the condition.

**TABLE 1.1**
**The General Categories of Brain Diseases**

| Category | Description | Example |
|---|---|---|
| Neurodegenerative disease | Neurodegenerative disease is a broad category including any condition in which neurons lose function and eventually die. This category encompasses movement disorders (such as Parkinson's disease), neuromuscular disorders, and most types of dementia. The clinical presentation depends on which neurons are first affected, e.g., motor neurons in motor neurone disease; neurons in the substantia nigra in Parkinson's disease (Shadfar et al. 2022). | Motor neurone disease. Amyotrophic lateral sclerosis. |
| Dementias | Neurodegenerative diseases affecting higher cortical function and causing the loss of cognitive function to the point that it interferes with daily life. It affects skills such as memory, problem solving, language, and other thinking abilities (Monzio Compagnoni et al. 2020). | Alzheimer's disease. Fronto-temporal dementia. Lewy body disease. |
| Movement disorders | Brain disorders that impair the ability to move in some way. A movement disorder could impair voluntary movements (hypermobility, reduced, or slowed movement) or cause involuntary movements. | Parkinson's disease. Dystonia. Huntington's disease. |
| Neuromuscular disorders | Disorders that affect the muscles, the nerves that control them, and communication between the nerves and muscles. Symptoms vary depending on the severity of the disease but can range from numbness (with involvement of sensory nerve fibres) to muscle weakness and wasting (with involvement of motor nerve fibres or muscle) (Bachiller et al. 2020). | Muscular dystrophies. Peripheral neuropathy. Charcot-Marie-Tooth disorder. |

*(Continued)*

**TABLE 1.1 (Continued)**
**The General Categories of Brain Diseases**

| Category | Description | Example |
|---|---|---|
| Brain tumours | Brain tumours may involve growths of brain tissue or secondary deposits that have spread to the brain from cancer elsewhere in the body. Primary brain tumours may be benign, as in a meningioma and acoustic neuroma, or malignant as in many forms of glioma. There are many types of brain tumours which vary in cause and severity (Masmudi-Martín et al. 2021). | Gliomas. Meningiomas. Acoustic neuroma. |
| Cerebrovascular disease | Conditions that affect blood flow or the blood vessels in the brain. These diseases can cause clots or ruptured blood vessels, which can result in brain damage or stroke. | Stroke. Aneurysm. Arteriovenous malformations (AVM). |
| Concussion and traumatic brain injury (TBI) | Injury caused by external forces, such as falls, car crashes, sports injuries, or domestic violence incidents. TBIs vary in severity from concussion ("bruising" of the brain) to bleeding in the brain or coma. | Concussion.TBI. |
| Epilepsy | A long-term neurological disorder in which groups of neurons become spontaneously active, leading to seizures or "fits." A seizure can affect consciousness and cause convulsions or involuntary movements (Tidball et al. 2020). | Epilepsy. |
| Migraine and headache disorders | Headaches can be a symptom of an underlying medical condition, but headache disorders (or primary headache) more commonly occur without a significant underlying abnormality of the brain. Some headache disorders can significantly impact a person's quality of life (Ashina et al. 2021). | Migraine. Tension-type headache. Cluster headache. |
| Infections | Neurological infections occur when viruses or bacteria get into the brain or spinal cord. Meningitis is an infection of the outer covering of the brain and spinal cord, and encephalitis is an infection of the brain itself. | Meningitis. Encephalitis. |
| Inflammatory diseases | Neuroinflammatory diseases happen when the immune system misfires and attacks healthy cells. This can occur in various parts of the central nervous system, including the brain, spinal cord, optic nerves (e.g., MS, transverse myelitis), peripheral nerve (Guillain-Barré syndrome), and neuromuscular junction (e.g., myasthenia gravis). | Multiple sclerosis. Transverse myelitis. Guillain-Barré syndrome. |
| Paediatric neurology | Paediatric neurology is the study of brain diseases, disorders, and injuries in children and adolescents. These conditions could also fall into other categories, but the causes, symptoms, and treatments are often differe nt for children. | Cerebral palsy. Autism. Dyslexia. |

## 1.4 MEASURES TO MAINTAIN HEALTHY BRAIN FUNCTIONS

- Adopting a healthy lifestyle. This includes a heart-healthy diet, regular exercise, quitting smoking, limiting alcohol consumption, and reducing stress (Erickson et al. 2019).
- Avoiding excessive exposure to X-rays and other sources of radiation.
- Ensuring you and your loved ones are vaccinated against bacterial meningitis.
- Knowing the warning signs of a stroke and seeking immediate emergency medical care. Managing chronic health conditions, such as high blood pressure, high cholesterol, diabetes, and obesity (Penney et al. 2020).
- Reducing your risk of head trauma by preventing falls, wearing your seatbelt, and wearing a helmet when cycling or playing contact sports.
- Staying mentally and socially active.

### 1.4.1 Diagnosis of Disease

There are several ways to diagnose brain diseases, including:

1. Biopsy: Your healthcare provider collects a small sample of tissue for laboratory analysis. Biopsies help determine whether a brain tumour is cancerous or non-cancerous.
2. Diagnostic testing: These can include an electroencephalogram (EEG) to measure the brain's electrical activity. Evoked potential testing assesses the transmission of nerve signals to the brain.
3. Imaging tests: CT, MRI, and PET scans provide detailed images of the brain. They can detect brain activity and areas of disease or damage.
4. Laboratory tests: Blood, urine, stool, or spinal aid testing can help the healthcare provider understand what might be causing the symptoms. Genetic testing can identify gene mutations known to cause some brain diseases.
5. Mental function tests: The patient completes these tests on paper or on a computer. These allow the healthcare provider to evaluate memory, thinking, and problem-solving abilities.
6. Neurological examination: The healthcare provider will check for changes in balance, coordination, hearing, eye-movement, and speech (Armstrong & Okun 2020, Koike et al. 2021, Sengoku 2020, Tiwari et al. 2020).

## REFERENCES

Arioli, Maria, Emiliano Ricciardi, and Zaira Cattaneo. "Social Cognition in the Blind Brain: A Coordinate-Based Meta-Analysis." *Human Brain Mapping* 42, no. 5 (2021): 1243–56. doi:10.1002/hbm.25289.

Armstrong, Melissa J., and Michael S. Okun. "Diagnosis and Treatment of Parkinson Disease: A Review: A Review." *JAMA: The Journal of the American Medical Association* 323, no. 6 (2020): 548–60. doi:10.1001/jama.2019.22360.

Ashina, Messoud, Gisela M. Terwindt, Mohammad Al-Mahdi Al-Karagholi, Irene de Boer, Mi Ji Lee, Debbie L. Hay, Laura H. Schulte, et al. "Migraine: Disease Characterisation, Biomarkers, and Precision Medicine." *Lancet* 397, no. 10283 (2021): 1496–1504. doi:10.1016/S0140-6736(20)32162-0.

Assaneo, M. Florencia, Pablo Ripollés, Joan Orpella, Wy Ming Lin, Ruth de Diego-Balaguer, and David Poeppel. "Spontaneous Synchronization to Speech Reveals Neural Mechanisms Facilitating Language Learning." *Nature Neuroscience* 22, no. 4 (2019): 627–32. doi:10.1038/s41593-019-0353-z.

Bachiller, Sara, Isabel M. Alonso-Bellido, Luis Miguel Real, Eva María Pérez-Villegas, José Luis Venero, Tomas Deierborg, José Ángel Armengol, and Rocío Ruiz. "The Ubiquitin Proteasome System in Neuromuscular Disorders: Moving beyond Movement." *International Journal of Molecular Sciences* 21, no. 17 (2020): 6429. doi:10.3390/ijms21176429.

Bazira, Peter J. "An Overview of the Nervous System." *Surgery* 39, no. 8 (2021): 451–62. doi:10.1016/j.mpsur.2021.06.012.

Bhushan, Rashmi, V. Ravichandiran, and Nitesh Kumar. "An Overview of the Anatomy and Physiology of the Brain." In *Nanocarriers for Drug-Targeting Brain Tumors*, 3–29. Elsevier, 2022.

Birey, Fikri, Jimena Andersen, Christopher D. Makinson, Saiful Islam, Wu Wei, Nina Huber, H. Christina Fan, et al. "Assembly of Functionally Integrated Human Forebrain Spheroids." *Nature* 545, no. 7652 (2017): 54–59. doi:10.1038/nature22330.

Bit, Arindam, Khemraj Deshmukh, and Shashikanta Tarai. "Brain Engineering Mechanics for Cognitive Modeling." In *Neurocognitive Perspectives of Prosocial and Positive Emotional Behaviours*. IOP Publishing, 2021.

Brion, Luc P., Roy Heyne, and Cheryl S. Lair. "Correction: Role of Zinc in Neonatal Growth and Brain Growth: Review and Scoping Review." *Pediatric Research* 89, no. 7 (2021): 1871. doi:10.1038/s41390-021-01425-6.

Budson, Andrew E., Kenneth A. Richman, and Elizabeth A. Kensinger. "Consciousness as a Memory System." *Cognitive and Behavioral Neurology: Official Journal of the Society for Behavioral and Cognitive Neurology* 35, no. 4 (2022): 263–97. doi:10.1097/WNN.0000000000000319.

Chandregowda, Adithya, Heather M. Clark, Joseph R. Duffy, Mary M. Machulda, Val J. Lowe, Jennifer L. Whitwell, and Keith A. Josephs. "Dynamic Aphasia as a Variant of Frontotemporal Dementia." *Cognitive and Behavioral Neurology: Official Journal of the Society for Behavioral and Cognitive Neurology* 34, no. 4 (2021): 303–18. doi:10.1097/WNN.0000000000000289.

Crowe-Riddell, Jenna M., and Harvey B. Lillywhite. "Sensory Systems." In *Health and Welfare of Captive Reptiles*, 45–91. Cham: Springer International Publishing, 2023.

Erickson, Kirk I., Charles Hillman, Chelsea M. Stillman, Rachel M. Ballard, Bonny Bloodgood, David E. Conroy, Richard Macko, David X. Marquez, Steven J. Petruzzello, and Kenneth E. Powell. "Physical Activity, Cognition, and Brain Outcomes: A Review of the 2018 Physical Activity Guidelines: A Review of the 2018 Physical Activity Guidelines." *Medicine and Science in Sports and Exercise* 51, no. 6 (2019): 1242–51. doi:10.1249/mss.0000000000001936.

Grant, Madison K., Anastasia M. Bobilev, Audrey Branch, and James D. Lauderdale. "Structural and Functional Consequences of PAX6 Mutations in the Brain: Implications for Aniridia." *Brain Research* 1756, no. 147283 (2021): 147283. doi:10.1016/j.brainres.2021.147283.

Gur, Ruben C., Ellyn R. Butler, Tyler M. Moore, Adon F. G. Rosen, Kosha Ruparel, Theodore D. Satterthwaite, David R. Roalf, et al. "Structural and Functional Brain Parameters Related to Cognitive Performance across Development: Replication and Extension of the Parieto-Frontal Integration Theory in a Single Sample." *Cerebral Cortex (New York, N.Y.: 1991)* 31, no. 3 (2021): 1444–63. doi:10.1093/cercor/bhaa282.

Hoppstädter, Mayra, Denise Püllmann, Robert Seydewitz, Ellen Kuhl, and Markus Böl. "Correlating the Microstructural Architecture and Macrostructural Behaviour of the Brain." *Acta Biomaterialia* 151 (2022): 379–95. doi:10.1016/j.actbio.2022.08.034.

Hou, Jinqian, and Fengxue Qi. "TU-120. Noninvasive Brain Stimulation Combined with Exercise Intervention: A New Perspective in Treatment of Pregnancy Depression." *Clinical Neurophysiology: Official Journal of the International Federation of Clinical Neurophysiology* 141 (2022): S9. doi:10.1016/j.clinph.2022.07.024.

Jensen, Nicole Jacqueline, Helena Zander Wodschow, Malin Nilsson, and Jørgen Rungby. "Effects of Ketone Bodies on Brain Metabolism and Function in Neurodegenerative Diseases." *International Journal of Molecular Sciences* 21, no. 22 (2020). doi:10.3390/ijms21228767.

Jorfi, Mehdi, Carla D'Avanzo, Doo Yeon Kim, and Daniel Irimia. "Three-Dimensional Models of the Human Brain Development and Diseases." *Advanced Healthcare Materials* 7, no. 1 (2018): 1700723. doi:10.1002/adhm.201700723.

Joseph, Vincent, Aida Bairam, and John L. Carroll. "Control of Breathing during Sleep and Wakefulness in the Fetus, Newborn, and Child." In *Pediatric Sleep Medicine*, 19–31. Cham: Springer International Publishing, 2021.

Koike, Shinsuke, Saori C. Tanaka, Tomohisa Okada, Toshihiko Aso, Ayumu Yamashita, Okito Yamashita, Michiko Asano, et al. "Brain/MINDS beyond Human Brain MRI Project: A Protocol for Multi-Level Harmonization across Brain Disorders throughout the Lifespan." *NeuroImage. Clinical* 30, no. 102600 (2021): 102600. doi:10.1016/j.nicl.2021.102600.

Masmudi-Martín, M., L. Zhu, M. Sanchez-Navarro, N. Priego, M. Casanova-Acebes, V. Ruiz-Rodado, E. Giralt, and M. Valiente. "Brain Metastasis Models: What Should We Aim to Achieve Better Treatments?" *Advanced Drug Delivery Reviews* 169 (2021): 79–99. doi:10.1016/j.addr.2020.12.002.

Mesman, Simone, and Marten P. Smidt. "Acquisition of the Midbrain Dopaminergic Neuronal Identity." *International Journal of Molecular Sciences* 21, no. 13 (2020): 4638. doi:10.3390/ijms21134638.

Monzio Compagnoni, Giacomo, Alessio Di Fonzo, Stefania Corti, Giacomo P. Comi, Nereo Bresolin, and Eliezer Masliah. "The Role of Mitochondria in Neurodegenerative Diseases: The Lesson from Alzheimer's Disease and Parkinson's Disease." *Molecular Neurobiology* 57, no. 7 (2020): 2959–80. doi:10.1007/s12035-020-01926-1.

Penney, Jay, William T. Ralvenius, and Li-Huei Tsai. "Modeling Alzheimer's Disease with IPSC-Derived Brain Cells." *Molecular Psychiatry* 25, no. 1 (2020): 148–67. doi:10.1038/s41380-019-0468-3.

Pistell, Paul J., Christopher D. Morrison, Sunita Gupta, Alecia G. Knight, Jeffrey N. Keller, Donald K. Ingram, and Annadora J. Bruce-Keller. "Cognitive Impairment Following High Fat Diet Consumption Is Associated with Brain Inflammation." *Journal of Neuroimmunology* 219, no. 1–2 (2010): 25–32. doi:10.1016/j.jneuroim.2009.11.010.

Rahimi-Balaei, Maryam, Hassan Marzban, and Richard Hawkes. "Early Cerebellar Development in Relation to the Trigeminal System." *Cerebellum (London, England)* 21, no. 5 (2022): 784–90. doi:10.1007/s12311-022-01388-2.

Risso, Gaia, and Giacomo Valle. "Multisensory Integration in Bionics: Relevance and Perspectives." *Current Physical Medicine and Rehabilitation Reports* 10, no. 3 (2022): 123–30. doi:10.1007/s40141-022-00350-x.

Schwartz, Kenneth A., Mary Noel, Michele Nikolai, Lawrence K. Olson, Norman G. Hord, Micheal Zakem, Justin Clark, Mohamed Elnabtity, Bryan Figueroa, and Howard T. Chang. "Long Term Survivals in Aggressive Primary Brain Malignancies Treated with an Adjuvant Ketogenic Diet." *Frontiers in Nutrition* 9 (2022): 770796. doi:10.3389/fnut.2022.770796.

Sciacca, Sara, Jeremy Lynch, Indran Davagnanam, and Robert Barker. "Midbrain, Pons, and Medulla: Anatomy and Syndromes." *Radiographics: A Review Publication of the Radiological Society of North America, Inc* 39, no. 4 (2019): 1110–25. doi:10.1148/rg.2019180126.

Sengoku, Renpei. "Aging and Alzheimer's Disease Pathology." *Neuropathology: Official Journal of the Japanese Society of Neuropathology* 40, no. 1 (2020): 22–29. doi:10.1111/neup.12626.

Shadfar, Sina, Mariana Brocardo, and Julie D. Atkin. "The Complex Mechanisms by Which Neurons Die Following DNA Damage in Neurodegenerative Diseases." *International Journal of Molecular Sciences* 23, no. 5 (2022): 2484. doi:10.3390/ijms23052484.

Tidball, Andrew M., Luis F. Lopez-Santiago, Yukun Yuan, Trevor W. Glenn, Joshua L. Margolis, J. Clayton Walker, Emma G. Kilbane, et al. "Variant-Specific Changes in Persistent or Resurgent Sodium Current in SCN8A-Related Epilepsy Patient-Derived Neurons." *Brain: A Journal of Neurology* 143, no. 10 (2020): 3025–40. doi:10.1093/brain/awaa247.

Timothy, Miky, and Paul M. Forlano. "Serotonin Distribution in the Brain of the Plainfin Midshipman: Substrates for Vocal-Acoustic Modulation and a Reevaluation of the Serotonergic System in Teleost Fishes." *The Journal of Comparative Neurology* 528, no. 18 (2020): 3451–78. doi:10.1002/cne.24938.

Tiwari, Arti, Shilpa Srivastava, and Millie Pant. "Brain Tumor Segmentation and Classification from Magnetic Resonance Images: Review of Selected Methods from 2014 to 2019." *Pattern Recognition Letters* 131 (2020): 244–60. doi:10.1016/j.patrec.2019.11.020.

Tucker, Don M., and Phan Luu. "Adaptive Control of Functional Connectivity: Dorsal and Ventral Limbic Divisions Regulate the Dorsal and Ventral Neocortical Networks." *Cerebral Cortex (New York, N.Y.: 1991)*, 2023. doi:10.1093/cercor/bhad085.

Zhang, Jiawei. "Secrets of the Brain: An Introduction to the Brain Anatomical Structure and Biological Function." *ArXiv [q-Bio.NC]*, 2019. http://arxiv.org/abs/1906.03314.

Zuperku, Edward J., Astrid G. Stucke, John G. Krolikowski, Jack Tomlinson, Francis A. Hopp, and Eckehard A. Stuth. "Inputs to Medullary Respiratory Neurons from a Pontine Subregion That Controls Breathing Frequency." *Respiratory Physiology & Neurobiology* 265 (2019): 127–40. doi:10.1016/j.resp.2018.06.011.

# 2 The Current Status of Cognitive Disorders and Their Diagnosis

*Priya Dev and Abhishek Pathak*
Banaras Hindu University, Varanasi, India

## 2.1 INTRODUCTION

The mental action or process of learning via experience, thought, and the senses is known as cognition. It includes a variety of high-level cognitive processes and activities, including language, planning, reasoning, judgement, perceptual comprehension, decision-making, and visuospatial function. Cognitive processes produce new information while also using current information.

The phrase "cognitive deficit" is all-inclusive and used to describe the impairment of several cognitive areas. A person's cognitive deficiency may be one of the symptoms of an underlying disorder; it is not specific to any one disease or condition. Additionally, the terms "cognitive impairment" as well as this one are interchangeable. It could be a transient ailment or a developing, long-lasting one. However, cognitive disorders, which are a subset of neurocognitive disorders, constitute a larger category (DSM-5). Any condition that severely damages a person's cognitive abilities to the point that it is hard for them to function normally in society without treatment is referred to as a cognitive disorder. The most well-known ailment linked to cognitive decline is Alzheimer's disease.

Age-related cognitive deficits can be brought on by disorders including stroke, delirium, dementia, depression, schizophrenia, persistent alcohol use, drug misuse, brain tumours, vitamin deficiencies, hormone imbalances, and some chronic illnesses. Cognitive deficiencies are a symptom of brain diseases such Alzheimer's disease, Parkinson's disease, Lewy body dementia, Huntington's disease, HIV dementia, and prion disease. Drugs including glucocorticoids, anticholinergics, sedatives, and tranquillizers are also linked to cognitive deficiencies. Cognitive abnormalities can occur at any age as a result of head trauma, brain infections, or meningeal infections (Belanoff et al. 2001; Kalachnik et al. 2002).

It is challenging to forecast and poorly documented how frequently cognitive deficiency arises from different sources. The most significant reason for cognitive deterioration, though, is ageing. The most well-known ailment linked to cognitive decline is Alzheimer's disease. In the USA, the condition affects around 5.5 million individuals, and more than 24 million people are thought to have it globally. The age-specific incidence of Alzheimer's disease rises markedly from less than 1% per year before the age of 65 to 6% per year beyond the age of 85 (Mayeux and Stern 2012; Rajan et al. 2019).

Neuronal tissue destruction is the main pathophysiology underlying cognitive decline or deficiencies. Damage to the white matter, which consists of the axon sheaths protecting the connections between the grey matter regions, as well as the grey matter itself, which includes the cortex, thalamus, and basal ganglia, is also included in this. Deficits in certain regions are the result of damage in those areas. For instance, impairment of visuospatial or dressing abilities may result from parietal lobe injury. Deficiencies in planning can result from injury to the frontal lobe systems, whereas deficits in language and memory can result from damage to the temporal lobes and abstract understanding (Dhakal and Bobrin 2023).


DOI: 10.1201/9781003245346-2

The causes of this damage include neurotoxicity brought on by metabolic problems, heavy metals, or other toxins like toluene, as well as infections, ischemia damage brought on by stroke or haemorrhage, direct traumas such as head trauma, malignancy, or surgery. Neurodegenerative conditions including Alzheimer's, Parkinson's, multiple sclerosis, or Huntington's disease can also result in damage. These conditions seem to interact immunologically with aberrant proteins to directly harm neural tissue. Therefore, we will cover the present state of several cognitive illnesses and their diagnosis in this chapter.

## 2.2 LEWY BODY DEMENTIA

After Alzheimer's disease (AD), Lewy body dementia (LBD) is the most common neurodegenerative condition confirmed to cause dementia. There is a huge discrepancy between the number of cases diagnosed clinically and those diagnosed by neuropathology. As a result, it is essential to correctly identify dementia with Lewy body (DLB) since these patients need a particular kind of care.

### 2.2.1 Epidemiology

In the USA, 1.4 million individuals are affected by LBD. According to prevalence estimates, DLB accounts for 4.2% of dementia diagnoses in community settings and 7.5% of diagnoses in healthcare. DLB has been demonstrated to contribute 3.8% of new dementia diagnoses (Jones and O'Brien 2014). The most important risk factor for DLB is age, with the majority of patients showing clinical symptoms between the ages of 70 and 85 (Sanford 2018). About 5% of all instances of dementia in adults over 75 are caused by DLB. It occurs 3.5/10,000 times per person-year (Marder et al. 2010). Men are more likely than women to have DLB.

### 2.2.2 Pathogenesis

The development of an unusual aggregation of α-synuclein proteins within the brain is a characteristic feature of LBD. The Lewy bodies and Lewy neurites are formed by these aggregations (Walker et al. 2015). LBD has a complex underlying pathogenic aetiology that can cause the neuronal reserve to rise or fall. These α-synuclein proteins build up, impairing the neurons' ability to function, and eventually killing them (Taylor et al. 2020). The presynaptic nerve terminals of the brain express α-synuclein, a 140 amino acid (AA) protein, in large amounts (Cheignon et al. 2018; Mehra et al. 2019). It occurs in the cytoplasm as an unfolded monomer, but when a lipid membrane is present, it is likely to fold and transform into dimers and oligomers, accounting for roughly 1% of the protein content in the cytosol. It is found in modest amounts in the glial cells and in higher concentrations in regions of the brain such as the hippocampus, thalamus, and cerebellum. The SNCA gene, located on 4q21, is responsible for encoding α-synuclein. There are two more spliced versions of this protein in addition to the 140-AA version – the 126-AA and the 112-AA – both of which are missing exons 3 and 5 (Šerý et al. 2013). Three major domains make up the α-synuclein protein, and they are: (1) an amphipathic N-terminal region with the sequence KTKEGV and 11 AA repeats, which are important for α-synucleintetramerization and are helpful for helix formation; (2) the central hydrophobic region, which includes the protein aggregation-helpful non-amyloid component area; And (3) the proline-rich, acidic C-terminal region (Mehra et al. 2021). Synuclein proteins that are phosphorylated, shortened, and nitrated abnormally produce oligomeric species that cluster into fibrils and are ubiquitinated. They also exhibit abnormal solubility (Meade et al. 2019). This causes neurons to malfunction or die. The loss of neurons causes severe dopamine malfunction, noticeable cholinergic disease, and other neurotransmitter problems (Caviness et al. 2011; Gomperts 2016; Brás et al. 2020). Memory and learning suffer from the loss of acetylcholine-producing neurons, whereas sleep, behaviour, cognition, movement, and mood suffer from the death of dopamine-producing neurons. The key diagnostic criteria for LBD are the destruction of these neurons and the subsequent symptoms (Siderowf et al. 2018).

### 2.2.3 Clinical Symptoms

- Decline in cognition that is severe enough to interfere with everyday functioning or regular social or occupational activities is referred to as dementia (McKeith et al. 2017).
- Memory dysfunction, with a prevalence of 57%, was the most common complaint reported by DLB patients, followed by visual hallucinations (44%), depression (34%), problem-solving challenges (33%), gait disturbances (28%), and tremor and stiffness (25%), according to a study by Auning et al. (2011) that distinguished the presenting complaints of DLB and AD.
- A key clinical characteristic of DLB is cognitive fluctuations with varying degrees of attention and attentiveness (McKeith et al. 2017).
- The primary cognitive domains that are compromised in pervasive developmental disorders (PDDs) and DLB are executive, visuospatial, constructional, and memory abilities (Milán-Tomás et al. 2021).
- Due to the overlapping symptoms with toxic metabolic disease processes, it has historically been difficult to diagnose and measure fluctuating cognition. REM sleep behaviour disorder (RBD) is common in 76% of DLB patients (Boot 2015). It is a type of sleep disorder marked by movements, vocalizations, and behaviours that mimic dreams. This happens because there isn't the typical REM sleep atonia, which controls the excessive motor activity when we sleep (McKeith et al. 2017; McCarter et al. 2012).
- Within 15 years, between 70 and 90% of RBD patients will eventually acquire dementia, more frequently DLB (Walker et al. 2015).

### 2.2.4 Diagnostic Standards

- Recent research has led to modifications in the criteria, such as: separating clinical features from biomarkers, getting rid of the category "suggestive feature," elevating RBD to a core clinical characteristic, and relegating antipsychotic (neuroleptic) hypersensitivity to a supporting element (McKeith et al. 2017).
- Currently, the presence of both suggestive biomarkers and core clinical symptoms is used by clinicians to make the diagnosis of DLB (McKeith et al. 2017).
- Patients and caregivers frequently report memory impairments as a presenting symptom, despite the fact that DLB diagnostic criteria emphasize that evident or permanent memory impairment may not appear in the early stages (Auning et al. 2011). While these conditions do not rule out DLB and may show mixed or multiple pathologies contributing to the clinical presentation, they are much less likely to occur than DLB to occur if parkinsonian signs are the only fundamental clinical symptoms and present for the first time at a stage of severe dementia.
- DLB is also much less likely to occur if any other physical condition or neurological dysfunction, including cerebrovascular disease, is sufficient to account for part or even the entire clinical picture (McKeith et al. 2017).
- LBD imaging helps clinicians to distinguish the overlapping symptoms of LBD and AD, such as:
  a. SPECT/PET: Results show reduced basal ganglia uptake of the dopamine transporter in LBD.
  b. 123 I-MIBG scintigraphy: Results in LBD-specific decreased myocardial uptake.
  c. Polysomnography: REM sleep analysis which is very particular to LBD.

d. CT/MRI: No or mild medial temporal lobe atrophy seen on brain images. This makes a distinction between AD, PDD, and LBD.
e. FDG-PET: This detects medial temporal lobe hypometabolism.
f. EEG: Detects predominant posterior slow-wave activity with periodic variations in the pre-alpha/theta region, which are extremely perceptive and precise.

### 2.2.5 Challenges

- According to estimates, DLB is overlooked in one out of every three cases, and AD is frequently misdiagnosed (Thomas et al. 2017; Galvin et al. 2010).
- As we work toward an early diagnosis, biomarkers for LBD may be necessary to increase diagnostic accuracy.
- Inadequate biomarker availability, under-utilization of the potential DLB diagnosis, poor neuropsychological screening, and the prevalence of uncommon presentations are all factors that might make it difficult to diagnose (Prasad et al. 2022).

## 2.3 ACUTE DISSEMINATED ENCEPHALOMYELITIS (ADEM)

A common acute demyelinating condition of the central nervous system (CNS) is called ADEM. Worldwide reports of ADEM state that it is frequent in paediatric emergencies. Typically, a previous viral infection or vaccine causes ADEM to develop. The white matter of the brain, the brain stem, the optic nerves, and less commonly the spinal cord are all heavily involved in ADEM, which typically has a monophasic course.

### 2.3.1 Epidemiology

Per year, 9.83 out of 1 million children were diagnosed with first acquired demyelinating syndrome with clinically isolated syndrome (66.4%), ADEM (32.0%), and neuromyelitisoptica (1.6%) (Absoud et al. 2013). According to one research study, the incidence of ADEM among California residents under the age of 20 was 0.4 per 100,000 per year (Leake et al. 2004). Due to a high prevalence of several viral and bacterial diseases, including measles, ADEM is widespread in underdeveloped and resource-constrained nations (Murthy et al. 1999a; Murthy et al. 1999b).

### 2.3.2 Aetiology of the Disease

The onset of ADEM is frequently accompanied by a wide range of viral or bacterial diseases, although an upper respiratory tract infection is the most common precursor. It is difficult to pinpoint the infectious agent that causes certain individuals' illnesses. The risk of ADEM increases after exposure to measles and rubella. One frequent viral cause of ADEM is the H1N1 influenza virus (Tenembaum 2013; Wingerchuk and Weinshenker 2013; Noorbakhsh et al. 2008). In endemic areas, ADEM can also be brought on by malaria and filaria (Mani et al. 2011; Paliwal et al. 2012). Newly emerging causes of ADEM include stem cell and allogeneic bone marrow transplants (Paisiou et al. 2013).

### 2.3.3 Pathogenesis

Patients with ADEM are likely to have a hereditary vulnerability. The major histocompatibility complex class II alleles HLA-DRB1*1501 and HLA-DRB5*0101 have been linked in a research study from Korea. ADEM was discovered to be connected to DRB1*01 and DRB1*017 in Russia. The HLA-DQB1*0602, DRB1*1501, and DRB1*1503 alleles were strongly related with genetic vulnerability to ADEM in Brazil (Oh et al. 2004; Idrissova et al. 2003; Alves-Leon et al. 2009).

According to the molecular mimicking idea, certain myelin antigens may have structural similarities to the antigenic determinants found on the virus that causes ADEM. It is believed that the antibodies produced against the causing bacterium cross-react with myelin antigens, triggering an immunological reaction against neural tissue (Pohl-Koppe et al. 1998; Cusick et al. 2012; Wucherpfennig and Strominger 1995). As an alternative, the inflammatory cascade theory proposes that a neurotropic viral infection of the CNS results in the release of myelin-based autoantigens into the bloodstream via a disturbed blood-brain barrier. In the peripheral blood circulation, the immune system responds to these autoantigens and starts a chain reaction of inflammatory reactions. During this procedure, autoreactive T-cell clones are produced. These T cells enter the brain parenchyma after breaking through the blood-brain barrier, causing damage to the brain tissue (Miller et al. 2001; Richards et al. 2011). IgG autoantibodies against myelin basic protein, proteolipid protein, myelin-associated oligodendrocyte basic glycoprotein, and a-B-crystallin are markers for ADEM. T lymphocytes, lipid-rich macrophages, and less commonly neutrophil, esinophil, or plasma cell infiltrates make up the inflammatory lesions of ADEM. Axons are largely intact. The demyelinating lesions exhibit astrocytic proliferation and gliosis in the latter stages of the illness. All demyelinating lesions in ADEM are typically the same age and mostly impact white matter. More often than not, vaccine-related neurological disorders involve the peripheral nervous system (Habek and Žarković 2011; Young et al. 2010).

### 2.3.4 Clinical Manifestation

- The majority of ADEM's clinical symptoms are polysymptomatic and multifocal;
- Non-specific prodromal symptoms like fever, malaise, headaches, nausea, and vomiting appear before the actual clinical symptoms;
- The primary hallmark of ADEM is encephalopathy (obtundation, stupor, decerebrate posture, and coma) which appears seven days post-prodromal symptoms;
- Behaviour changes, such as bewilderment, impatience, and restlessness;
- Neurologic abnormalities such as vision loss, hemiparesis, paraparesis, ataxia, bladder dysfunction, sensory loss, and a range of mobility difficulties;
- Children are particularly susceptible to ataxia;
- In seriously afflicted individuals, a tentorial herniation may raise intracranial pressure and cause mortality;
- The peripheral nervous system may occasionally be affected as well (Marin and Callen 2013; Garg 2003).

### 2.3.5 Diagnostic Evaluation

- MRI findings that include meningismus, cerebrospinal fluid (CSF) pleocytosis, or multifocal enhancing lesions (Young et al. 2010).
- The CSF may show a small amount of lymphocytosis in severe and fulminant cases. In the acute stage, cells may be mostly polymorphonuclear. CSF protein levels are often high but rarely exceed 100 mg/dL.
- Up to 25% of cases may start out with oligoclonalIgG bands, although these may fade away later.
- Almost all ADEM patients can have white matter abnormalities shown on an MRI. The centrum semiovale, which connects the cerebellum, brainstem, spinal cord, and cortical white and grey matter, is where lesions are most frequently seen. The putamen is the structure of grey matter that is most commonly affected (Zhang et al. 2014).
- Demyelinating lesions in ADEM may exhibit a variety of patterns of enhancement, including patchy and fluffy, single or multiple ring-shaped, open ringed, nodular, gyral, and diffused. It may be necessary to biopsy a massive, mass-effect brain lesion (a tumefactive demyelinating lesion) in order to rule out an infectious or cancerous condition.

- The lesions can be identified and their stage determined using quantitative MRI methods including proton magnetic resonance spectroscopy and diffusion-weighted imaging. In the acute stage of ADEM lesions, there is limited diffusion; in the subacute stage, there is free diffusion and a decline in the N-acetyl aspartate/choline ratios (Balasubramanya et al. 2007).

## 2.4 ATTENTION DEFICIT HYPERACTIVITY DISORDER (ADHD)

One of the most prevalent neurodevelopmental disorders of non-age is ADHD. This is commonly diagnosed for the first time at a young age and continues throughout adulthood. Children with ADHD may struggle to focus, restrain impulsive behaviour, or behave excessively (Jaeschke et al. 2021). According to the DSM-IV, consideration, hyperactivity, and impulsivity are symptoms of ADHD. Although the World Health Organization (WHO) uses a different term for the complaint – hyperkinetic disorder – it cites comparable functional benchmarks. ADHD/HD, as it is commonly known, is one of the medical field's most in-depth disorders (Goldman et al. 1998). It has been linked to a broader variety of negative difficulties for those who are impacted as well as a grave burden on families and society. A comprehension of the epidemiological aspect of ADHD/HD may provide insight into its distribution and origin specifically (aetiology), as well as familiarity for convening the allocation of funds for internal health services over a period of ten years especially (decades), in which researchers across all countries around the world have made significant contributions (Bakare 2012).

### 2.4.1 Clinical Variants of ADHD

Depending on which symptoms are most prominent in a given person, there are three basic forms of ADHD:

- Predominantly inattentive presentation: It is challenging for the individual to control or overcome an activity. The individual is constantly nervous or forgets specific things of a mundane nature (Magnin and Maurs 2017).
- Predominantly impulsive-hyperactive presentation: The person develops suddenness and a talkative personality. Long-term immobility is challenging. Children may continually run, jump, or climb. The individual struggles with impulsivity and feels restless.
- Combined presentation: This has the combined or inverse forms of the previous two presentations (Wamulugwa et al. 2017).

### 2.4.2 Symptoms

Different types of ADHD present with various symptoms, some of which are:

- Talking excessively;
- Depression;
- Sleep problems;
- Anxiety;
- Daydreaming often;
- Specific learning disabilities;
- Struggling to get along with others;
- Hyperactivity-impulsivity. The American Academy of Pediatrics (AAP) advises that health care professionals inquire about a child's growing-up in a variety of contexts, including at home, school, or with peers, parents, preceptors, and other adults who monitor the child. The doctor should check what kinds of symptoms the youngster is experiencing (Faraone et al. 2021).

### 2.4.3 Diagnosis

The disorder of ADHD is particularly prevalent in non-age groups. It is a neurodevelopmental disorder characterized by age-inappropriate inattentiveness, hyperactivity, and impulsivity. Any youngster affected by this ailment will find it difficult to focus or pay attention. It is both a hereditary and environmental issue. At a young age, under 12, it is often introduced to the youngster. Some of the disease's very effective symptoms include children who have trouble playing and controlling their behaviour.

## 2.5 ALZHEIMER'S DISEASE (AD)

The Alzheimer's Association assigns 60–80% of dementia cases to AD, a degenerative brain illness. Depression, confusion, difficulty swallowing and walking, poor judgement, diminished interaction, and changes in behaviour are only a few of the characteristics of the condition that worsen to make it harder to do daily tasks (Alzheimer's Association 2021). Age, genetics, and sex are only a few examples of the variables that affect how long it takes for a continuum of these symptoms to emerge (Vermunt et al. 2019).

### 2.5.1 Prevalence

Approximately 13.8 million Americans aged 65 and older are expected to develop AD by the year 2060, according to current estimates, and the COVID-19 pandemic has seen a 16% rise in the number of deaths (Alzheimer's Association 2021). The overall cost of care payments for AD patients and associated disorders, excluding informal caring, was estimated at $355 billion in 2021.

### 2.5.2 Pathogenesis

Amyloid-beta (Ab) and tau protein aggregation is linked to the gradual cognitive deterioration in AD (Selkoe and Hardy 2016). Beta-secretase and gamma-secretase cleave the amyloid precursor protein (APP) in order to produce Ab. Ab aggregates into toxic oligomers that harm neurons as a result (Haass and Selkoe 2007). The alternative splicing of the micro-tubule-associated protein tau (MAPT) gene yields tau, which is then converted into soluble protein isoforms (Goedert et al. 1989). Ab and tau have a number of functional interactions that have been linked to cognitive decline and neuronal circuit destruction in AD (Tripathi and Kalita 2019; Busche and Hyman 2020).

Two theories are well known regarding the pathogenesis of AD: the neuronal intracellular accumulation of hyperphosphorylated tau protein to form neurofibrillary tangles (NFTs); and the neuronal extracellular deposition of Ab peptides (senile/amyloid plaques). However, synaptic disruption is the main underlying cause of the cognitive and behavioural impairment seen in AD. For instance, elevated Ab is linked to human neural dysfunction, and phosphorylated tau weakens synapses by aggregating in the dendritic spine and internalizing N-methyl-d-aspartic acid receptors (NMDARs) as a result (Sperling et al. 2009; Palop and Mucke 2010; Wesson et al. 2011). The development of AD has also been linked to elevated levels of inflammatory cytokines and related genes (Wesson et al. 2011; Hollingworth et al. 2011). Below is a discussion of some newly discovered neuromechanistic signalling pathways that have been linked to the pathophysiology of AD.

#### 2.5.2.1 The Metabolic Pathway of Nerve Growth Factor (NGF)

The neurotrophin family, which includes NGF, is essential for the proper operation of the central and peripheral neurological systems (PNSs). NGF is primarily released into the extracellular environment as a precursor protein (proNGF), which plasmin, a serine protease, subsequently cleaves to produce mature NGF (mNGF) (Bruno and Cuello 2006). The physiological functions of NGF are carried out by binding to two distinct cell-surface receptors, the tropomyosin-related kinase A (TrkA) receptor and the p75 neurotrophin receptor, following the release of proNGF by the post-synaptic neurons of the cortex and hippocampus and its conversion to mNGF (p75NTR). NGF travels retrogradely to the cell bodies of the innervating neurons, the BFCN, where it binds to its receptor, namely TrkA on pre-synaptic cholinergic neurons. This triggers a signalling cascade that leads to the release of acetylcholine. Plasmin-induced NGF maturation is positively regulated by the activators that turn plasminogen into plasmin – tissue plasminogen activator (tPA) and urokinase plasminogen activator (uPA) – and negatively regulated by the inhibitors of the activators – plasminogen activator inhibitor 1 (PAI-1) and neuroserpin. On the other hand, the tissue inhibitor of metalloproteinases 1 controls the breakdown of mNGF by activated matrix metalloproteinases (MMPs), such as MMP-9 release during neural activation (TIMP-1). ProMMP-9's conversion to MMP-9 is also caused by plasmin. It has also been demonstrated that MMP-3, a protease generated in response to cholinergic stimulation in cortical cells, degrades mNGF both *in vitro* and *in vivo* (Pentz et al. 2021).

At several points along the process, this coordinated set of actions is changed in AD. Inflammatory response brought on by decreased acetylcholine synthesis and elevated Ab levels altered the conversion of proNGF to mNGF, downregulated the TrkA receptor, impaired retrograde signalling and transport, increased mNGF degradation, amongst other factors (Mitra et al. 2019).

#### 2.5.2.2 The Signal Transducer and Activator of the Transcription Pathway: Janus Kinase

A direct method is provided by the Janus kinase/signal transducer and activator of transcription (JAK/STAT) pathways to ensure that an extracellular signal is converted into a transcriptional response. By transferring extracellular signals from ligands like cytokines, hormones, and growth factors to the nucleus, the JAK/STAT signalling system controls the expression of genes that respond to cytokines. This route is well recognized for controlling cellular processes like differentiation, apoptosis, and cell growth and proliferation. These ligands attach to their receptors and activate the four members of the JAK family: JAK1, JAK2, JAK3, and Tyk2 (tyrosine kinase 2). This will phosphorylate the JAKs and the receptors in turn. There are seven STAT proteins: STAT1, STAT2, STAT3, STAT4, STAT5, STAT6, and STAT7. As a result, STAT4, STAT5A, STAT5B, and STAT6 are recruited to the sites that the phosphorylated JAKs create. The STATs were phosphorylated, activated, and formed dimers as a result. Dimerized STATs go to the nucleus where they bind to certain regulatory regions to control gene expression (Kisseleva et al. 2002; Rawlings et al. 2002).

The significance of reactive oxygen species in activating the JAK/STAT signalling pathway strengthens the evidence that oxidative stress is connected to the aetiology of AD (Simon et al. 1998). Additionally, it has been demonstrated that inhibiting the JAK/STAT pathway through the control of Nrf2 signalling has a protective impact in AD (Sharma et al. 2020).

#### 2.5.2.3 The FGF7/FRFR2/PI3K/AKT Pathway

Growth factors for the fibroblast (FGFs) family are known to have 22 ligands, which is a huge family of proteins. They exercise their cellular and physiological effects, which include proliferation, angiogenesis, invasion, and migration, via binding to high-affinity tyrosine kinase receptors, or FGFRs. By phosphorylating certain tyrosine residues, this interaction activates the FGFR's intracellular tyrosine kinase domain. PI3K/AKT signalling is one of the downstream intracellular signalling pathways that the FGFR couple once it is active.

The mRNA levels of FGF7, a member of the FGF family, have been found to be increased in AD patients and cells treated with b-amyloid peptides (Ab). To further support this, it was demonstrated that overexpression of FGF7 in cells exposed to Ab was linked to a decrease in cell survival and proliferation rate. MiRNA expression has been found to be different in studies on the aetiology of AD and in AD experimental models (Samadian et al. 2021).

### 2.5.3 Clinical Symptoms

Clinical symptoms of AD are divided into three stages depending on the severity of the disease.

#### 2.5.3.1 Mild Alzheimer's Disease Symptoms

A person with mild AD may appear to be in good condition, but they will have increasing difficulty in understanding what is going on around them. The individual and his or her family frequently become aware that something is wrong over time. Issues may include:

- Loss of memory;
- Repeating enquiries;
- Poor decision-making due to poor judgement;
- Putting items in strange locations or losing things;
- Taking longer to finish routine everyday chores;
- Decline in initiative and spontaneity;
- Difficulty managing finances and paying debts;
- Changes in mood and personality;
- Wandering and being disoriented;
- Increased aggressiveness or anxiousness.

#### 2.5.3.2 Moderate Alzheimer's Disease Symptoms

For many spouses and families, this period requires more extensive monitoring and care, which can be challenging. Some signs might be:

- Forgetfulness;
- Inability to pick up new skills;
- Reduced duration of attention;
- Increased confusion and memory loss;
- Having trouble properly thinking and arranging one's ideas;
- Language challenges as well as issues with reading, writing, and dealing with numbers;
- Delusions, paranoia, and hallucinations;
- Difficulties adjusting to new circumstances;
- Having trouble distinguishing friends and relatives;
- Impulsive actions, such as changing into new clothes at unsuitable times or locations or using foul words;
- Difficulty doing complex chores, such as dressing;
- Wandering, crying, agitation, and restlessness, especially in the late afternoon or evening;
- Inappropriate outbursts of fury;
- Repetition of words or actions, as well as sporadic twitching of the muscles.

#### 2.5.3.3 Warning Signs of Advanced Alzheimer's

People who have advanced AD are fully reliant on others for their care and are unable to communicate. As the illness closes, the person may spend most of the time in bed. Their signs frequently consist of:

- Lack of communication.
- Lack of bladder and bowel control.
- Loss of weight.
- An increase in sleep.
- Skin maladies.
- Moaning, writhing, or gurgling.
- Seizures.
- Having trouble swallowing.

- Aspiration pneumonia is a common cause of mortality in patients with AD. When a person cannot swallow properly, food or liquids enter the lungs instead of air, leading to the development of this kind of pneumonia (Iqbal et al. 2013).

## 2.6 FRONTOTEMPORAL DEMENTIA (FTD)

Progressive abnormalities in behaviour, executive function, and language are hallmarks of FTD, a subtle neurodegenerative clinical condition. The condition is a prominent cause of early onset dementia and is the third most prevalent kind of dementia across all age groups, after AD and dementia with Lewy bodies.

### 2.6.1 Epidemiology

According to the WHO, the number of people with dementia will double every 20 years, reaching 115.4 million by 2050. FTD is the second or third most frequent dementia subtype in most studies, with a prevalence ranging from 3 to 26% in a meta-analysis of 73 publications on early onset dementia (patient age 65 years) (Knopman and Roberts 2011; Lambert et al. 2014; Hodges et al. 2003).

### 2.6.2 Symptoms

Three clinical types of FTD can present themselves, depending on the symptoms that may converge as an originally localized degeneration extends to vast areas of the frontal and temporal lobes. Patients gradually manifest global cognitive decline, motor impairments, including Parkinsonism, and in certain cases motor neurone disease. Patients with the advanced illness have trouble swallowing, moving, and eating. Pneumonia or other secondary infections are frequently the cause of death, which normally occurs approximately eight years after the beginning of symptoms. Three clinical types of FTD include the following.

#### 2.6.2.1 FTD with Behavioural Variants

Personality changes, disinhibition, and apathy characterize behavioural-variant FTD are its most evident early signs. Behavioural disinhibition can lead to impolite and socially inappropriate behaviour, such as: approaching strangers without acknowledging their physical and social boundaries; impulsive or careless actions, such as reckless spending; new criminal behaviours, such as theft, public urination, sexual advances, or hit-and-run accidents; as well as embarrassing personal remarks. Reduced inhibition frequently leads to poor financial judgement that can cause financial loss. Despite the possibility that they may express improper sexual comments, patients often have low libido. Apathy can be misinterpreted as depression since it shows itself as a loss of interest in cleanliness, social contact, hobbies, and employment. Patients display a lack of compassion and empathy for their loved ones, as well as a decline in social interest and receptivity to the feelings and needs of others. Patients often lack self-awareness and may not be able to identify many of the changes that an informant reports. Some people have reduced pain sensitivity (Miller and Boeve 2016).

#### 2.6.2.2 Primarily Progressive Non-fluent Aphasia

Non-fluent primary progressive aphasia is characterized by the omission or improper use of grammar as well as slow, laboured, and halting speech output (agrammatism). Including insertions, deletions, replacements, transpositions, and distortions, patients frequently create inconsistent speech problems. Mild grammatical mistakes are detected in written language output and syntactic comprehension tests early in the illness. Some people continue to write clearly despite having obvious spoken language difficulties (Gorno-Tempini et al. 2011).

#### 2.6.2.3 Primary Progressive Aphasia with Semantic Variation

The combination of semantic aphasia with associative agnosia is referred to as semantic dementia (Neary et al. 1998). Early asymmetrical degeneration of the amygdala and anterior temporal lobes causes the symptoms. Word difficulty, reduced word understanding, and anomia for persons, places, and objects are all symptoms of semantic loss. The right temporal lobe variation manifests with behavioural alterations, whereas the left temporal lobe version mostly exhibits language semantic loss (semantic-variant primary progressive aphasia) (Seeley et al. 2005). Surface dyslexia and dysgraphia, deficits in which words with unusual sounds or spelling are regularized, are present in patients. They also preserve good grammar and fluent speaking, and other language domains are spared, particularly in the early stages of the illness.

Behaviour changes, such as irritability, emotional disengagement, sleeplessness, and rigid or selective eating, sometimes centred around one particular food type, happen when the illness advances from the temporal lobes into the orbitofrontal cortex. Sometimes sadness also appears (Seeley et al. 2005). Although semantics are lost in the left temporal lobe version, right-side functions like visual attention are occasionally enhanced. As a result, those who have a left temporal lobe variation are more likely to acquire visual compulsions, such as the need to constantly solve puzzles, bead jewellery, collect money, garden, paint, and collect things that are brilliantly coloured. Contrarily, those who have a right temporal lobe variation experience linguistic compulsions involving words and symbols, such as the need to write down phone numbers, addresses, and notes, make puns, or play Solitaire.

### 2.6.3 Diagnosis

A number of procedures can be utilized to aid in the diagnosis of FTD. Structural MRI and CT indicate patterns of atrophy (Rosen et al. 2002). Single-photon-emission CT, functional MRI, and fluorodeoxyglucose PET all demonstrate disproportionate hypoperfusion and hypometabolism in the predominance of frontal or temporal atrophy, and atrophy in the frontoinsular areas (Le Ber et al. 2006).

Some people who match the diagnostic criteria for behavioural-variant FTD have a very delayed disease development (over decades) with gradual cognitive decline and frequently normal MRI and PET tests. FTD phenocopy is the name of their illness. Some of these people suffer from a main mental illness such as bipolar disorder, Asperger's syndrome, or a factitious disease (Davies et al. 2006; Kipps et al. 2010) whilst others may have a slow-moving sporadic or hereditary type of FTD (Khan et al. 2012).

A thorough history that considers the evolution of behavioural abnormalities, laboratory work, neuroimaging, family history, and performance in neuropsychological tests is required for the differential diagnosis of FTD.

Consideration should be given to inflammatory (autoimmune, paraneoplastic), toxic (heavy metals, illegal substances), or infectious (syphilis, HIV) causes. Obstructive sleep apnoea screenings for patients are recommended. Dementia that resembles behavioural-variant FTD may be brought on by normal pressure hydrocephalus and low intracranial pressure disorders. Low levels of β-amyloid in the cerebrospinal fluid are indicative of Alzheimer's disease, but extremely high levels of tau in the cerebrospinal fluid may be indicative of dementia that is quickly progressing. Although AD and FTD neuropathology can co-occur, β-amyloid imaging is useful, especially in young patients, to rule out AD. It may be necessary to seek genetic counselling and conduct a search for FTD-causing genes if there is a family history of dementia, movement abnormalities, or psychosis. The majority of instances with hereditary frontotemporal lobar degeneration (approximately 60%) are caused by mutations in the genes C9orf72, MAPT, and GRN (Le Ber 2013; Goldman et al. 2011).

Nearly all instances of frontotemporal lobar degeneration are caused by either the microtubule-associated protein tau (MAPT), the TAR DNA-binding protein with molecular weight 43 kDa (TDP-43), or the fused-in-sarcoma (FUS) protein. Frontotemporal lobar degeneration-tau, frontotemporal lobar degeneration-TDP, and frontotemporal lobar degeneration-FUS are the related pathogenic subgroups. There are several instances of frontotemporal lobar degeneration that feature inclusions that are positive solely for ubiquitin, only for p62, or not at all (Mackenzie et al. 2010).

## 2.7 EPILEPSY

### 2.7.1 Epidemiology

Epilepsy is a brain condition that can be distinguished by any of the following symptoms: at least two unprovoked (or reflex) seizures occurring more than 24 hours apart; one unprovoked (or reflex) seizure and a likelihood of subsequent seizures equal to the general recurrence risk (at least 60%) after two unprovoked seizures occurring within the next ten years; and a diagnosis of an epilepsy syndrome (Fisher et al. 2005; Fisher et al. 2014). The global lifetime prevalence of epilepsy is 7.6 per 1000 people, according to Fiest et al.'s meta-analysis (Fiest et al. 2017). Men are somewhat more likely to experience the incidence and prevalence than women.

### 2.7.2 Pathogenesis

Voltage-gated and transmitter-gated ion channels, which have the potential to make neurons electrically hyperactive, are the cause of epileptic seizures. Frequent seizures, especially status epilepticus, often result in oxidative stress, neuronal death (mostly in the entorhinal cortex, a brain region also directly linked to cognitive processing), neurogenesis, alterations in growth factors like BDNF, and inflammation (Van Rijckevorsel 2006; Holmes 2015).

### 2.7.3 Epilepsy's Cognitive Impairment Mechanisms

Complex interactions exist between aetiology, seizures, and cognition (Lenck-Santini and Scott 2015). The anatomical site of the epileptic activity has a considerable impact on cognitive abilities. This is the region of the brain where the primary focus of epileptic seizures is very strongly linked to cognitive impairment in adulthood. A region of the brain where the epileptic seizure's primary focus is very strongly linked to cognitive impairment in adulthood (Lenck-Santini and Scott 2015; Saniya et al. 2017). As a result, it is not surprising that individuals with temporal lobe epilepsy have the worst memory (Bell et al. 2011). The hippocampus is crucial in the development of memory. The threshold of aberrant excitability in the brain during an epileptic seizure is the lowest of all brain structures (Lin et al. 2009). Long-term, short-term, and spatial memories are all compromised as a result of the aberrant hippocampal circuitry formed by surviving pyramidal cells (Lenck-Santini and Scott 2015).

When it comes to epilepsy syndromes, such as those categorized as epileptic encephalopathies, cognitive impairment is frequently most severe in patients with early onset epilepsy (Lenck-Santini and Scott 2015). The term "epileptic encephalopathy" refers to a category of severe epilepsies that can be present from birth, produce recurrent epileptic seizures, as well as cognitive, neurological, and behavioural impairments, and may exacerbate children's developmental issues (Nickels and Wirrell 2017).

Additionally, genetic factors frequently play a role in the underlying aetiology of epileptic encephalopathies. A genetic connection to the mechanism of cognitive impairment in epilepsy has been investigated in four separate investigations. Several genes, including the sodium voltage-gated channel alpha subunit 1 (SCN1A) (Frank et al. 2006), the gamma-aminobutyric acid type A receptor subunit alpha1 (GABRA1) (Macdonald et al. 2010), the tuberous sclerosis-1 gene (TSC1) (Bateup et al. 2011), and the potassium sodium-activated channel subfamily T member 1 (KCNT1)

(Imran et al. 2019), have been found to cause ion channel failure or abnormal cortical development. Through a number of processes, including abnormalities in synaptic functioning, changes in neural connections, reduced metabolism, and impaired homeostasis, the deficiencies lead to hyperexcitation of some brain regions (Staley 2015).

### 2.7.4 Cognitive Impairment and Epileptiform Activity

Electroencephalography (EEG) exhibits distinctive graphoelements that represent epileptiform activity (sharp waves, spikes, spike-and-wave complexes). This activity may be categorized simply into three types: ictal (during a seizure), postictal (after a seizure), and interictal (between two seizures). Epileptiform activity is frequently linked to memory loss, mental retardation, behavioural and communication problems, and attention deficits (Stafstrom and Carmant 2015).

Additionally, depending on a variety of variables, epileptiform activity may lead to short-term or long-term impairments. For instance, they include the number of recurrences, the severity, the patient's age, the sort of medicine used to prevent seizures, and how well it works. Interictal epileptic discharges can have long-lasting consequences that over time can significantly alter cognitive functioning, including learning and memory (Landi et al. 2019). Additionally, the intensity and frequency of theta waves diminish with repeated seizures (Lin et al. 2009; Zhou et al. 2007).

### 2.7.5 Symptoms

- Symptoms may generally be categorized as focal, generalized, or undetermined onset seizures (Fisher et al. 2017).
- There are several epileptic seizure types, which can manifest as small or spectacular, brief or prolonged, frequent or uncommon events.
- They may manifest from being a severe widespread tonic-clonic seizure to a little myoclonic flashing of the eyelids or a focused numbness of the thumb and lips (Panayiotopoulos 2010).
- Disorientation usually happens after the seizure has ended and the patient has regained consciousness. This time frame might be anything from a few minutes to several hours.
- People who have epilepsy (PWE) have typical symptoms, which include speech issues, exhaustion, odd behaviour, headaches, and decreased focus and memory (Kuks and Snoek 2018).
- Co-morbidity often causes more stress than actual seizures do for many people.
- There are cognitive and neuropsychological problems (Helmstaedter and Witt 2017).
- There are epileptic encephalopathies.
- Cognitive impairment may last anywhere from a few minutes to many days after the symptoms of tiredness and disorientation have subsided.
- A cumulative decline in spatial memory function is shown when seizures are frequent (Lin et al. 2009).
- Persistent seizures decrease long-term potentiation (LTP).

### 2.7.6 Diagnosis

- EEG examination gauges the brain's electrical activity. Seizures are associated with certain aberrant electrical patterns.
- Brain scans using MRI is used to check for anomalies in blood vessels, tumours, and infections.
- Clinical symptoms include loss of consciousness, jerky movements of the muscles, a blank stare, stiffness of the muscles, change in breathing, loss of bladder or bowel control (urinated or defecated during the seizure), pale skin tone, and difficulty speaking or understanding what is being said.

## 2.8 POSTERIOR CORTICAL ATROPHY (PCA)

PCA is a progressive neurodegenerative condition which is characterized by a high level of visual impairment. PCA is frequently regarded as an unusual manifestation of AD, because most PCA patients at autopsy indicate AD pathology. The frequency of PCA is unclear. α-synucleinopathy associated with LBD, corticobasal degeneration, prion disease, and non-specific pathologies are some other diseases that have been identified alone or in conjunction with Alzheimer's pathology.

### 2.8.1 Clinical Features

- Difficulty reading;
- Memory issues;
- Contextual disorientation;
- Constructional dyspraxia;
- Agraphia/dysgraphia;
- Apperceptive visual agnosia;
- Blurred vision;
- Anomia;
- Prosopagnosia;
- Clothing apraxia;
- Acalculia;
- Limb apraxia;
- Left/right disorientation;
- Finger agnosia;
- Visual hallucinations.

### 2.8.2 Diagnosis

- Posterior atrophy can be seen in CT brain scans using MR and CT.
- Occipitoparietal hypometabolism can be identified in cases with fluorodeoxyglucose (FDG) positron emission tomography (PET) imaging.
- CSF biomarkers tests can be done for phosphorylated tau and amyloid beta 42 levels.
- Core cognitive features (at least three of which must be early or present) are alexia, left/right disorientation, acalculia, limb apraxia (not limb-kinetic), apperceptive prosopagnosia, agraphia, homonymous visual field defect, finger agnosia, constructional dyspraxia, environmental agnosia, oculomotor apraxia, dressing apraxia, optic ataxia, and finger agnosia.
- Non-posterior cortical features are decreased anterograde memory functions (like speech and non-visual language) (Olds et al. 2020).

## 2.9 PARKINSON'S DISEASE (PD)

Following AD, PD is the most prevalent neurodegenerative condition. Neuronal loss in the substantia nigra, which results in striatal dopaminergic insufficiency, and α-synuclein buildup in intraneuronal inclusions are the neuropathological hallmarks of PD. However, a number of processes and pathway dysregulation, including as oxidative stress, malfunctioning mitochondria, an imbalance in cellular calcium, neuroinflammation, and other deficiencies in the neurotransmitter system, contribute to the pathophysiology of PD (Zaman et al. 2021). In addition to its hallmark motor characteristics, including as bradykinesia (slowness of movement), stiffness, and resting tremor, PD is accompanied with a wide range of non-motor symptoms that significantly increase the burden of the illness. One of the most significant non-motor symptoms of PD, cognitive impairment, is up to six times more frequent than in the general population (Aarsland et al. 2001) and is essential to the disease's natural course. Even in the early stages of PD, cognitive impairment has been proven to have major economic effects beyond the motor symptoms, which makes it a top concern for both patients and care partners. Cognitive decline can negatively impact quality of life (QOL) and function (Leroi et al. 2012; Vossius et al. 2011; Chandler et al. 2021).

### 2.9.1 Epidemiology

Patients with PD are 2.5–6.0 times more likely to acquire dementia than people without PD of the same age (Aarsland et al. 2001; Perez et al. 2012). AD affects 24–31% of persons with PD (Aarsland et al. 2005). The cumulative prevalence of PDD in patients with a mean age at diagnosis of between 54.0 and 70.2 years is 17% at five years after diagnosis, 46% at ten years after diagnosis, and 83% at 14 years after diagnosis (Hely et al. 2008; Buter et al. 2008). Furthermore, the pace of cognitive deterioration in PDD is comparable to that in AD, and many patients with PDD will require nursing home placement and become totally dependent on outside care and assistance (Aarsland et al. 2004).

Globally, 6.1 million people were predicted to have PD in 2016, up from 2.5 million in 1990, and by 2040 this figure is projected to more than quadruple (Dorsey et al. 2018).

### 2.9.2 Pathophysiology

There are many different theoretical ideas put out to explain the tissue alterations connected to cognitive loss in PD, and there is evidence to suggest that a number of degenerative processes and mechanisms may be at play.

#### 2.9.2.1 Systemic Neurotransmitter Decline and Larger Dopaminergic Deficiencies throughout the Brain

A moderate-to-severe loss of dopaminergic neurons in the nigrostriatal projection pathway characterizes all PD patients by definition. In comparison to those with PD without cognitive impairment, those with Parkinson's Disease – Mild Cognitive Impairment (PD-MCI) experience more extensive dopaminergic terminal degeneration in the striatum, notably denervation of dopaminergic terminals in the associative dorsal caudate nucleus (Sasikumar and Strafella 2020). However, other dopaminergic systems in the brain are somewhat preserved in PD-MCI patients, but those with PDD show a significant loss of the lateral dopaminergic pathway reaching frontal, parietal, and temporal cortical regions (Sasikumar and Strafella 2020). Dopamine may have a significant role in cognitive function, as evidenced by the fact that in healthy persons, cortical dopamine modulation can improve working memory, as well as visuospatial and attentional processing, and boosts cognitive effort (Ranganath and Jacob 2016; Westbrook et al. 2020).

#### 2.9.2.2 Sympathetic and Noradrenergic Nervous Systems

Neurons in the locus coeruleus that synthesize noradrenaline also create neuromelanin pigment as a byproduct in humans (Keren et al. 2015). The sensory signal detection and regulation of several areas of cognition, but notably in attention, behavioural flexibility, working memory, and long-term memory, are mediated by these neurons, which also support waking and arousal (Borodovitsyna et al. 2017). The frontal cortex and hippocampus are two regions with high noradrenergic innervation that originate in the locus coeruleus and are crucial for cognitive behaviors (Borodovitsyna et al. 2017). There is a correlation between the existence of PD-MCI and a decrease in the neuromelanin-sensitive MRI signal of the locus at the time of the initial diagnosis of PD (Li et al. 2019).

#### 2.9.2.3 Basic Cholinergic Systems in the Forebrain

The neocortex, hippocampus, and amygdala get the majority of their cholinergic innervation from the basal forebrain cholinergic neurons (Ballinger et al. 2016; Pillet et al. 2020). These neurons have a significant role in controlling the circuit dynamics that underlie cognitive processing, particularly those related to executive, memory, and attention functions (Ballinger et al. 2016). A decrease in the volume and density of the basal forebrain cholinergic region, as well as their projections to the neocortex, hippocampus, and amygdala, is linked to cognitive decline over a two-year period in both newly diagnosed PD patients and those who are further along in the disease (Schulz et al. 2018; Bohnen et al. 2015; Pereira et al. 2020). Loss of basal forebrain cholinergic projections to the hippocampus corresponds with memory problems and the development of PDD in terms of memory dysfunction (Pereira et al. 2020; Gargouri et al. 2019).

### 2.9.3 Genetic Influences

Risk factors for PD include mutations in the genes SNCA (encoding α-synuclein), TMEM (encoding lysosomal potassium channel) 175, and GBA (encoding α-glucosylceramidase), which increase α-synuclein, decrease potassium currents that impair lysosomal and mitochondrial function, and decrease glucocerebrosidase and lysosomal activity, respectively (Wang et al. 2015). Glucocerebrosidase expression, enzymatic activity, and α-synuclein deposition are all affected by a specific single nucleotide polymorphism in GBA that is connected to PD-MCI and PDD (Jiang et al. 2020). The APOE 4 (encoding apolipoprotein E) allele, but not any other genetic variations, are linked to progression and worsening cognitive impairment in PD (Tan et al. 2021; Iwaki et al. 2019; D'Souza and Rajkumar 2020). The APOE 4 allele may make these people more likely than the general population to accumulate beta-amyloid over time (D'Souza and Rajkumar 2020).

### 2.9.4 Clinical Features

- **Tremor**. A tremor, or rhythmic shaking, usually begins in a limb, often a hand or fingers. Patients may rub their thumb and forefinger back and forth. This is known as a pill-rolling tremor. A patient's hand may tremble when it's at rest. The shaking may decrease when performing tasks.
- **Slowed movement (bradykinesia)**. Over time, PD may slow movement, making simple tasks difficult and time-consuming. Steps may become shorter when walking. It may be difficult to get out of a chair. The patient may drag or shuffle their feet as they try to walk.
- **Rigid muscles**. Muscle stiffness may occur in any part of the body. The stiff muscles can be painful and limit the range of motion.
- **Impaired posture and balance**. Posture may become stooped or the patient may fall or have balance problems as a result of PD.
- **Loss of automatic movements**. Decreased ability to perform unconscious movements, including blinking, smiling, or swinging the arms when walking.
- **Speech changes**. Speech is not clear and patient mumbles.

### 2.9.5 Diagnosis

- Imaging tests: These – such as MRI, ultrasound of the brain, and PET scans – also may be used to help rule out other disorders. A single-photon emission computerized tomography (SPECT) scan called a dopamine transporter (DAT) scan is specific for PD. Cognitive profile: The Montreal Cognitive Assessment (MoCA), the Mattis Dementia Rating Scale Second Edition (MDRS-2), and the Parkinson's Disease – Cognitive Rating Scale (PD-CRS) were classified as three scales for screening cognitive function based on their clinimetric properties in PD.
- Neuropsychological testing for each of the domains of working memory and attention; executive capabilities; linguistic, memory, and visuospatial skills.
- Neuropsychiatric characteristics: Apathy, depression, hallucination with images, and mental illness (Skorvanek et al. 2018).

## 2.10 ACUTE DISSEMINATED ENCEPHALOMYELITIS (ADEM)

The CNS demyelinating illness known as ADEM is uncommon and often has a monophasic course. Post-infectious, post-vaccination, and idiopathic encephalomyelitis are all included under the umbrella term ADEM (Johnson 1987). In ADEM, symptoms such as headache, fever, nausea, and vomiting can occur with or without an altered mental state and have an immediate start.

### 2.10.1 Epidemiology

The yearly incidence of ADEM ranges from 0.07 to 0.60 per 100,000 people per year (Torisu et al. 2010; Pohl et al. 2007; Xiong et al. 2014). Between 0.47/100,000 and 0.64/100,000 children were thought to have paediatric ADEM in Asian nations (Torisu et al. 2010; Xiong et al. 2014) compared to 0.07/100,000 to 0.30/100,000 in San Diego and Europe (Pohl et al. 2007; Leake et al. 2004; Gudbjornsson et al. 2015). Even while ADEM can strike at any age, it usually happens in children. The male to female ratio in the child population is 1.8:1.0, and the median age of onset is between five and eight years (Tenembaum et al. 2002). Adult instances occur between the ages of 33 and 41, with neither gender predominating.

### 2.10.2 Etiopathogenesis

In terms of pathology, ADEM is characterized by perivenular sleeves of demyelination, edoema, and perivenous inflammation, as well as foamy macrophages that contain myelin products (Esposito et al. 2015; Pohl et al. 2016). T and B lymphocytes, neutrophils, plasma cells, microglial cells, and eosinophilic granulocytes may also be present. Occasionally these confluent regions may occur as perivenous lesions merge. Axons in demyelinating lesions are typically comparatively spared, although in ADEM deaths, substantial axonal damage has been seen. Increased levels of phosphorylated microtubule-associated protein (TAU), which is typically found in neuronal axons, in the cerebrospinal fluid are a sign of axonal injury (CSF). Glial nodules in the grey matter (GM), perivascular necrosis, infiltration of the meninges, and vasculitic-like lesions are examples of abnormal findings (Young et al. 2010). In addition to this mechanism, the infection may cause the release of cytokines and non-specific self-sensitization of T lymphocytes towards myelin autoantigens (Kothur et al. 2016). The breakdown of T-cell tolerance may be triggered by this event, known as "bystander activation". Therefore, the immune-mediated harm to the CNS in ADEM may be caused by both cell-mediated and humoral effector pathways.

### 2.10.3 Clinical Signs and Symptoms

- Classic ADEM is a monophasic sickness that develops after an earlier illness or, less frequently, a vaccine. The latency phase can be anywhere from a few days to a few months, and the usual presentation comprises the abrupt development of several neurologic symptoms, frequently accompanied by a sharp decline in mental status.
- Children and adults both have the same prodromal symptoms, which include headache, malaise, irritability, fever, nausea, and vomiting. Neurological symptoms often appear two to five days after initial presentation (Pohl et al. 2016).
- Changes in behaviour and/or awareness, ranging in severity from lethargy to coma, are all part of encephalopathy. Consciousness impairment affects 46–73% of paediatric patients and 20–56% of adult patients (Marchioni et al. 2013), and it may need critical care hospitalization (43%) or the use of mechanical breathing (16%) (Tenembaum et al. 2002). Additionally, some individuals may display agitation, disorientation, and psychosis.
- Focal neurological symptoms. Depending on the part of the brain affected, individuals may exhibit various symptoms. When the occipital lobes are damaged, the same visual field

deficits and, if they are severe and bilateral, cortical blindness may ensue. Higher deficiencies in brain function, such as agraphia, alexia, aphasia, and acalculia, may also be present in patients. Patients may have pyramidal symptoms when the motor cortex is involved (i.e., Babinski sign, spastic hypertonus, and hyperreflexia). Astereognosis and agraphesthesia, or loss of proprioception, as well as a decrease in pain and temperature perception, are examples of sensory symptoms. Patients who have brainstem involvement may have cranial nerve palsy. The following are the most typical symptoms: hearing loss, decreased taste and smell sensitivity, respiratory failure, dysphagia, dysarthria, vertigo, nystagmus, and diplopia (both cranial nerve palsies and/or inflammation of the gaze-control centres) (Pohl et al. 2016). The prognosis is often worse and there is a greater likelihood of a fulminant disease course when the brainstem is involved (Tenembaum 2008).

- Meningitis occurs in 26–31% of cases and is brought on by lymphocyte infiltration of the meninges.

### 2.10.4 Diagnostic Criteria

Pediatric acquired demyelinating diseases of the CNS, including ADEM, were given diagnostic criteria by the International Pediatric Multiple Sclerosis Study Group (IPMSSG) in 2007. The initial criteria were revised in 2013. However ADEM is still a diagnosis of exclusion. Once other potential neurological disorders have been reliably ruled out, all of the criteria listed below must be met (Krupp et al. 2013) to determine whether someone has ADEM:

1. A first multifocal clinical CNS episode with a suspected demyelinating inflammation cause;
2. Encephalopathy, which is characterized by stupor, lethargy, or behavioural modifications without a fever, underlying disease, or postictal signs;
3. An acute phase (three months) where the brain MRI is abnormal.

## REFERENCES

Aarsland, Dag, K. Andersen, J. P. Larsen, A. Lolk, H. Nielsen, and P. Kragh-Sørensen. "Risk of dementia in Parkinson's disease: a community-based, prospective study." *Neurology* 56, no. 6 (2001): 730–736.

Aarsland, Dag, Kjeld Andersen, Jan Petter Larsen, Robert Perry, Tore Wentzel-Larsen, Anette Lolk, and Per Kragh-Sørensen. "The rate of cognitive decline in Parkinson disease." *Archives of Neurology* 61, no. 12 (2004): 1906–1911.

Aarsland, Dag, Julia Zaccai, and Carol Brayne. "A systematic review of prevalence studies of dementia in Parkinson's disease." *Movement Disorders: Official Journal of the Movement Disorder Society* 20, no. 10 (2005): 1255–1263.

Absoud, Michael, Ming J. Lim, Wui K. Chong, Christian G. De Goede, Katharine Foster, Roxana Gunny, Cheryl Hemingway et al. "Paediatric acquired demyelinating syndromes: incidence, clinical and magnetic resonance imaging features." *Multiple Sclerosis Journal* 19, no. 1 (2013): 76–86.

Alves-Leon, Soniza Vieira, Maria Lucia Veluttini-Pimentel, Maria Emmerick Gouveia, Fabíola Rachid Malfetano, Emerson L. Gaspareto, Marcos P. Alvarenga, Izabel Frugulhetti, and Thereza Quirico-Santos. "Acute disseminated encephalomyelitis: clinical features, HLA DRB1* 1501, HLA DRB1* 1503, HLA DQA1* 0102, HLA DQB1* 0602, and HLA DPA1* 0301 allelic association study." *Arquivos de Neuro-psiquiatria* 67 (2009): 643–651.

Alzheimer's Association (2021). 2021 Alzheimer's disease facts and figures. *Alzheimers Dement* 17, 327–406. doi:10.1002/alz.12328.

American Psychiatric Association. *Diagnostic and Statistical Manual of Mental Disorders DSM 4 TR* (Text Revision). American Psychiatric Association; 2003.

Auning, Eirik, Arvid Rongve, Tormod Fladby, Jan Booij, Tibor Hortobágyi, Françoise J. Siepel, Clive Ballard, and Dag Aarsland. "Early and presenting symptoms of dementia with Lewy bodies." *Dementia and Geriatric Cognitive Disorders* 32, no. 3 (2011): 202–208.

Bakare, M. O. "Attention deficit hyperactivity symptoms and disorder (ADHD) among African children: a review of epidemiology and co-morbidities: original." *African Journal of Psychiatry* 15, no. 5 (2012): 358–361.

Balasubramanya, K. S., J. M. E. Kovoor, P. N. Jayakumar, S. Ravishankar, R. B. Kamble, J. Panicker, and D. Nagaraja. "Diffusion-weighted imaging and proton MR spectroscopy in the characterization of acute disseminated encephalomyelitis." *Neuroradiology* 49, no. 2 (2007): 177–183.

Ballinger, Elizabeth C., Mala Ananth, David A. Talmage, and Lorna W. Role. "Basal forebrain cholinergic circuits and signaling in cognition and cognitive decline." *Neuron* 91, no. 6 (2016): 1199–1218.

Bateup, Helen S., Kevin T. Takasaki, Jessica L. Saulnier, Cassandra L. Denefrio, and Bernardo L. Sabatini. "Loss of Tsc1 in vivo impairs hippocampal mGluR-LTD and increases excitatory synaptic function." *Journal of Neuroscience* 31, no. 24 (2011): 8862–8869.

Belanoff, Joseph K., Kristin Gross, Alison Yager, and Alan F. Schatzberg. "Corticosteroids and cognition." *Journal of Psychiatric Research* 35, no. 3 (2001): 127–145.

Bell, Brian, Jack J. Lin, Michael Seidenberg, and Bruce Hermann. "The neurobiology of cognitive disorders in temporal lobe epilepsy." *Nature Reviews Neurology* 7, no. 3 (2011): 154–164.

Ber, Isabelle Le, Eric Guedj, Audrey Gabelle, Patrice Verpillat, Magali Volteau, Catherine Thomas-Anterion, Marielle Decousus et al. "Demographic, neurological and behavioural characteristics and brain perfusion SPECT in frontal variant of frontotemporal dementia." *Brain* 129, no. 11 (2006): 3051–3065.

Bohnen, Nicolaas I., Roger L. Albin, Martijn L.T.M. Müller, Myria Petrou, Vikas Kotagal, Robert A. Koeppe, Peter J.H. Scott, and Kirk A. Frey. "Frequency of cholinergic and caudate nucleus dopaminergic deficits across the predemented cognitive spectrum of Parkinson disease and evidence of interaction effects." *JAMA Neurology* 72, no. 2 (2015): 194–200.

Boot, Brendon P. "Comprehensive treatment of dementia with Lewy bodies." *Alzheimer's Research & Therapy* 7, no. 1 (2015): 1–8.

Borodovitsyna, Olga, Matthew Flamini, and Daniel Chandler. "Noradrenergic modulation of cognition in health and disease." *Neural Plasticity* (2017).

Brás, Inês Caldeira, Antonio Dominguez-Meijide, Ellen Gerhardt, David Koss, Diana F. Lázaro, Patrícia I. Santos, Eftychia Vasili, Mary Xylaki, and Tiago Fleming Outeiro. "Synucleinopathies: Where we are and where we need to go." *Journal of Neurochemistry* 153, no. 4 (2020): 433–454.

Bruno, Martin A., and A. Claudio Cuello. "Activity-dependent release of precursor nerve growth factor, conversion to mature nerve growth factor, and its degradation by a protease cascade." *Proceedings of the National Academy of Sciences* 103, no. 17 (2006): 6735–6740.

Busche, Marc Aurel, and Bradley T. Hyman. "Synergy between amyloid-β and tau in Alzheimer's disease." *Nature Neuroscience* 23, no. 10 (2020): 1183–1193.

Buter, T. C., A. Van Den Hout, F. E. Matthews, J. P. Larsen, C. Brayne, and D. Aarsland. "Dementia and survival in Parkinson disease: a 12-year population study." *Neurology* 70, no. 13 (2008): 1017–1022.

Caviness, John N., Lih Fen Lue, Charles H. Adler, and Douglas G. Walker. "Parkinson's disease dementia and potential therapeutic strategies." *CNS Neuroscience & Therapeutics* 17, no. 1 (2011): 32–44.

Chandler, Julie M., Radhika Nair, Kevin Biglan, Erin A. Ferries, Leanne M. Munsie, Tich Changamire, and Nick Patel. "Characteristics of Parkinson's Disease in Patients with and without Cognitive Impairment." *Journal of Parkinson's Disease* 11, no. 3 (2021): 1381–1392.

Cheignon, Clémence, M. Tomas, D. Bonnefont-Rousselot, Peter Faller, Christelle Hureau, and Fabrice Collin. "Oxidative stress and the amyloid beta peptide in Alzheimer's disease." *Redox Biology* 14 (2018): 450–464.

Cusick, Matthew F., Jane E. Libbey, and Robert S. Fujinami. "Molecular mimicry as a mechanism of autoimmune disease." *Clinical Reviews in Allergy & Immunology* 42, no. 1 (2012): 102–111.

D'Souza, Tyrra, and Anto P. Rajkumar. "Systematic review of genetic variants associated with cognitive impairment and depressive symptoms in Parkinson's disease." *Acta Neuropsychiatrica* 32, no. 1 (2020): 10–22.

Daley, David, and Chris P. Hollis. "The World Federation of ADHD international consensus statement: 208 evidence-based conclusions about the disorder." (2021).

Davies, Rhys R., Christopher M. Kipps, Joanna Mitchell, Jillian J. Kril, Glenda M. Halliday, and John R. Hodges. "Progression in frontotemporal dementia: identifying a benign behavioral variant by magnetic resonance imaging." *Archives of Neurology* 63, no. 11 (2006): 1627–1631.

Dhakal, A., and Bobrin, B.D. *Cognitive deficits*. StatPearls Publishing, 2023.

Dorsey, E. Ray, Alexis Elbaz, Emma Nichols, Nooshin Abbasi, Foad Abd-Allah, Ahmed Abdelalim, Jose C. Adsuar et al. "Global, regional, and national burden of Parkinson's disease, 1990–2016: a systematic analysis for the Global Burden of Disease Study 2016." *The Lancet Neurology* 17, no. 11 (2018): 939–953.

Dugger, Sarah Anne. *Evaluation of a Precision Medicine Approach for hnRNP U-Related Developmental Epileptic Encephalopathy Using a Mouse Model of Disease*. Columbia University, 2020.

Esposito, Susanna, Giada Maria Di Pietro, Barbara Madini, Maria Vincenza Mastrolia, and Donato Rigante. "A spectrum of inflammation and demyelination in acute disseminated encephalomyelitis (ADEM) of children." *Autoimmunity Reviews* 14, no. 10 (2015): 923–929.

Faraone, Stephen V., Tobias Banaschewski, David Coghill, Yi Zheng, Joseph Biederman, Mark A. Bellgrove, Jeffrey H. Newcorn et al. "The world federation of ADHD international consensus statement: 208 evidence-based conclusions about the disorder." *Neuroscience & Biobehavioral Reviews* 128 (2021): 789–818.

Fiest, Kirsten M., Khara M. Sauro, Samuel Wiebe, Scott B. Patten, Churl-Su Kwon, Jonathan Dykeman, Tamara Pringsheim, Diane L. Lorenzetti, and Nathalie Jetté. "Prevalence and incidence of epilepsy: a systematic review and meta-analysis of international studies." *Neurology* 88, no. 3 (2017): 296–303.

Fisher, Robert S., Carlos Acevedo, Alexis Arzimanoglou, Alicia Bogacz, J. Helen Cross, Christian E. Elger, Jerome Engel Jr et al. "ILAE official report: a practical clinical definition of epilepsy." *Epilepsia* 55, no. 4 (2014): 475–482.

Fisher, Robert S., J. Helen Cross, Jacqueline A. French, Norimichi Higurashi, Edouard Hirsch, Floor E. Jansen, Lieven Lagae et al. "Operational classification of seizure types by the International League Against Epilepsy: Position Paper of the ILAE Commission for Classification and Terminology." *Epilepsia* 58, no. 4 (2017): 522–530.

Fisher, Robert S., Walter Van Emde Boas, Warren Blume, Christian Elger, Pierre Genton, Phillip Lee, and Jerome Engel Jr. "Epileptic seizures and epilepsy: definitions proposed by the International League Against Epilepsy (ILAE) and the International Bureau for Epilepsy (IBE)." *Epilepsia* 46, no. 4 (2005): 470–472.

Frank, C.A., Kennedy, M.J., Goold, C.P., Marek, K.W., and Davis, G.W. "Mechanisms underlying the rapid induction and sustained expression of synaptic homeostasis." *Neuron* 52, no. 4 (2006): 663–677. doi:10.1016/j.neuron.2006.09.029.

Galvin, James E., John E. Duda, Daniel I. Kaufer, Carol F. Lippa, Angela Taylor, and Steven H. Zarit. "Lewy body dementia: the caregiver experience of clinical care." *Parkinsonism & Related Disorders* 16, no. 6 (2010): 388–392.

Garg, Raj Kumar. "Acute disseminated encephalomyelitis." *Postgraduate Medical Journal* 79, no. 927 (2003): 11–17.

Gargouri, Fatma, Cécile Gallea, Marie Mongin, Nadya Pyatigorskaya, Romain Valabregue, Claire Ewenczyk, Marie Sarazin, Lydia Yahia-Cherif, Marie Vidailhet, and Stéphane Lehéricy. "Multimodal magnetic resonance imaging investigation of basal forebrain damage and cognitive deficits in Parkinson's disease." *Movement Disorders* 34, no. 4 (2019): 516–525.

Goedert, M. G. S. M., M. G. Spillantini, R. Jakes, D. Rutherford, and R. A. Crowther. "Multiple isoforms of human microtubule-associated protein tau: sequences and localization in neurofibrillary tangles of Alzheimer's disease." *Neuron* 3, no. 4 (1989): 519–526.

Goldman, Larry S., Myron Genel, Rebecca J. Bezman, and Priscilla J. Slanetz. "Diagnosis and treatment of attention-deficit/hyperactivity disorder in children and adolescents." *JAMA* 279, no. 14 (1998): 1100–1107.

Goldman, J. S., R. Rademakers, E. D. Huey, A. L. Boxer, R. Mayeux, B. L. Miller, and B. F. Boeve. "An algorithm for genetic testing of frontotemporal lobar degeneration." *Neurology* 76, no. 5 (2011): 475–483.

Gomperts, Stephen N. "Lewy body dementias: dementia with Lewy bodies and Parkinson disease dementia." *Continuum: Lifelong Learning in Neurology* 22, no. 2 Dementia (2016): 435.

Gorno-Tempini, Maria Luisa, Argye E. Hillis, Sandra Weintraub, Andrew Kertesz, Mario Mendez, Stefano F. Cappa, Jennifer M. Ogar et al. "Classification of primary progressive aphasia and its variants." *Neurology* 76, no. 11 (2011): 1006–1014.

Gudbjornsson, Brynjar Thor, Ásgeir Haraldsson, Hildur Einarsdóttir, and Ólafur Thorarensen. "Nationwide incidence of acquired central nervous system demyelination in Icelandic children." *Pediatric Neurology* 53, no. 6 (2015): 503–507.

Haass, Christian, and Dennis J. Selkoe. "Soluble protein oligomers in neurodegeneration: lessons from the Alzheimer's amyloid β-peptide." *Nature Reviews Molecular Cell Biology* 8, no. 2 (2007): 101–112.

Habek, Mario, and Kamelija Žarković. "Pathology of acute disseminated encephalomyelitis." *Translational Neuroscience* 2, no. 3 (2011): 252–255.

Hatipoğlu, Hasan, and Sibel Canbaz Kabay. "Periodontal Ve Sistemik Hastaliklar: Bilişsel Bozukluklar." *Dental and Medical Journal-Review* 4, no. 1: 8–20.

Helmstaedter, Christoph, and Juri-Alexander Witt. "Epilepsy and cognition–a bidirectional relationship?" *Seizure* 49 (2017): 83–89.

Hely, Mariese A., Wayne G.J. Reid, Michael A. Adena, Glenda M. Halliday, and John G.L. Morris. "The Sydney multicenter study of Parkinson's disease: the inevitability of dementia at 20 years." *Movement Disorders* 23, no. 6 (2008): 837–844.

Hodges, J. R., R. Davies, J. Xuereb, J. Kril, and G. Halliday. "Survival in frontotemporal dementia." *Neurology* 61, no. 3 (2003): 349–354.

Hollingworth, Paul, Denise Harold, Lesley Jones, Michael J. Owen, and Julie Williams. "Alzheimer's disease genetics: current knowledge and future challenges." *International Journal of Geriatric Psychiatry* 26, no. 8 (2011): 793–802.

Holmes, Gregory L. "Cognitive impairment in epilepsy: the role of network abnormalities." *Epileptic Disorders* 17, no. 2 (2015): 101–116.

Idrissova, Z. R., M. N. Boldyreva, E. P. Dekonenko, N. A. Malishev, I. Y. Leontyeva, I. N. Martinenko, and A. S. Petrukhin. "Acute disseminated encephalomyelitis in children: clinical features and HLA-DR linkage." *European Journal of Neurology* 10, no. 5 (2003): 537–546.

Imran, T., Ahmed, R.R., Streimikiene, D., Soomro, R.H., Parmar, V., and Vveinhardt, J. "Assessment of entrepreneurial traits and small-firm performance with entrepreneurial orientation as a mediating factor." *Sustainability* 11, no. 19 (2019): 5301. doi:10.3390/su11195301.

Iqbal, Khalid, Michael Flory, and Hilkka Soininen. "Clinical symptoms and symptom signatures of Alzheimer's disease subgroups." *Journal of Alzheimer's Disease* 37, no. 3 (2013): 475–481.

Iwaki, H., C. Blauwendraat, H.L. Leonard, J.J. Kim, G. Liu, J. Maple-Grødem, J.C. Corvol, L. Pihlstrøm, M. van Nimwegen, S.J. Hutten, and H.N. Khanh-Dung. Genome-wide association study of Parkinson's disease progression biomarkers in 12 longitudinal patients' cohorts. *bioRxiv*, (2019) 585836.

Jaeschke, Rafał R., Ewelina Sujkowska, and Magdalena Sowa-Kućma. "Methylphenidate for attention-deficit/hyperactivity disorder in adults: a narrative review." *Psychopharmacology* 238, no. 10 (2021): 2667–2691.

Jellinger, Kurt A., and Amos D. Korczyn. "Are dementia with Lewy bodies and Parkinson's disease dementia the same." (2018).

Jiang, Zhiqiang, Yilin Huang, Piao Zhang, Chongyin Han, Yueer Lu, Zongchao Mo, Zhanyu Zhang et al. "Characterization of a pathogenic variant in GBA for Parkinson's disease with mild cognitive impairment patients." *Molecular Brain* 13, no. 1 (2020): 1–10.

Johnson, Richard T. "The pathogenesis of acute viral encephalitis and postinfectious encephalomyelitis." *The Journal of Infectious Diseases* (1987): 359–364.

Jones, S. A. Vann, and J. T. O'Brien. "The prevalence and incidence of dementia with Lewy bodies: a systematic review of population and clinical studies." *Psychological Medicine* 44, no. 4 (2014): 673–683.

Kalachnik, John E., Thomas E. Hanzel, Robert Sevenich, and Stuart R. Harder. "Benzodiazepine behavioral side effects: review and implications for individuals with mental retardation." *American Journal on Mental Retardation* 107, no. 5 (2002): 376–410.

Keren, Noam I., Saeid Taheri, Elena M. Vazey, Paul S. Morgan, Ann-Charlotte E. Granholm, Gary S. Aston-Jones, and Mark A. Eckert. "Histologic validation of locus coeruleus MRI contrast in post-mortem tissue." *Neuroimage* 113 (2015): 235–245.

Khan, Baber K., Jennifer S. Yokoyama, Leonel T. Takada, J. Sha Sharon, Nicola J. Rutherford, Jamie C. Fong, Anna M. Karydas et al. "Atypical, slowly progressive behavioural variant frontotemporal dementia associated with C9ORF72 hexanucleotide expansion." *Journal of Neurology, Neurosurgery & Psychiatry* 83, no. 4 (2012): 358–364.

Kipps, Christopher M., John R. Hodges, and Michael Hornberger. "Nonprogressive behavioural frontotemporal dementia: recent developments and clinical implications of the 'bvFTD phenocopy syndrome'." *Current Opinion in Neurology* 23, no. 6 (2010): 628–632.

Kisseleva, Tatiana, S. Bhattacharya, J. Braunstein, and C. W. Schindler. "Signaling through the JAK/STAT pathway, recent advances and future challenges." *Gene* 285, no. 1–2 (2002): 1–24.

Knopman, David S., and Rosebud O. Roberts. "Estimating the number of persons with frontotemporal lobar degeneration in the US population." *Journal of Molecular Neuroscience* 45, no. 3 (2011): 330–335.

Kothur, Kavitha, Louise Wienholt, Shekeeb S. Mohammad, Esther M. Tantsis, Sekhar Pillai, Philip N. Britton, Cheryl A. Jones et al. "Utility of CSF cytokine/chemokines as markers of active intrathecal inflammation: comparison of demyelinating, anti-NMDAR and enteroviral encephalitis." *PLoS One* 11, no. 8 (2016): e0161656.

Krupp, Lauren B., Marc Tardieu, Maria Pia Amato, Brenda Banwell, Tanuja Chitnis, Russell C. Dale, Angelo Ghezzi et al. "International Pediatric Multiple Sclerosis Study Group criteria for pediatric multiple sclerosis and immune-mediated central nervous system demyelinating disorders: revisions to the 2007 definitions." *Multiple Sclerosis Journal* 19, no. 10 (2013): 1261–1267.

Kuks, Joannes Bernardus Maria, and J. W. Snoek. *Textbook of clinical neurology*. Bohn Stafleu van loghum, 2018.

Kumawat, A.R., Singh, K., and Mangal, G. 'Scope of panchakarma in neuro-developmental disorders', *International Ayurvedic Medical Journal*, 8, no. 7 (2020): 3951–3958. doi:10.46607/iamj0807212020.

Lambert, Matthew A., Horst Bickel, Martin Prince, Laura Fratiglioni, Eva Von Strauss, Dorota Frydecka, Andrzej Kiejna, Jean Georges, and E. L. Reynish. "Estimating the burden of early onset dementia; systematic review of disease prevalence." *European Journal of Neurology* 21, no. 4 (2014): 563–569.

Landi, Silvia, Luigi Petrucco, Federico Sicca, and Gian Michele Ratto. "Transient cognitive impairment in epilepsy." *Frontiers in Molecular Neuroscience* 11 (2019): 458.

Le Ber, I. "Genetics of frontotemporal lobar degeneration: an up-date and diagnosis algorithm." *Revue neurologique* 169, no. 10 (2013): 811–819.

Leake, John A. D., Salvatore Albani, Annie S. Kao, Melvin O. Senac, Glenn F. Billman, Mark P. Nespeca, Amy D. Paulino, Eileen R. Quintela, Mark H. Sawyer, and John S. Bradley. "Acute disseminated encephalomyelitis in childhood: epidemiologic, clinical and laboratory features." *The Pediatric Infectious Disease Journal* 23, no. 8 (2004): 756–764.

Lenck-Santini, Pierre-Pascal, and Rodney C. Scott. "Mechanisms responsible for cognitive impairment in epilepsy." *Cold Spring Harbor Perspectives in Medicine* 5, no. 10 (2015): a022772.

Leroi, Iracema, Kathryn McDonald, Hiranmayi Pantula, and Vijay Harbishettar. "Cognitive impairment in Parkinson disease: impact on quality of life, disability, and caregiver burden." *Journal of Geriatric Psychiatry and Neurology* 25, no. 4 (2012): 208–214.

Li, Yuanfang, Changpeng Wang, Jian Wang, Ying Zhou, Fang Ye, Yong Zhang, Xiaoqin Cheng et al. "Mild cognitive impairment in de novo Parkinson's disease: a neuromelanin MRI study in locus coeruleus." *Movement Disorders* 34, no. 6 (2019): 884–892.

Lin, Hai, Gregory L. Holmes, John L. Kubie, and Robert U. Muller. "Recurrent seizures induce a reversible impairment in a spatial hidden goal task." *Hippocampus* 19, no. 9 (2009): 817–827.

Macdonald, Robert L., Jing-Qiong Kang, and Martin J. Gallagher. "Mutations in GABAA receptor subunits associated with genetic epilepsies." *The Journal of Physiology* 588, no. 11 (2010): 1861–1869.

Mackenzie, Ian R. A., Manuela Neumann, Eileen H. Bigio, Nigel J. Cairns, Irina Alafuzoff, Jillian Kril, Gabor G. Kovacs et al. "Nomenclature and nosology for neuropathologic subtypes of frontotemporal lobar degeneration: an update." *Acta neuropathologica* 119 (2010): 1–4.

Magnin, Eloi, and C. Maurs. "Attention-deficit/hyperactivity disorder during adulthood." *Revue neurologique* 173, no. 7–8 (2017): 506–515.

Mani, Siddhartha, Soumya Sarathi Mondal, Goutam Guha, Subhabrata Gangopadhyay, Adyapad Pani, Sumanta Das Baksi, Debjoy Sau, and Koushik Bhattacharjee. "Acute disseminated encephalomyelitis after mixed malaria infection (Plasmodium falciparum and Plasmodium vivax) with MRI closely simulating multiple sclerosis." *The Neurologist* 17, no. 5 (2011): 276–278.

Marchioni, Enrico, Sabrina Ravaglia, Cristina Montomoli, Eleonora Tavazzi, Lorenzo Minoli, Fausto Baldanti, Milena Furione et al. "Postinfectious neurologic syndromes: a prospective cohort study." *Neurology* 80, no. 10 (2013): 882–889.

Marder, S.R., Sorsaburu, S., Dunayevich, E., Karagianis, J.L., Dawe, I.C., Falk, D.M., Dellva, M.A., Carlson, J.L., Cavazzoni, P.A., and Baker, R.W. "Case reports of postmarketing adverse event experiences with olanzapine intramuscular treatment in patients with agitation." *The Journal of Clinical Psychiatry* 71, no. 4 (2010):433–441.

Marin, Samantha E., and David J. A. Callen. "The magnetic resonance imaging appearance of monophasic acute disseminated encephalomyelitis: an update post application of the 2007 consensus criteria." *Neuroimaging Clinics* 23, no. 2 (2013): 245–266.

Mayeux, Richard, and Yaakov Stern. "Epidemiology of Alzheimer disease." *Cold Spring Harbor Perspectives in Medicine* 2, no. 8 (2012): a006239.

McCarter, Stuart J., Erik K. St. Louis, and Bradley F. Boeve. "REM sleep behavior disorder and REM sleep without atonia as an early manifestation of degenerative neurological disease." *Current Neurology and Neuroscience Reports* 12 (2012): 182–192.

McKeith, Ian G., Bradley F. Boeve, Dennis W. Dickson, Glenda Halliday, John-Paul Taylor, Daniel Weintraub, Dag Aarsland et al. "Diagnosis and management of dementia with Lewy bodies: Fourth consensus report of the DLB Consortium." *Neurology* 89, no. 1 (2017): 88–100.

Meade, Richard M., David P. Fairlie, and Jody M. Mason. "Alpha-synuclein structure and Parkinson's disease–lessons and emerging principles." *Molecular Neurodegeneration* 14, no. 1 (2019): 1–14.

Mehra, Surabhi, Laxmikant Gadhe, Riya Bera, Ajay Singh Sawner, and Samir K. Maji. "Structural and functional insights into α-synuclein fibril polymorphism." *Biomolecules* 11, no. 10 (2021): 1419.

Mehra, Surabhi, Shruti Sahay, and Samir K. Maji. "α-Synuclein misfolding and aggregation: Implications in Parkinson's disease pathogenesis." *Biochimica et Biophysica Acta (BBA)-Proteins and Proteomics* 1867, no. 10 (2019): 890–908.

Milán-Tomás, Ángela, Marta Fernández-Matarrubia, and María Cruz Rodríguez-Oroz. "Lewy body dementias: a coin with two sides?" *Behavioral Sciences* 11, no. 7 (2021): 94.

Miller, Bruce L., and Bradley F. Boeve, eds. *The behavioral neurology of dementia.* Cambridge University Press, 2016.

Miller, Stephen D., Yael Katz-Levy, Katherine L. Neville, and Carol L. Vanderlugt. "Virus-induced autoimmunity: epitope spreading to myelin autoepitopes in Theiler's virus infection of the central nervous system." *Advances in Virus Research* 56 (2001): 199–217.

Mitra, Sumonto, Homira Behbahani, and Maria Eriksdotter. "Innovative therapy for Alzheimer's disease-with focus on biodelivery of NGF." *Frontiers in Neuroscience* 13 (2019): 38.

Murthy, J. M. K., Ravi Yangala, A. K. Meena, and J. Jaganmohan Reddy. "Acute disseminated encephalomyelitis: clinical and MRI study from South India." *Journal of the Neurological Sciences* 165, no. 2 (1999a): 133–138.

Murthy, J. M., R. Yangala, A. K. Meena, and J. J. Reddy. "Clinical, electrophysiological and magnetic resonance imaging study of acute disseminated encephalomyelitis." *The Journal of the Association of Physicians of India* 47, no. 3 (1999b): 280–283.

Neary, David, Julie S. Snowden, Lars Gustafson, Ulla Passant, Donald Stuss, S. A. S. A. Black, M. Freedman et al. "Frontotemporal lobar degeneration: a consensus on clinical diagnostic criteria." *Neurology* 51, no. 6 (1998): 1546–1554.

Nickels, Katherine C., and Elaine C. Wirrell. "Cognitive and social outcomes of epileptic encephalopathies." *Seminars in Pediatric Neurology*, vol. 24, no. 4 (2017): 264–275.

Noorbakhsh, Farshid, Richard T. Johnson, Derek Emery, and Christopher Power. "Acute disseminated encephalomyelitis: clinical and pathogenesis features." *Neurologic Clinics* 26, no. 3 (2008): 759–780.

Oh, Hyun Hee, Soon Hak Kwon, Chang Woo Kim, Byung Ho Choe, Cheol Woo Ko, Hee Du Jung, Jang Soo Suh, and Jun Hwa Lee. "Molecular analysis of HLA class ll-associated susceptibility to neuroinflammatory diseases in Korean children." *Journal of Korean Medical Science* 19, no. 3 (2004): 426–430.

Olds, Jennifer J., William L. Hills, Judith Warner, Julie Falardeau, Lori Haase Alasantro, Mark L. Moster, Robert A. Egan et al. "Posterior cortical atrophy: characteristics from a clinical data registry." *Frontiers in Neurology* 11 (2020): 358.

Paisiou, Anna, Evgenios Goussetis, Maria Dimopoulou, Vassiliki Kitra, Ioulia Peristeri, Giorgos Vessalas, Maria Gavra, Virginia A. Theodorou, and Stelios Graphakos. "Acute disseminated encephalomyelitis after allogeneic bone marrow transplantation for pure red cell aplasia–A case report and review of the literature." *Pediatric Transplantation* 17, no. 2 (2013): E41–E45.

Paliwal, Vimal K., G. Goel, R. Vema, S. Pradhan, and R. K. Gupta. "Acute disseminated encephalomyelitis following filarial infection." *Journal of Neurology, Neurosurgery & Psychiatry* 83, no. 3 (2012): 347–349.

Palop, Jorge J., and Lennart Mucke. "Amyloid-β–induced neuronal dysfunction in Alzheimer's disease: from synapses toward neural networks." *Nature neuroscience* 13, no. 7 (2010): 812–818.

Panayiotopoulos, Chrysostomos P. "The epilepsies: seizures, syndromes and management." (2010).

Pentz, Rowan, M. Florencia Iulita, Maya Mikutra-Cencora, Adriana Ducatenzeiler, David A. Bennett, and A. Claudio Cuello. "A new role for matrix metalloproteinase-3 in the NGF metabolic pathway: proteolysis of mature NGF and sex-specific differences in the continuum of Alzheimer's pathology." *Neurobiology of Disease* 148 (2021): 105150.

Pereira, Joana B., Sara Hall, Mattis Jalakas, Michel J. Grothe, Olof Strandberg, Erik Stomrud, Eric Westman, Danielle van Westen, and Oskar Hansson. "Longitudinal degeneration of the basal forebrain predicts subsequent dementia in Parkinson's disease." *Neurobiology of Disease* 139 (2020): 104831.

Perez, Florian, Catherine Helmer, Alexandra Foubert-Samier, Sophie Auriacombe, Jean-François Dartigues, and François Tison. "Risk of dementia in an elderly population of Parkinson's disease patients: a 15-year population-based study." *Alzheimer's & Dementia* 8, no. 6 (2012): 463–469.

Pillet, Laure-Elise, Camille Taccola, Justine Cotoni, Hervé Thiriez, Karine André, and Romain Verpillot. "Correlation between cognition and plasma noradrenaline level in Alzheimer's disease: a potential new blood marker of disease evolution." *Translational Psychiatry* 10, no. 1 (2020): 1–10.

Pohl, Daniela, Gulay Alper, Keith Van Haren, Andrew J. Kornberg, Claudia F. Lucchinetti, Silvia Tenembaum, and Anita L. Belman. "Acute disseminated encephalomyelitis: updates on an inflammatory CNS syndrome." *Neurology* 87, no. 9 Supplement 2 (2016): S38–S45.

Pohl, Daniela, Isabell Hennemuth, Rüdiger Von Kries, and Folker Hanefeld. "Paediatric multiple sclerosis and acute disseminated encephalomyelitis in Germany: results of a nationwide survey." *European Journal of Pediatrics* 166, no. 5 (2007): 405–412.

Pohl-Koppe, Annette, Sandra K. Burchett, Elizabeth A. Thiele, and David A. Hafler. "Myelin basic protein reactive Th2 T cells are found in acute disseminated encephalomyelitis." *Journal of Neuroimmunology* 91, no. 1–2 (1998): 19–27.

Prasad, Sakshi, Maanya Rajasree Katta, Shuchi Abhishek, Rishala Sridhar, Sai Sudha Valisekka, Maha Hameed, Jasneet Kaur, and Namrata Walia. "Recent advances in Lewy body dementia: A comprehensive review." *Disease-a-Month* (2022): 101441.

Quraishi, Imran H., Shani Stern, Kile P. Mangan, Yalan Zhang, Syed R. Ali, Michael R. Mercier, Maria C. Marchetto et al. "An epilepsy-associated KCNT1 mutation enhances excitability of human iPSC-derived neurons by increasing Slack KNa currents." *Journal of Neuroscience* 39, no. 37 (2019): 7438–7449.

Rajan, Kumar B., Jennifer Weuve, Lisa L. Barnes, Robert S. Wilson, and Denis A. Evans. "Prevalence and incidence of clinically diagnosed Alzheimer's disease dementia from 1994 to 2012 in a population study." *Alzheimer's & Dementia* 15, no. 1 (2019): 1–7.

Ranganath, Ajit, and Simon N. Jacob. "Doping the mind: dopaminergic modulation of prefrontal cortical cognition." *The Neuroscientist* 22, no. 6 (2016): 593–603.

Rawlings, D. J., R. J. Korsch, B. R. Goleby, G. M. Gibson, D. W. Johnstone, and M. Barlow. "TheJAK/STATsignaling pathway." (2002).

Richards, Maureen H., Meghann Teague Getts, Joseph R. Podojil, Young-Hee Jin, Byung S. Kim, and Stephen D. Miller. "Virus expanded regulatory T cells control disease severity in the Theiler's virus mouse model of MS." *Journal of Autoimmunity* 36, no. 2 (2011): 142–154.

Rosen, Howard J., Maria Luisa Gorno-Tempini, W. P. Goldman, R. J. Perry, N. Schuff, Michael Weiner, R. Feiwell, J. H. Kramer, and Bruce L. Miller. "Patterns of brain atrophy in frontotemporal dementia and semantic dementia." *Neurology* 58, no. 2 (2002): 198–208.

Samadian, Mohammad, Mahdi Gholipour, Mohammadreza Hajiesmaeili, Mohammad Taheri, and Soudeh Ghafouri-Fard. "The eminent role of microRNAs in the pathogenesis of Alzheimer's disease." *Frontiers in Aging Neuroscience* 13 (2021): 641080.

Sanford, A. M. Lewy Body Dementia. *Clinics in Geriatric Medicine* 34, no. 4 (2018): 603–615.

Saniya, K., B. G. Patil, Madhavrao D. Chavan, K. G. Prakash, Kumar Sai Sailesh, R. Archana, and Minu Johny. "Neuroanatomical changes in brain structures related to cognition in epilepsy: an update." *Journal of Natural Science, Biology, and Medicine* 8, no. 2 (2017): 139.

Sasikumar, Sanskriti, and Antonio P. Strafella. "Imaging mild cognitive impairment and dementia in Parkinson's disease." *Frontiers in Neurology* 11 (2020): 47.

Schulz, Jonathan, Gennaro Pagano, Juan Alberto Fernández Bonfante, Heather Wilson, and Marios Politis. "Nucleus basalis of Meynert degeneration precedes and predicts cognitive impairment in Parkinson's disease." *Brain* 141, no. 5 (2018): 1501–1516.

Seeley, W. W., A. M. Bauer, B. L. Miller, M. L. Gorno-Tempini, J. H. Kramer, M. Weiner, and H. J. Rosen. "The natural history of temporal variant frontotemporal dementia." *Neurology* 64, no. 8 (2005): 1384–1390.

Selkoe, Dennis J. "Toward a comprehensive theory for Alzheimer's disease. Hypothesis: Alzheimer's disease is caused by the cerebral accumulation and cytotoxicity of amyloid β-protein." *Annals of the New York Academy of Sciences* 924, no. 1 (2000): 17–25.

Selkoe, D.J., and Hardy, J. "The amyloid hypothesis of Alzheimer's disease at 25 years." *EMBO Molecular Medicine* 8, no. 6 (2016): 595–608. doi: 10.15252/emmm.201606210.

Šerý, Omar, Jana Povová, Ivan Míšek, Lukáš Pešák, and Vladimír Janout. "Molecular mechanisms of neuropathological changes in Alzheimer's disease: a review." *Folia Neuropathologica* 51, no. 1 (2013): 1–9.

Sharma, Veerta, Amarjot Kaur, and Thakur Gurjeet Singh. "Counteracting role of nuclear factor erythroid 2-related factor 2 pathway in Alzheimer's disease." *Biomedicine & Pharmacotherapy* 129 (2020): 110373.

Siderowf, Andrew, Dag Aarsland, Brit Mollenhauer, Jennifer G. Goldman, and Bernard Ravina. "Biomarkers for cognitive impairment in Lewy body disorders: status and relevance for clinical trials." *Movement Disorders* 33, no. 4 (2018): 528–536.

Simon, Amy R., Usha Rai, Barry L. Fanburg, and Brent H. Cochran. "Activation of the JAK-STAT pathway by reactive oxygen species." *American Journal of Physiology-Cell Physiology* 275, no. 6 (1998): C1640–C1652.

Skorvanek, Matej, Jennifer G. Goldman, Marjan Jahanshahi, Connie Marras, Irena Rektorova, Ben Schmand, Erik van Duijn et al. "Global scales for cognitive screening in Parkinson's disease: Critique and recommendations." *Movement Disorders* 33, no. 2 (2018): 208–218.

Sperling, Reisa A., Peter S. LaViolette, Kelly O'Keefe, Jacqueline O'Brien, Dorene M. Rentz, Maija Pihlajamaki, Gad Marshall et al. "Amyloid deposition is associated with impaired default network function in older persons without dementia." *Neuron* 63, no. 2 (2009): 178–188.

Stafstrom, Carl E., and Lionel Carmant. "Seizures and epilepsy: an overview for neuroscientists." *Cold Spring Harbor Perspectives in Medicine* 5, no. 6 (2015): a022426.

Staley, Kevin. "Molecular mechanisms of epilepsy." *Nature Neuroscience* 18, no. 3 (2015): 367–372.

Tan, Manuela M. X., Michael A. Lawton, Edwin Jabbari, Regina H. Reynolds, Hirotaka Iwaki, Cornelis Blauwendraat, Sofia Kanavou et al. "Genome-wide association studies of cognitive and motor progression in Parkinson's disease." *Movement Disorders* 36, no. 2 (2021): 424–433.

Taylor, John-Paul, Ian G. McKeith, David J. Burn, Brad F. Boeve, Daniel Weintraub, Claire Bamford, Louise M. Allan, Alan J. Thomas, and John T O'Brien. "New evidence on the management of Lewy body dementia." *The Lancet Neurology* 19, no. 2 (2020): 157–169.

Tenembaum, Silvia N. "Disseminated encephalomyelitis in children." *Clinical Neurology and Neurosurgery* 110, no. 9 (2008): 928–938.

Tenembaum, Silvia N. "Acute disseminated encephalomyelitis." *Handbook of Clinical Neurology* 112 (2013): 1253–1262.

Tenembaum, Silvia, Nestor Chamoles, and Natalio Fejerman. "Acute disseminated encephalomyelitis: a long-term follow-up study of 84 pediatric patients." *Neurology* 59, no. 8 (2002): 1224–1231.

Thomas, Alan J., John Paul Taylor, Ian McKeith, Claire Bamford, David Burn, Louise Allan, and John O'Brien. "Development of assessment toolkits for improving the diagnosis of the Lewy body dementias: feasibility study within the DIAMOND Lewy study." *International Journal of Geriatric Psychiatry* 32, no. 12 (2017): 1280–1304.

Torisu, Hiroyuki, Ryutaro Kira, Yoshito Ishizaki, Masafumi Sanefuji, Yui Yamaguchi, Sawa Yasumoto, Yoshihiko Murakami et al. "Clinical study of childhood acute disseminated encephalomyelitis, multiple sclerosis, and acute transverse myelitis in Fukuoka Prefecture, Japan." *Brain and Development* 32, no. 6 (2010): 454–462.

Tripathi, Timir, and Parismita Kalita. "Synergistic effect of amyloid-β and tau disrupts neural circuits." *ACS Chemical Neuroscience* 10, no. 3 (2019): 1129–1130.

van den Toren, Suzanne J., Amy van Grieken, Wico C. Mulder, Yvonne T. M. Vanneste, Marjolein Lugtenberg, Marlou L. A. de Kroon, Siok Swan Tan, and Hein Raat. "School absenteeism, Health-Related Quality of Life [HRQOL] and happiness among young adults aged 16–26 years." *International Journal of Environmental Research and Public Health* 16, no. 18 (2019): 3321.

Van Rijckevorsel, K. "Cognitive problems related to epilepsy syndromes, especially malignant epilepsies." *Seizure* 15, no. 4 (2006): 227–234.

Vermunt, Lisa, Sietske A. M. Sikkes, Ardo Van Den Hout, Ron Handels, Isabelle Bos, Wiesje M. Van Der Flier, Silke Kern et al. "Duration of preclinical, prodromal, and dementia stages of Alzheimer's disease in relation to age, sex, and APOE genotype." *Alzheimer's & Dementia* 15, no. 7 (2019): 888–898.

Vossius, Corinna, Jan P. Larsen, Carmen Janvin, and Dag Aarsland. "The economic impact of cognitive impairment in Parkinson's disease." *Movement Disorders* 26, no. 8 (2011): 1541–1544.

Walker, Zuzana, Katherine L. Possin, Bradley F. Boeve, and Dag Aarsland. "Lewy body dementias." *The Lancet* 386, no. 10004 (2015): 1683–1697.

Wamulugwa, Joan, Angelina Kakooza, Sabrina Bakeera Kitaka, Joyce Nalugya, Mark Kaddumukasa, Shirley Moore, Martha Sajatovic, and Elly Katabira. "Prevalence and associated factors of attention deficit hyperactivity disorder (ADHD) among Ugandan children; a cross-sectional study." *Child and Adolescent Psychiatry and Mental Health* 11, no. 1 (2017): 1–7.

Wang, Hui-Fu, Jin-Tai Yu, Shao-Wen Tang, Teng Jiang, Chen-Chen Tan, Xiang-Fei Meng, Chong Wang, Meng-Shan Tan, and Lan Tan. "Efficacy and safety of cholinesterase inhibitors and memantine in cognitive impairment in Parkinson's disease, Parkinson's disease dementia, and dementia with Lewy bodies: systematic review with meta-analysis and trial sequential analysis." *Journal of Neurology, Neurosurgery & Psychiatry* 86, no. 2 (2015): 135–143.

Wesson, Daniel W., Ralph A. Nixon, Efrat Levy, and Donald A. Wilson. "Mechanisms of neural and behavioral dysfunction in Alzheimer's disease." *Molecular Neurobiology* 43, no. 3 (2011): 163–179.

Westbrook, Andrew, R. Van Den Bosch, J. I. Määttä, L. Hofmans, D. Papadopetraki, Roshan Cools, and M. J. Frank. "Dopamine promotes cognitive effort by biasing the benefits versus costs of cognitive work." *Science* 367, no. 6484 (2020): 1362–1366.

Wingerchuk, Dean M., and Brian G. Weinshenker. "Acute disseminated encephalomyelitis, transverse myelitis, and neuromyelitis optica." *CONTINUUM: Lifelong Learning in Neurology* 19, no. 4 (2013): 944–967.

World Health Organization. *The ICD-10 classification of mental and behavioural disorders: clinical descriptions and diagnostic guidelines*. World Health Organization, 1992.

Wucherpfennig, Kai W., and Jack L. Strominger. "Molecular mimicry in T cell-mediated autoimmunity: viral peptides activate human T cell clones specific for myelin basic protein." *Cell* 80, no. 5 (1995): 695–705.

Xiong, Chang-Hui, Yan Yan, Zhen Liao, Shi-Hui Peng, Hai-Rong Wen, Yan-Xia Zhang, Shu-Hua Chen et al. "Epidemiological characteristics of acute disseminated encephalomyelitis in Nanchang, China: a retrospective study." *BMC Public Health* 14, no. 1 (2014): 1–6.

Young, Nathan P., Brian G. Weinshenker, Joseph E. Parisi, B. Scheithauer, C. Giannini, Shanu F. Roemer, Kristine M. Thomsen, Jayawant N. Mandrekar, Bradley J. Erickson, and Claudia F. Lucchinetti. "Perivenous demyelination: association with clinically defined acute disseminated encephalomyelitis and comparison with pathologically confirmed multiple sclerosis." *Brain* 133, no. 2 (2010): 333–348.

Zaman, V. et al. Cellular and molecular pathophysiology in the progression of Parkinson's disease. *Metabolic Brain Disease* 36, 815–827 (2021).

Zhang, L., Wu, A., Zhang, B., Chen, S., Men, X., Lin, Y., et al. Comparison of deep gray matter lesions on magnetic resonance imaging among adults with acute disseminated encephalomyelitis, multiple sclerosis, and neuromyelitis optica. *MultScler* 20 no. 4 (2014): 418–423.

Zhou, Jun-Li, Tatiana N. Shatskikh, Xianzeng Liu, and Gregory L. Holmes. "Impaired single cell firing and long-term potentiation parallels memory impairment following recurrent seizures." *European Journal of Neuroscience* 25, no. 12 (2007): 3667–3677.

# 3 Current Cognitive Medical Tests and Available Therapies

*Priya Dev and Abhishek Pathak*
Banaras Hindu University, Varanasi, India

## 3.1 INTRODUCTION

As we know, MRIs and other techniques can spot noticeable abnormalities in brain health, but they are neither simple nor risk-free to use. The void is filled by cognitive exams, which offer a very simple, non-invasive way to evaluate cognitive condition. In actual practice, we see that the diagnostic knowledge now gleaned from MRI data does not fully replace that which may be discovered by cognitive examination. In contrast to utilising only MRI data, Lebedeva et al. discovered that adding mini-mental state examination (MMSE) input to a random-forest classifier increased test accuracy, sensitivity, and specificity (Lebedeva et al. 2017). Significant neurocognitive disorders (NCDs) are not uniform medical illnesses. Despite being the primary factor in major NCDs, AD is not the main cause (Alzheimer's Association 2019; Falk et al. 2018). Although AD makes up between 60 and 80% of instances of major NCDs, frontotemporal, vascular, and Parkinson-related major NCDs are also common (Falk et al. 2018). Due to the absence of a universal physiological marker for all major and minor NCD variations, assessments that focus on the cognitive symptoms of major NCDs are helpful for screening individuals for additional, more in-depth investigation. In fact, minor NCDs are defined by the Diagnostic and Statistical Manual of Mental Disorders (DSM)-5 criteria as the existence of a noticeable decreased cognitive ability, as noted by an informant or a cognitive test, that does not yet interfere with the subject's day-to-day activities and that is not explained by delirium or a mental disorder (Alzheimer's Association 2019).

## 3.2 COMPARABLE COGNITIVE EVALUATIONS

### 3.2.1 Mini-Mental State Examination

The most widely used cognitive test at the moment is the MMSE. It consists of 11 questions with a combined score of 30, and it is used to classify a subject's level of cognitive impairment from mild to severe. The tests evaluate the cognitive functions of language, direction, registration, focus, calculations, and attention (Folstein et al. 1975). The cut-offs for cognitive normality typically vary depending on education level since, when assessing highly educated participants, the traditional cut-off score of roughly 23 must be adjusted to attain equivalent sensitivity/specificity (O'Bryant et al. 2008).

This exam has undergone many variations, some of which have been modified for patients with unique needs. The modified MMSE (3MS), which broadens scoring to 100 points and includes a few questions to evaluate different areas of cognition, the hearing/vision-impaired MMSE, and the normal MMSE are some examples of modifications (Teng and Chui 1987).

Indian clinicians most frequently employ the MMSE (Folstein et al. 1975) as a quick global cognitive assessment, both in the outpatient setting and at the bedside. The maximum score on the MMSE, a test administered using pencil and paper, is 30, with lower values indicating more serious cognitive issues. In the MMSE, a score of 24 is regarded as the cut-off to identify cognitive


DOI: 10.1201/9781003245346-3

impairment. Prior to post-anathesia recovery (PAR)'s copyright enforcement, it was frequently utilised for research as well. It has been shown to have low sensitivity and specificity (Creavin et al. 2016), particularly when used in mild or early disease conditions, and to overestimate cognitive impairment. Despite this, it is still used to obtain a standard index of cognitive dysfunction severity that is simple for clinicians to understand across the spectrum of neurocognitive disorders.

The Hindi mental state examination (HMSE) (Ganguli et al. 1995), a translation and adaptation of the MMSE, is used to screen the elderly, illiterate, Hindi-speaking population in rural areas. Like the MMSE, 30 is the highest possible score if all questions are correctly answered. It is openly accessible.

#### 3.2.1.1 Advantages

The popularity of the MMSE is arguably its biggest asset. Since it is the most widely used cognitive exam, data from a sizable patient pool are available for analysis for test scoring calibration and patient comparison. The ease of use of the MMSE is another benefit. It can be administered and scored with little training in under ten minutes. It has a rather high accuracy and specificity when it comes to detecting people with serious NCDs, despite its simplicity. When used to distinguish between educated individuals who were either normal or had relatively severe major NCDs, the MMSE had an accuracy of 89%, a sensitivity of 66%, and a specificity of 99%, according to an assessment of data that included MMSE scores from 1141 people with 16+ years of schooling (O'Bryant et al. 2008). In a similar vein, the MMSE covers a wide range of cognitive abilities despite its ease of use, with each area covering at least three points of the test. This enables both a preliminary screen for the cognitive domains in which the patient has the largest deficits as well as a reasonably comprehensive assessment of the patient's cognition. The MMSE scores were found to be correlated with morphological features of the brain, particularly the hippocampus (Dinomais et al. 2016), which is known to play a role in episodic and spatial memory (Eichenbaum et al. 1999), as well as the amygdala, cingulate gyrus, and parahippocampal gyrus (Dinomais et al. 2016), demonstrating that the MMSE produces results that are comparable to those of much more expensive tests.

#### 3.2.1.2 Disadvantages

Currently, the MMSE's associated intellectual property problems are a drawback. Clinicians must pay royalties to MiniMental, the current patent holders, for each occurrence of MMSE administration, at least for the official, current version, even though the material cost of administration is, in theory, negligible because the MMSE is patented. The creation of royalty-free cognitive tests has been prompted by this inconvenience (Folstein et al. 1975). While the MMSE concentrates on a number of distinct cognitive domains, it is constrained in its evaluation of other crucial features, such as visuospatial reasoning, for which there is only one question. This is another drawback of the test. This is a serious flaw because impaired visuospatial navigation is a well-known sign of AD and amnestic mild NCDs (Hort et al. 2007). The test also strongly relies on language, which can skew findings if the participant has poor reading and language skills (Park et al. 2018; Albert and Teresi 1999; Weiss et al. 1995; Mayeaux et al. 1995). Additionally, because of the assessment's low sensitivity, individuals who can achieve reasonably high MMSE scores but still show symptoms of serious NCDs must undergo a secondary evaluation (O'Bryant et al. 2008). The test's capacity to predict future decline is constrained in addition to its low sensitivity; however, analytical approaches like the COmputational Model to Predict the Development of Alzheimer's diSease Spectrum (COMPASS) are being developed to address this flaw (Zhu et al. 2016).

### 3.2.2 Clock-Drawing Test

One of the most conceptually straightforward cognitive tests that is frequently used is the clock-drawing exam. Although numerous scoring methods have been used for the test, they all generally provide points for various aspects of the clock, such as its design and the placement of the hands and numerals (Palsetia et al. 2018). At a specific time, typically 11:10, the patient is given the assignment of drawing an analogue clockface. This particular moment was selected because it requires the use of both visual fields and inhibits the "frontal pull" of the number 10 at the same time. Drawing the minute hand pointing to the number 10 on the clockface rather than the number 2 is a common error in serious NCD patients (Ryan et al. 2009). There are several scoring criteria for the clock, but the traditional one emphasises visuospatial skills and employs a ten-point scale (Sunderland et al. 1989).

#### 3.2.2.1 Advantages

The clock-drawing test's simplicity may be its biggest plus. With little preparation, the test can be given in under two minutes. The test's capacity to assess several cognitive processes, especially visuospatial reasoning, is a considerable advantage. Drawing intricate details helps the test to evaluate praxis. The requirement to place the minute hand at the proper time during the test evaluates calculation skills. The test measures visuospatial reasoning by comparing the relative sizes and positions of the clock face's numerals.

#### 3.2.2.2 Disadvantages

The clock-drawing test's primary flaw is inconsistent scoring. Since the prompt is so open-ended, each rater may provide a different score. The test also suffers from floor and ceiling effects since it is so straightforward; some patients with only mild NCDs are able to draw the clock properly, while others with serious NCDs are not able to draw even the circle of the face.

Secondary evaluation will be necessary to distinguish between these two patient groups. The clock-drawing exam is also limited by several important areas of cognition due to its simplicity, notably those that are connected to language. The clock-drawing exam may function best as a component of a larger test in order to reduce the impact of scoring variation on the overall score, attenuate floor and ceiling effects, and enlarge the cognitive domains tested. These three drawbacks point to this. Last but not least, this test can be unfair to people without a formal education. A Brazilian investigation of confounding variables that can affect a subject's performance on the clock-drawing test, for instance, discovered an association between education level and performance on the test (de Paula et al. 2013).

### 3.2.3 Addenbrooke's Cognitive Examinations

In order to include questions that assessed cognitive abilities not covered by the MMSE, such as visuospatial reasoning, the Addenbrooke's cognitive examination (ACE) was created as an extension of the MMSE. The MMSE is included in the evaluation verbatim in order to provide a 30-point MMSE sub-score. The ACE served as the basis for numerous variations, such as the ACE-Revised (ACE-R), which was created so that subdomain scores could be clearly defined, and the ACE-III, which was created to strengthen certain components of the ACE-R, such as repetition and comprehension, and which takes the place of the MMSE portion of the ACE and ACE-R (Noone 2015). The common cut-off for serious NCDs is between 82 and 88 out of 100 on the ACE-III composite score (Noone 2015).

The ACE-III (Mathuranath et al. 2000) is a 100-point, short, paper-and-pencil test that can be performed at the bedside to assess overall cognitive function. It is available in several other languages, including Marathi, Tamil, Telugu, Hindi, Indian English, and Kannada. This exam is free to take, and the clinical and research use cut-off scores are 88 and 82, respectively (Zhu et al. 2016). The ACE was previously available in some other Indian languages, including Bengali and Malayalam (known as MACE with established population-derived norms for an urban Malayalam-speaking population; Palsetia et al. 2018). However, these adaptations are of the ACER, which is no longer used in clinical and research settings and has been taken down from the NeuRA Research Institute's website (https://www.neura.edu.au/).

#### 3.2.3.1 Advantages

One of the benefits of the ACE is its capacity to assess visuospatial ability in both 2D and 3D, encompassing tasks like putting together broken letters and spatial reasoning with a wire Necker cube, while maintaining the variety of cognitive domains examined by the MMSE. The ACE performs better than the MMSE in terms of diagnostic ability since it fills various gaps left by the MMSE. The authors of the mini-ACE (M-ACE), a 30-point shortened version of the ACE, compared their test to the MMSE and discovered that the M-ACE was both more sensitive and less vulnerable to ceiling effects than the MMSE. Patients who received less than 21/30 on the M-ACE probably had a significant NCD, according to research (Hsieh et al. 2015). Also less vulnerable to floor effects is the ACE. The test was able to distinguish between different phases of Alzheimer's disease, according to a 2000 study evaluating ACE's capacity to identify mild or major NCDs, AD, and frontotemporal significant NCDs (Mathuranath et al. 2000). The ACE also has the benefit of being simple to administer and requiring little training. Finally, it appears that the test is still reliable even after being translated into different languages. For instance, a Japanese version of the ACE with a 74/100 threshold achieved a sensitivity of 0.889 and a specificity of 0.987.

#### 3.2.3.2 Disadvantages

The ACE versions that incorporate questions from the MMSE are susceptible to the same patent issues as the ACE-III, which stands apart from the MMSE. Additionally, because the ACE was created in the United Kingdom (UK), some of the questions are slanted in favour of people who are familiar with British culture or other European nations with comparable political structures. The name of the prime minister or head of the opposition party, for instance, is requested in some of the inquiries (Callow et al. 2015).

### 3.2.4 General Practitioner Cognition Assessment

Doctors working in primary care settings can use the General Practitioner Assessment of Cognition (GPCOG), which was created for this purpose. Two interviews – one with the patient and the other with an informant, a close friend, or relative of the patient – make up the test format. There are two different ways to complete the nine-question patient interview: in writing or online (Brodaty et al. 2002). The clock-drawing test, address recall, and a recent news item are all included in the patient interview. Six questions are asked during the informant interview on the patient's capacity to carry out daily activities such as finding things, speaking, and handling money (Brodaty et al. 2002).

#### 3.2.4.1 Advantages

The GPCOG assesses the patient's orientation, visual spatial ability, executive function, retrieval of recent information, and delayed recollection in just nine questions (Brodaty et al. 2002). The test has equivalent sensitivity and specificity to the MMSE, taking around four minutes for the patient interview and two minutes for the informant interview (Brodaty et al. 2002). The physician can now focus on other tasks because there are written and online choices for the patient assessment. The GPCOG is also free to use, unlike the MMSE which is patented. Finally, it appears that the GPCOG has no preference for educational attainment or cultural background (Basic et al. 2009).

#### 3.2.4.2 Disadvantages

The test's dependence on an informant's presence is one of its drawbacks. The patient's age was also found to be a significant (correlation = 0.187, P = 0.01) predictor of their score on the cognitive assessment portion of the GPCOG, despite not being a factor in the informant-based section (Brodaty et al. 2004).

### 3.2.5 Montreal Cognitive Assessment

The Montreal Cognitive Assessment (MoCA) was created as a screening tool to replace the MMSE that is better suited to the detection of mild NCDs. The initial test achieved better sensitivity for both mild NCDs and AD, though with less specificity (Nasreddine et al. 2005); however, with fine-tuning of the cut-off scores, the MoCA can achieve better sensitivity and specificity in detecting mild NCDs than the MMSE (Ciesielska et al. 2016). In addition to the MMSE, it can be used to evaluate people who score within the normal cognitive range but show other indicators of cognitive impairment, such as difficulty with daily tasks. It can also be used to examine people whose illness is minor enough that it has no impact on their daily lives. The paper-based exam can be taken for no cost. It includes inquiries and other cognitive exams that cover a wide range of typical domains. The clock-drawing exam is also included, and a modified trail-making test is used to evaluate visuomotor, visuoperceptual, and task-switching abilities. Language proficiency, conceptual thinking, recall/memory, and orientation are all tested as part of the MoCA (Julayanont and Nasreddine 2017).

The MoCA (Nasreddine et al. 2005) is a free, quick, and easy-to-use global cognitive screening tool that is growing in popularity because it is available in a variety of languages, including Bengali, Kannada, Malayalam, Marathi, Tamil, Telugu, Hindi, and Urdu, which are all spoken in India. It has been approved for usage in Parkinson's disease patients who speak Malayalam (Krishnan et al. 2015). There are measures to adjust the score for low levels of schooling, visual impairments, and physical disabilities, and the highest score is 30. For repeated evaluations, it offers strong test–retest reliability. The threshold score of 26 is used to separate persons with mild cognitive impairment from normal subjects. When compared to the MMSE, the MoCA demonstrates greater sensitivity and specificity. The computerised test is currently being developed.

#### 3.2.5.1 Advantages

Even though it only lasts for around ten minutes and may be completed in a typical clinical environment, the exam measures a wide range of critical cognitive abilities. Additionally, the test is freely accessible (Julayanont and Nasreddine 2017). It has also been discovered that the MoCA more accurately predicts cognitive reserve than the MMSE, which may contribute to the MoCA's increased sensitivity to early stage AD (Kang et al. 2018); people with higher cognitive reserves have been found to have a lower risk of developing major NCDs (Valenzuela and Sachdev 2006).

#### 3.2.5.2 Disadvantages

The MoCA's disadvantage with regard to sensory impairment is noteworthy. In a study comparing the MoCA scores of 301 older adults, of whom 50% had no sensory impairments and 38, 5, and 7% had hearing, vision, or dual-sense impairments, it was discovered that, despite modifying the scores of the sensory-impaired individuals, those who had no impairments were more likely to pass (Dupuis et al. 2015). Although, as with other examinations, the overall score was obtained and compared to a current one, there were some questions with noticeably higher failure rates among 2653 older people with cardiovascular disease (Rossetti et al. 2011). The test also needs to be adjusted for age and educational level.

### 3.2.6 A Tool for Dementia Screening in the Community

The 10/66 research battery of tests uses the Community Screening Instrument for Dementia (CSI-D) (Hall et al. 1993) as a cognitive screening instrument to assess general cognitive function (Sosa et al. 2009). A global cognitive score is produced using a 32-item cognitive test. Additionally, it incorporates the results of a 26-item informant interview regarding the patient's daily activities and overall health into a single predictive algorithm (Prince et al. 2011). The CSI-D has also been produced in a condensed form for non-specialist healthcare professionals to use in primary care settings (Prince et al. 2011).

#### 3.2.6.1 Cognitive Testing in Kolkata

The population of Kolkata possesses normative data thanks to the Kolkata cognitive screening (Prince et al. 2011), a global cognitive screening battery. Bengali is the test language used. The translated test battery is openly accessible and free.

#### 3.2.6.2 The Adult Health Survey Conducted by the World Health Organization's Study on AGEing

A culture-sensitive screening instrument known as the World Health Organization's Study on AGEing and Adult Health survey (SAGE) was created as part of the household health survey that was conducted in Ghana, India, and Tanzania. The pilot study comprises normative data for the word list learning test, category fluency (animals), and digit span from 469 Indian adults (forward and backward). The SAGE data and cognitive tests are openly available (Das et al. 2006).

#### 3.2.6.3 Indian Variant of Cognistat

The short cognitive screening tool Cognistat, originally known as the neurobehavioural cognitive status examination, has been modified for use in the Indian population and has demonstrated good validity for use in patients with traumatic brain injury. Normative data produced from the population have not yet been established, despite the fact that it has shown strong reliability and validity on a small scale. The test's publishers' website does not mention the Indian version as a purchasing option, therefore it is uncertain if it is currently offered for sale (Gupta and Kumar 2009).

#### 3.2.6.4 Multi-domain Cognitive Screening Test (MDCST)

The MDCST (Hota et al. 2012) is a sensitive and user-friendly global cognitive screening tool designed to identify early mild cognitive impairment (MCI). It has also demonstrated strong psychometric features that will allow it to be used in future demographic research. It has been approved for usage on the population of lowlanders who are acclimated and stay at elevations higher than 4300 m.

#### 3.2.6.5 Rapid Test for Dementia Assessment

The four test items on the dementia assessment by rapid test (DART) (Swati et al. 2015) – the repetition of three words, category fluency (vegetables), recall of words, and drawing a clock – are graded on a scale from 0 to 4. When compared to the MMSE, it has been proven to have low specificity but strong concurrent validity. This brief screening exam is freely accessible.

#### 3.2.6.6 Mattis Dementia Rating Scale Translation into Hindi

The 36 tasks divided into five components make up the Hindi version of the Mattis Dementia rating scale (Gopaljee et al. 2011), which has a maximum score of 144. For assessing dementia in the Hindi-speaking Indian population, it has demonstrated good validity and reliability.

#### 3.2.6.7 Universal Dementia Assessment Scale (Rowland)

The application of the Rowland Universal Dementia Assessment Tool in the Malayalam-speaking community has been verified (Iype et al. 2006). The cut-off score was 23, and the test has a maximum score of 30. When compared to the Malayalam MMSE, it was discovered that the Rowland Universal Dementia Assessment Scale (RUDAS) had similar sensitivity but greater specificity.

#### 3.2.6.8 A Screen for Impaired Picture Memory

The Picture-based Memory Impairment Screen (Verghese et al. 2012) is a non-specialist-administered cognitive test that uses pictures to assess culture-fairness. It can be delivered in four minutes and is an efficient screening tool. It was created for use in persons 55 years and older with little to no formal education, and it exhibits strong reliability and validity. Twelve digital photos are grouped into three sets of four for this test. The subject is shown any one group of images, and after completing an interference task, they are required to recall as many images as they can. If the participant is unable to recall the information on their own, category cues are provided and rated accordingly.

#### 3.2.6.9 Available Domain-Wise Tests with Indian Benchmarks

In the clinical environment, speech-language pathologists frequently perform a thorough evaluation of language function. There are aphasia test batteries available for the Indian population, including the Indian Aphasia Battery (Nehra et al. 2013) and the Western Aphasia Battery with Indian norms (Chengappa and Kumar 2008). The Bilingual Aphasia Test battery is available in variants in Hindi, Kannada, Oriya, Tamil, and Urdu (Chengappa and Kumar 2008); however, population-derived criteria have not been developed for the test battery in each of these languages.

#### 3.2.6.10 Designed and Standardised Batteries for the Indian Population

##### *3.2.6.10.1 The Postgraduate Institute of Medical Education and Research (PGI) Battery of Brain Malfunction*

The five subtests that make up the PGI battery of brain dysfunction include the PGI Memory Scale, Bhatia's Short Scale, the Verbal Adult Intelligence Scale, the Nahor–Benson Perceptual Acuity Test, and the Bender Visual Motor Gestalt Test. Based on 19 test factors, this test battery provides an overall assessment of cognitive impairment. It was created in 1990 and has established guidelines for people aged 20–59.

##### *3.2.6.10.2 A Memory Scale for PGI*

Ten subtests of the PGI memory scale (Pershad and Verma 1990) measure verbal and non-verbal memory, remote memory, recent memory, short-term memory, and long-term memory. The examination was created at Chandigarh's Postgraduate Institute of Medical Education and Research. It has been standardised for adults aged 20–45.

##### *3.2.6.10.3 The Neuropsychological Test Battery of the National Institute of Mental Health and Neurosciences (NIMHANS)*

The first neuropsychological test battery created in India was the NIMHANS (Pershad and Wig 1978). Based on Luria's theories of brain localisation and lateralization of higher mental functions, it is a battery of lobe function tests. It has around 20 tests, including a few modified western tests and a native delayed reaction test to rate working memory (Pershad and Wig 1978).

##### *3.2.6.10.4 Adult NIMHANS Cognitive Test*

The 19 commonly used western neuropsychological tests that have been modified and standardised for the Indian population make up the NIMHANS Neuropsychological Battery for Adults (Mukundan and Murthy 1979). It has been approved for treatment in several neurocognitive disorders and has population-derived standards for individuals aged 16–65.

##### *3.2.6.10.5 Children's NIMHANS Neuropsychological Test*

The NIMHANS neuropsychological battery for children (Rao et al. 2004) was validated for use in children with brain injuries and has norms for ages 5–15.

##### *3.2.6.10.6 The Senior NIMHANS Neuropsychological Battery*

A thorough test battery called the NIMHANS neuropsychological battery for the elderly (NNB-E) (Kar et al. 2011) was created for use with Indian seniors between the ages of 55 and 80. It has been demonstrated to have strong discriminant validity for detecting elderly people with Alzheimer's disease.

###### *3.2.6.10.7 The Comprehensive Neuropsychological Battery in Hindi (Adult Form) from the All India Institute of Medical Sciences*

The comprehensive neuropsychological battery in Hindi (adult form) (Tripathi et al. 2013) developed by the All India Institute of Medical Sciences is a battery of tests with age ranges of 15–80. The Luria Nebraska Neuropsychological Battery served as its foundation. There are 160 items in total, distributed across ten fundamental scales and four auxiliary scales. It is the only locally created Hindi test battery in India.

###### *3.2.6.10.8 10/66 Battery of Cognitive Tests from the Dementia Research Group*

The 10/66 Dementia Research Group trials, which include measures of general cognitive function, verbal fluency, and memory, use the cognitive test battery developed by the group (Gupta et al. 2000). It was created using data from the Consortium to Establish a Registry for Alzheimer's Disease and the Community Screening Instrument for Dementia (CSID). It provides site-specific standards for people aged 65–80. Given that the same battery has been normed across seven countries, it is helpful for cross-cultural studies (Cuba, Dominican Republic, Venezuela, Peru, Mexico, China, and India).

###### *3.2.6.10.9 HIV Battery of Cognitive Tests*

The cognitive domains that are known to be susceptible to the effects of HIV were assessed using the HIV cognitive test battery (Sosa et al. 2009). It includes examinations that were adapted for evaluation in Tamil and Telugu from those used in the United States. For this battery, there are no recognised standards.

#### 3.2.6.11 Commercially Available Test Batteries

The Wechsler Intelligence Scale for Children, Fourth Edition, India and Wechsler Adult Intelligence Scale, Fourth Edition, India, which are recognised as the gold standard evaluations globally, are now offered by publishers with adaptations, standards, and norms tailored specifically for the Indian population. Additionally, the publishers offer the Wechsler Memory Scale, Third Edition, India, which is utilised all over the country to evaluate verbal and non-verbal learning and memory. The publisher recently made the Wechsler Abbreviated Scale of Intelligence, Second Edition, India available as a quick and accurate test of cognitive aptitude (Yepthomi et al. 2006). Although some of the tests in the test batteries and their pertinent norms can be used independently in clinical and research settings, making them valuable for a thorough cognitive assessment, they are more frequently used only in larger academic and medical institutions by clinical psychologists and neuropsychologists due to their high cost of acquisition. A thorough battery of computerised neuropsychological tests called CNS Vital Signs is offered in a variety of languages, including Bengali, Gujarati, Hindi, Kannada, Malayalam, Marathi, Punjabi, Tamil, Telugu, and Urdu. It consists of ten exams that have been normed, although it's not apparent if there are any norms based on the Indian population.

## 3.3 VIRTUAL REALITY APPLICATIONS FOR DIAGNOSING AND TREATING COGNITIVE DISORDERS

### 3.3.1 Diagnostics in Virtual Reality

#### 3.3.1.1 Context

Virtual reality (VR) is a concept that entails submerging a person in a simulated setting. In some cases, tactile feedback can be transmitted to the user through other systems, such as controllers. Users are able to interact with this environment through some set of physical sensors, and typically perceive that environment through a headset that provides visuals and audio for the environment (Park et al. 2019a). In the context of major NCDs, the allure of VR comes from its ability to assess and improve spatial reasoning, along with other cognitive abilities, depending on the focus and design of the programme (Park et al. 2019b; Zucchella et al. 2018). The distinctive features of VR systems have generated considerable interest in the medical and psychiatric fields. Alzheimer's disease and even mild amnestic NCDs are both characterised by a decline in visuospatial thinking (Hort et al. 2007). While it is possible to test spatial cognition with straightforward visuospatial tests, including some paper and pencil methods, these tests tend to correlate only partially, if at all, with spatial navigation in large-scale environments (Hegarty et al. 2006). This is a flaw in the current state-of-the-art diagnostic examinations for major NCDs. Setting the test environment in virtual reality is one potential approach for including large-scale spatial reasoning questions in 3D. The capacity to properly navigate virtual reality environments has been found to coincide with that of their real-world equivalents (Van Schaik et al. 2008), and the MMSE score is correlated with that ability.

#### 3.3.1.2 Egocentric and Allocentric Navigation

The positioning of items relative to the individual's location (egocentric navigation) and the positioning of objects relative to one another (allocentric navigation) are the two main kinds of navigation strategies. Weniger et al. asked patients to memorise a VR park environment in order to identify deficiencies in egocentric navigation in Alzheimer's and mild NCDs. The authors also asked patients to memorise a VR maze in order to characterise any deficiencies in allocentric navigation. Although the study was unable to distinguish between mild NCD patients and controls on egocentric and allocentric navigation tasks, mild NCD patients performed worse than controls in both of these tests (Weniger et al. 2011). Using moderate amnestic NCD, Serino et al. (2015) evaluated the allocentric and egocentric spatial ability.

A virtual room comprising particular things, including a target object, was entered by the AD patient and the control players. One of two tests was run during the second phase. In the first, patients saw a top-down image of the room with other objects present, but the target object absent. In the second, patients entered an empty VR room with only an arrow for directional guidance; this room was approached from a different side than the first. Although these differences depended on the task and the angle from which the participants entered the virtual space, there were significant disparities between AD patients and the controls (Serino et al. 2015). Alzheimer's, mild NCD, and normal older people were assessed on their ability to navigate virtual and physical surroundings, measuring their memory and navigation skills. In particular, there was no discernible difference between real-world and VR performances, demonstrating the effectiveness of both the real-world and virtual assessments in discriminating across groups (Cushman et al. 2008).

#### 3.3.1.3 Navigational Memory

To assess spatial working memory, Lee et al. developed a non-immersive virtual rendition of the traditional radial arm maze (RAM). Six arms of the maze, one of which has a goal, are joined to a central platform. After leaving one arm, a person must first go to the central platform before visiting another arm. Remembering which arms have been visited and which have not is the maze's main challenge. The maze can be revisited, and some of the arms won't ever contain treasure because of how the mazes are made. "Spatial reference memory" is the process of learning and remembering which arms will never contain riches. Working memory and spatial reference memory were both shown to be impaired in AD patients, according to Lee et al., whereas only spatial reference memory was reported to be affected in moderate NCD patients (Lee et al. 2014). Plancher et al. (2012) used the active and passive vehicular exploration of a VR city setting to test the episodic memories of amnestic mild NCD patients, AD patients, and controls.

Allocentric and egocentric navigational memory (remembering the position/sequence of items, for example) as well as other route-related details were among the details that participants were asked to recall. The participant's cognitive health was a significant predictor of poor performance, albeit this effect was significantly more pronounced in AD patients than in people with moderate amnestic NCDs (Plancher et al. 2012).

#### 3.3.1.4 Activities of Daily Life (ADL)

The ability to perform everyday tasks is essential to the classification of significant NCDs, which are characterised as cognitive deficits that make performing daily activities challenging. Although many surveys and questionnaires have been developed, using this criterion in diagnosis is challenging because it relies on patient and/or caregiver interviews, which can be subjective and affected by the subject's interpretation of a question. Furthermore, reliable administration is largely restricted to outpatient settings (Sikkes et al. 2009; Bucks et al. 1996; Johnson et al. 2004). In particular, VR makes it possible to simulate tasks that participants would actually encounter so that they can be graded on how well they handle them. In order to screen for early significant NCDs, Tarnanas et al. (2013) developed an unconventional VR setup that included a treadmill and curved screen. Participants had to navigate fire-building situations that varied in difficulty.

The Bristol ADL and Blessed ADL tests were found to be less accurate predictors of moderate NCD to AD conversion than individuals' performance scores (Tarnanas et al. 2013). "A Day to Remember," a VR experience made by Dulau et al., including gamified cognitive exams as well as real-world activities. Most players found the VR game to be simple to play and said it was less stressful than the direct screening exams. The test's precision was considerably weak, even if it was functionally associated with the paper MMSE, and it was indicated that a participant's difficulty using the new technology might be a confounding factor (Dulau et al. 2019). A low-immersion virtual supermarket was developed by Zygouris et al. to test many aspects of task completion, including the amount of time needed to finish a shopping list, the accuracy of the products purchased, the amount of money spent, and the kinds of items purchased. All participants were successful in finishing the exercise and administering the exam on the given tablet at home (Zygouris et al. 2015, 2017). The aforementioned performance criteria were first utilised in a research to separate 34 mild NCD patients from a sample of 55. Based on the errors made and specific age/performance limits, a decision tree was built. It was possible to attain a sensitivity of 82% and a specificity of 95%. In a follow-up study, the same methodology was used, and a Naive Bayes classifier was trained using data from 20 of the participants' trials. The classifier successfully identified those with moderate NCD with a sensitivity of 94% and a specificity of 89% (Zygouris et al. 2017).

#### 3.3.1.5 Advantages

The fundamental benefit of VR-based cognitive examinations is the potential to examine visuospatial reasoning in 3D, a crucial sign of cognitive loss caused by AD and other NCDs that standard tests fall short of fully capturing (Karr et al. 2018). Additionally, computer-based testing streamlines cloud data storage and significantly reduces test administration variability; provided patients have the necessary tools, tests can even be given by patients themselves (Zygouris et al. 2017). The tests are simple to perform, allowing data from numerous trials to be collected, enhancing the sensitivity/specificity and accuracy of classifiers (Zygouris et al. 2015, 2017). Furthermore, because the settings of the controlled environment may be easily adjusted as needed (Bohil et al. 2011), it is possible to address more complex queries that would not be practical or viable to perform in a real environment. Additionally, the "gamification" of the testing work might reduce the stress associated with traditional testing by transforming the activity into a more enjoyable one (Clay et al. 2020). A person's ability to successfully accomplish the activities of daily life, which are crucial for determining a person's capacities and whether they can live independently, has only a limited relationship to neuropsychological tests (Farias et al. 2003). VR tools have been found to closely resemble their physical equivalents, particularly in navigation (Cushman et al. 2008), and they can be used to assess particular characteristics, including episodic memory, in a more realistic, practical setting (Plancher et al. 2012). Compared to their paper and pen counterparts, VR exams show higher ecological validity (Tarnanas et al. 2013; Dulau et al. 2019). Such assessments of instrumental daily activities are crucial in the diagnosis of instances of pre-major NCDs and can aid in the prediction of the development of mild NCDs into AD (Tarnanas et al. 2013). Dual task tests that evaluate a person's intellect and ability to sustain gait are also made easier with the help of VR.

#### 3.3.1.6 Disadvantages

VR-based diagnosis has the drawback of having a somewhat greater fixed cost for obtaining the necessary equipment than other testing. However, as the price of VR headsets and equipment goes down over time, the usefulness of VR-based tests and treatments increases (Castelvecchi 2016). Additionally, compared to present assessments, VR-based tests demand greater administrative skills. Evaluation of social cues is another area of cognition where VR may have limitations. In contrast to VR, traditional cognitive examinations entail a conversation between the patient and the test supervisor. The lack of direct verbal connection between the administrator and patient when using contemporary cognitive assessment tools like the MMSE in VR may result in results that are inconsistent with those of the original versions. Additionally, some VR system users experience motion sickness, which can impair their performance and make using the VR system uncomfortable (Sikkes et al. 2009). Certain aspects of the VR experience, such as the number of graphic frames per second and the restriction of sharp turns, can be tuned to reduce discomfort (Dulau et al. 2019). Tests like the "Simulator Sickness Questionnaire" can be used to identify people who are prone to feeling sick in the VR environment in a way that could affect their results (Kennedy et al. 1993). The use of VR and other digital exams may potentially be hampered by general technophobia (Tarnanas et al. 2013; Dulau et al. 2019). Recent research appears to have addressed some of these accessibility concerns, such as motion sickness, possibly as a result of technological advancements (Clay et al. 2020). These drawbacks might be more effectively offset as VR technology develops and spreads.

### 3.3.2 Virtual Reality-based Therapy

#### 3.3.2.1 Context

For severe or mild NCDs, there is currently no known pharmaceutical treatment or preventive measure. However, certain actions and way of life decisions might lessen a person's likelihood of being cognitively impaired, and research has shown that AD is negatively connected with mental stimulation and education (Geerlings et al. 1997). Therefore, it would be desirable to invest in the creation of mental exercises that might be able to halt the trend of cognitive deterioration as the hunt for an effective medication treatment goes on. It has been proven to be beneficial to use computer environments to enhance cognitive function, and this has been done in the context of mild NCDs. Computerised cognitive training includes exercises for honing particular cognitive skills, especially created video games, nicknamed "serious games", and virtual reality experiences. Despite not always taking place in a VR setting, these programmes show that gamified exercises have several benefits. Following computerised training sessions, cognitive advantages as well as certain emotional and wellbeing gains have been noted (Lampit et al. 2014; Hill et al. 2017; Barnes et al. 2009). It has been discovered that both specially created and commercially available "exergames" (like those for the Nintendo Wii) help elderly people with their balance (Schwenk et al. 2016; Williams et al. 2011). Serious games, like "Kitchen and Cooking", that require users to perform cognitively taxing tasks or simulate actual events that are crucial to daily living are typically well-liked by the older population and have significant positive effects on cognition and independence (Manera et al. 2015). Virtual reality games hold particular promise for teaching 3D navigation. Depression is also a significant risk factor for the emergence of major NCDs. Immersing patients in imaginary worlds with the aim of elevating mood is one potential use of VR.

#### 3.3.2.2 Exercises in Virtual Reality

For people with mild NCDs, Lee (2016) created a 12-week virtual reality workout programme. Three gaming sessions each week were held with the patients, for a total of 36 sessions. Balance, depression, and quality of life were monitored in the patients throughout this time, and all three measures showed considerable improvement. A control group attending conventional therapy sessions did not experience any appreciable improvement (Lee 2016). Although the specifics of the VR training programme used are unknown, Hwang and Lee used a VR training programme on 24 older people with mild NCD and discovered that their balance and cognitive test scores had improved in comparison to controls (Hwang and Lee 2017). VR video-game-based exercise, according to Htut et al., can concurrently enhance cognitive function while being less helpful than regular physical activity in tests of physical ability but better than controls (Htut et al. 2018). It has been discovered that combining virtual worlds with popular training methods, including stationary cycling, is suitable for both younger and older people and is evaluated as fun by users, encouraging long-term adherence to the exercise programme (Sakhare et al. 2019; Ben-Sadoun et al. 2016).

#### 3.3.2.3 Online Cognitive Training Exercises

Since VR tests are effective in assessing a patient's navigational skills, they might be helpful for rehabilitating those skills. A VR navigation simulation based on Graz, Austria, was used by Kober et al. Participants showed brain damage with obvious impairments in spatial orientation rather than moderate NCDs or Alzheimer's disease. Following the VR training session, it was discovered that users' overall performance on spatial cognition tests had improved (Kober et al. 2013). Man et al. discovered that VR-based memory training resulted in higher memory improvements in relation to cognitive problems than participating in therapist-led memory training (Man et al. 2012). Although the study's participants only played the game for a short period of time overall, Fasilis et al. found that major NCD patients who played serious VR games did not significantly improve: the training programme lasted ten hours over four to five weeks (Fasilis et al. 2018).

#### 3.3.2.4 Dual-task Training

In dual-task training, a mentally taxing job is carried out while the subject is moving. These tasks are helpful for measuring gait control, whose loss is typical of mild NCDs and is particularly prevalent in Parkinson's disease cases (Belghali et al. 2017). Liao et al. developed a dual-task VR exercise programme combining physical and cognitive training, and they discovered that the programme significantly improved dual-task performance in the VR group compared to the non-VR group while also improving executive function and gait performance. VR systems' special capacity to combine physical exercise with an interactive setting appears to be a big help in addressing issues with dual-task performance (Liao et al. 2019).

#### 3.3.2.5 Benefits

Users of VR-based therapy may be able to train in their homes if they have the necessary equipment (Dockx et al. 2016). VR-based therapy enables patients to practise cognitive function without supervision. Additionally, they offer patients the chance to practise routine chores with little risk. It is simple to store patient performance data for tasks in the cloud for analysis. Additionally, some VR exercise programmes are more well-liked than traditional physical activity regimens (Htut et al. 2018) and users of some VR training programmes describe them as "fun", which can encourage adherence to a VR-based cognitive training programme (Liao et al., 2019). As previously mentioned, VR exercise makes it simple to incorporate a cognitive component (Eggenberger et al. 2015), which can provide simultaneous physical and cognitive benefits that may benefit from the promotion of neuroplastic processes induced by exercise (Eggenberger et al. 2015; Foster et al. 2011). Additionally, research shows that VR's sense of immersion plays a significant role in sharpening spatial skills.

Over the course of four weeks, 33 participants with an average age of 62 were evaluated to determine the impact of immersive (VR) and non-immersive versions of the video game "Fruit Ninja". Inhibition and task switching were improved in the VR exergaming participants but not in the non-VR group (Huang 2020).

#### 3.3.2.6 Negative Aspects

Once more, the initial cost of equipment procurement is a large fixed cost. Although VR has the potential to allow patients to train their mental faculties independently of clinicians, in reality it's possible that the VR equipment would be too expensive for most people to invest in at home; as a result, the doctor would still be responsible for supervising the training. Additionally, it's possible that VR has limitations when it comes to developing social skills. The aforementioned studies note that participants largely tolerated and enjoyed VR systems, but sample sizes were relatively small; larger studies with more rigorously explained inclusion and exclusion criteria are necessary for further analysis of the prevalence of tolerability issues. Additionally, as previously mentioned, some people experience motion sickness from virtual environments, and the discomfort may limit or prevent their use of therapeutic VR (Sikkes et al. 2009). Additionally, serious games are generally thought to be better suited for people with milder NCDs rather than AD and major NCDs; people with major NCDs also need caregiver assistance more than people with mild NCDs (Manera et al. 2017).

### 3.3.3 Mixed and Augmented Reality

Virtual elements are added to the real world rather than a fully virtual area being created in augmented reality (AR), which is different from VR. A projection of the real environment is typically used, with virtual information and features superimposed on it to increase the user's sense of reality. "True" AR is generally restricted to information displays and non-interactive components, with the addition of interactive, entirely virtual components falling under the mixed reality umbrella (MR). On the reality continuum, mixed reality sits between VR and AR, with virtual, interactive features added to a presentation of the real world (Farshid et al. 2018). In order to recognise what is in the user's environment and how the user is interacting with it, cameras and other tracking mechanisms are required for both MR and AR applications. Systems can be stationary or mobile, though the computing power of mobile systems can be constrained.

Because these systems are "in" and have gained social acceptance, their practical applications in daily life are somewhat constrained. Complex interactions sometimes need a significant amount of computational power, and performing voice and gesture interactions in public can be obtrusive or uncomfortable (Carmigniani et al. 2011). Mobile augmented reality (MAR) systems have been used in a number of applications, including navigation, education, and entertainment, thanks to the nearly universal use of mobile devices and the introduction of cloud computing (Chatzopoulos et al. 2017).

Although research demonstrating this have generally involved relatively young pupils rather than older and/or cognitively impaired persons, AR systems have been shown to improve learning (Albrecht et al. 2013; Kucuk et al. 2016). MAR applications that work with a phone have also been suggested for the gamification of specific tasks, such as helping older people stay hydrated (Lehman et al. 2018).

MAR for major NCDs and AD with numerous AR applications were created with AD patients in mind. A daily living activity assistant for AR was studied by Rohrbach et al. The researchers evaluated the ability of AD patients to brew a cup of tea using a Microsoft HoloLens and their application, Therapy Lens. Holographic cues that described the necessary steps were included in the programme. The processes could be advanced by the use of voice commands. The programme's overall value was not clear because participants who received AR support did not perform any better and actually took longer to complete each task overall. Researchers noted that some participants had trouble recalling how to operate the system and speculated that this may be due to people with neurodegenerative illnesses having poor learning abilities. Although some participants complained that the AR system was uncomfortable and others claimed not to have noticed or remembered the holograms, participants still expressed interest in it (Rohrbach et al. 2019). Other methods, such as the Cooperative for Assistance and Relief Everywhere (cARe), have been suggested as a way to train patients with serious NCDs on daily activities using AR predictions. Notably, cARe has the option to "time out", which prompts the user once again and provides instructions for the current step. This feature can be useful if the patient gets sidetracked or forgets their duty. Incentives based on praise were also used to encourage patients. Although research on cARe is still in progress, preliminary findings indicate that it is more useful than written directions when it comes to cooking. Like Therapy Lens, there were issues with the audio communication, and the system failed to take into account patients changing the order of stages (Wolf et al. 2018).

An MR cognitive trainer built for HoloLens was developed by Aruanno et al. The trainer was tested using two different prototypes; the first was gesture-controlled, and the second – which was updated in response to input from the first prototype – was voice- and gesture-controlled. Both included a variety of text-based exercises designed to improve short-term and spatial memory that involved finding specific things in boxes projected around the user's environment. Despite the absence of controls from the study, participants found the trainer to be interesting and the second prototype to be user-friendly, even for those who were not familiar with technology. The HoloLens itself is meant to lessen the motion sickness and weariness that are common to VR systems, therefore there was very little discomfort reported. Additionally, by forgoing VR's total immersion, MR enables the user to maintain awareness of the real world. The study sheds light on various issues that must be addressed in the creation of MR cognitive trainers, such as where and how to place textual instructions, what feedback (sound, visual, etc.) to supply the user, and interaction techniques – the response was generally good. Using the Consortium to Establish a Registry for Alzheimer's Disease, Park et al. studied the effects of an MR cognitive trainer and discovered that the programme significantly enhanced visuospatial working memory compared to conventional cognitive training (Aruanno et al. 2017; Park et al. 2019b).

## 3.4 RECOMMENDATIONS

Even though there is currently no pharmaceutical treatment for major NCDs, an early diagnosis of the condition is still useful for helping patients manage it and for advancing research that could lead to a cure. Also useful for enhancing and maintaining cognitive functions are non-pharmacological therapies like VR-based cognitive training and serious games. The decision-making process for a patient's present and future alternatives for assistive care can currently be facilitated by an early diagnosis. Consequently, a useful cognitive test for serious NCDs is required. A test's pragmatism and scientific quality must both be taken into account.

The clock-drawing test may be the most practical cognitive test, but it does not adequately assess language skills. The MMSE, which has grown in popularity and is now the norm for use in cognitive investigations, may be the test with the most present utility. However, to maximise accuracy, sensitivity, and specificity, perhaps a more comprehensive assessment such as ACE should be taken into consideration due to its associated intellectual property issues and shortcomings in testing visuospatial abilities. It might be helpful to use a straightforward test without a corresponding patent, like the General Practioner Assessment of Cognition (GPCOG), to resolve the intellectual property issues. However, there is currently no test in widespread use that can evaluate visuospatial reasoning in three dimensions, a critical deficit in amnestic mild NCDs and AD.

The diagnosis of serious NCDs, as well as the development of cognitive skills and the reduction of depressive symptoms, may all benefit from the use of VR-based 3D environments. It is more practical to use virtual, augmented, and mixed realities in both hospital and at-home settings as the technology enabling them becomes more widely available. We suggest that VR spatial assessments, such as virtual mazes, be developed and examined because it is clear how important the capacity to use spatial thinking is for identifying one's primary NCD condition. These VR programmes could act as cognitive training tools as well as tests. As they allow the user to preserve environmental awareness while still allowing for a 3D spatial component to games and activities, AR and MR techniques may be best for usage at home. ADL tasks also offer a test that is fairly simple to comprehend and complete and that can be used to assess the severity of someone's cognitive impairment. Patients with mild and severe NCDs may be encouraged to complete tasks that are essential to maintaining their mental faculties due to the increased engagement seen with AR and MR activities.

## REFERENCES

Albert, Steven M., and Jeanne A. Teresi. "Reading ability, education, and cognitive status assessment among older adults in Harlem, New York City." *American Journal of Public Health* 89, no. 1 (1999): 95–97.

Albrecht, Urs-Vito, Kristian Folta-Schoofs, Marianne Behrends, and Ute Von Jan. "Effects of mobile augmented reality learning compared to textbook learning on medical students: randomized controlled pilot study." *Journal of Medical Internet Research* 15, no. 8 (2013): e2497.

Alzheimer's Association. "2019 Alzheimer's disease facts and figures." *Alzheimer's & Dementia* 15, no. 3 (2019): 321–387.

Aruanno, Beatrice, Franca Garzotto, and Mario Covarrubias Rodriguez. "Hololens-based mixed reality experiences for subjects with Alzheimer's disease." In *Proceedings of the 12th Biannual Conference on Italian SIGCHI Chapter*, pp. 1–9. 2017.

Barnes, Deborah E., Kristine Yaffe, Nataliya Belfor, William J. Jagust, Charles DeCarli, Bruce R. Reed, and Joel H. Kramer. "Computer-based cognitive training for mild cognitive impairment: results from a pilot randomized, controlled trial." *Alzheimer Disease and Associated Disorders* 23, no. 3 (2009): 205.

Basic, David, Angela Khoo, David Conforti, Jeffrey Rowland, Freda Vrantsidis, Dina Logiudice, Keith Hill, Jan Harry, Katherine Lucero, and Robert Prowse. "Rowland Universal Dementia Assessment Scale, Mini-Mental State Examination and General Practitioner Assessment of Cognition in a multicultural cohort of community-dwelling older persons with early dementia." *Australian Psychologist* 44, no. 1 (2009): 40–53.

Belghali, Maroua, Nathalie Chastan, Fabien Cignetti, Damien Davenne, and Leslie M. Decker. "Loss of gait control assessed by cognitive-motor dual-tasks: pros and cons in detecting people at *risk* of developing Alzheimer's and Parkinson's diseases." *Geroscience* 39, no. 3 (2017): 305–329.

Ben-Sadoun, Grégory, Guillaume Sacco, Valeria Manera, Jérémy Bourgeois, Alexandra König, Pierre Foulon, Baptiste Fosty, François Bremond, Fabienne d'Arripe-Longueville, and Philippe Robert. "Physical and cognitive stimulation using an exergame in subjects with normal aging, mild and moderate cognitive impairment." *Journal of Alzheimer's Disease* 53, no. 4 (2016): 1299–1314.

Bohil, Corey J., Bradly Alicea, and Frank A. Biocca. "Virtual reality in neuroscience research and therapy." *Nature Reviews Neuroscience* 12, no. 12 (2011): 752–762.

Brodaty, Henry, Nicola M. Kemp, and Lee-Fay Low. "Characteristics of the GPCOG, a screening tool for cognitive impairment." *International Journal of Geriatric Psychiatry* 19, no. 9 (2004): 870–874.

Brodaty, Henry, Dimity Pond, Nicola M. Kemp, Georgina Luscombe, Louise Harding, Karen Berman, and Felicia A. Huppert. "The GPCOG: a new screening test for dementia designed for general practice." *Journal of the American Geriatrics Society* 50, no. 3 (2002): 530–534.

Bucks, R. S., D. L. Ashworth, G. K. Wilcock, and K. Siegfried. "Assessment of activities of daily living in dementia: development of the Bristol Activities of Daily Living Scale." *Age and Ageing* 25, no. 2 (1996): 113–120.

Callow, Lauren, Fiona Alpass, Janet Leathem, and Christine Stephens. "Normative data for older New Zealanders on the Addenbrooke's Cognitive Examination-Revised." *New Zealand Journal of Psychology (Online)* 44, no. 3 (2015): 29.

Carmigniani, Julie, Borko Furht, Marco Anisetti, Paolo Ceravolo, Ernesto Damiani, and Misa Ivkovic. "Augmented reality technologies, systems and applications." *Multimedia Tools and Applications* 51, no. 1 (2011): 341–377.

Castelvecchi, Davide. "Low-cost headsets boost virtual reality's lab appeal." *Nature* 533, no. 7602 (2016): 153–154.

Chatzopoulos, Dimitris, Carlos Bermejo, Zhanpeng Huang, and Pan Hui. "Mobile augmented reality survey: From where we are to where we go." *IEEE Access* 5 (2017): 6917–6950.

Chengappa, Shyamala K., and Ravi Kumar. "Normative & Clinical Data on the Kannada Version of Western Aphasia Battery (WAB-K)." *Language in India* 8, no. 6 (2008): 6–8.

Ciesielska, Natalia, Remigiusz Sokołowski, Ewelina Mazur, Marta Podhorecka, Anna Polak-Szabela, and Kornelia Kędziora-Kornatowska. "Is the Montreal Cognitive Assessment (MoCA) test better suited than the Mini-Mental State Examination (MMSE) in mild cognitive impairment (MCI) detection among people aged over 60? Meta-analysis." *Psychiatria Polska* 50, no. 5 (2016): 1039–1052.

Clay, Felix, David Howett, James FitzGerald, Paul Fletcher, Dennis Chan, and Annabel Price. "Use of immersive virtual reality in the assessment and treatment of Alzheimer's disease: a systematic review." *Journal of Alzheimer's Disease* 75, no. 1 (2020): 23–43.

Creavin, Sam T., Susanna Wisniewski, Anna H. Noel-Storr, Clare M. Trevelyan, Thomas Hampton, Dane Rayment, Victoria M. Thom et al. "Mini-Mental State Examination (MMSE) for the detection of dementia in clinically unevaluated people aged 65 and over in community and primary care populations." *Cochrane Database of Systematic Reviews* 1 (2016).

Cushman, Laura A., Karen Stein, and Charles J. Duffy. "Detecting navigational deficits in cognitive aging and Alzheimer disease using virtual reality." *Neurology* 71, no. 12 (2008): 888–895.

Das, Shyamal Kumar, Tapas Kumar Banerjee, Chandra Shekhar Mukherjee, Paramita Bose, Atanu Biswas, Avijit Hazra, A. Dutt et al. "An urban community-based study of cognitive function among non-demented elderly population in India." *Neurology Asia* 11 (2006): 37–48.

Dinomais, Mickael, Sebastien Celle, Guillaume T. Duval, Frederic Roche, Samir Henni, Robert Bartha, Olivier Beauchet, and Cedric Annweiler. "Anatomic correlation of the mini-mental state examination: a voxel-based morphometric study in older adults." *PloS one* 11, no. 10 (2016): e0162889.

Dockx, K., Bekkers, E.M., Van den Bergh, V., Ginis, P., Rochester, L., Hausdorff, J.M., Mirelman, A., and Nieuwboer, A. "Virtual reality for rehabilitation in Parkinson's disease." *Cochrane Database of Systematic Reviews* 12 (2016).

Dulau, Eva, Chrisna R. Botha-Ravyse, Mika Luimula, Panagiotis Markopoulos, Evangelos Markopoulos, and Kimmo Tarkkanen. "A virtual reality game for cognitive impairment screening in the elderly: a user perspective." In *2019 10th IEEE International Conference on Cognitive Infocommunications (CogInfoCom)*, pp. 403–410. IEEE, 2019.

Dupuis, Kate, M. Kathleen Pichora-Fuller, Alison L. Chasteen, Veronica Marchuk, Gurjit Singh, and Sherri L. Smith. "Effects of hearing and vision impairments on the Montreal Cognitive Assessment." *Aging, Neuropsychology, and Cognition* 22, no. 4 (2015): 413–437.

Eggenberger, Patrick, Vera Schumacher, Marius Angst, Nathan Theill, and Eling D. de Bruin. "Does multi-component physical exercise with simultaneous cognitive training boost cognitive performance in older adults? A 6-month randomized controlled trial with a 1-year follow-up." *Clinical Interventions in Aging* 10 (2015): 1335.

Eichenbaum, Howard, Paul Dudchenko, Emma Wood, Matthew Shapiro, and Heikki Tanila. "The hippocampus, memory, and place cells: is it spatial memory or a memory space?" *Neuron* 23, no. 2 (1999): 209–226.

Falk, Nathan, Ariel Cole, and T. Jason Meredith. "Evaluation of suspected dementia." *American Family Physician* 97, no. 6 (2018): 398–405.

Farias, Sarah Tomaszewski, Ernest Harrell, Craig Neumann, and Andrew Houtz. "The relationship between neuropsychological performance and daily functioning in individuals with Alzheimer's disease: ecological validity of neuropsychological tests." *Archives of Clinical Neuropsychology* 18, no. 6 (2003): 655–672.

Farshid, Mana, Jeannette Paschen, Theresa Eriksson, and Jan Kietzmann. "Go boldly!: Explore augmented reality (AR), virtual reality (VR), and mixed reality (MR) for business." *Business Horizons* 61, no. 5 (2018): 657–663.

Fasilis, T., P. Patrikelis, A. Siatouni, A. Alexoudi, A. Veretzioti, L. Zachou, and S. St. Gatzonis. "A pilot study and brief overview of rehabilitation via virtual environment in patients suffering from dementia." *Psychiatrike= Psychiatriki* 29, no. 1 (2018): 42–51.

Folstein, M. F., S. E. Folstein, and P. R. McHugh. "'Mini-mental state.' A practical method for grading the cognitive state of patients for the clinician." *Journal of Psychiatric Research* 12, no. 3 (1975): 189–198.

Foster, Philip P., Kevin P. Rosenblatt, and Rodrigo O. Kuljiš. "Exercise-induced cognitive plasticity, implications for mild cognitive impairment and Alzheimer's disease." *Frontiers in Neurology* 2 (2011): 28.

Ganguli, Mary, Graham Ratcliff, Vijay Chandra, Sujatha Sharma, Joanne Gilby, Rajesh Pandav, Steven Belle et al. "A Hindi version of the MMSE: the development of a cognitive screening instrument for a largely illiterate rural elderly population in India." *International Journal of Geriatric Psychiatry* 10, no. 5 (1995): 367–377.

Geerlings, M. I., D. J. H. Deeg, B. Schmand, J. Lindeboom, and C. Jonker. "Increased risk of mortality in Alzheimer's disease patients with higher education? A replication study." *Neurology* 49, no. 3 (1997): 798–802.

Gopaljee, S., C. B. Dwivedi, and Rakesh Pandey. "Psychometric evaluation of the Hindi adaptation of Mattis Dementia Rating Scale (HMDRS)." *The Indian Journal of social Science Research* 9 (2011): 82–90.

Gupta, Ashum, and Natasha Khullar Kumar. "Indian adaptation of the Cognistat: Psychometric properties of a cognitive screening tool for patients of traumatic brain injury." *Indian Journal of Neurotrauma* 6, no. 02 (2009): 123–132.

Gupta, Surya, S. K. Khandelwal, P. N. Tandon, M. C. Maheshwari, V. S. Mehta, K. R. Sundaram, A. K. Mahapatra, and S. Jain. "The development and standardization of comprehensive neuropsychological battery in Hindi (adult form)." *Journal of Personality and Clinical Studies* 16, no. 2 (2000): 75–108.

Hall, Kathleen S., Hugh C. Hendrie, Harry M. Brittain, and James A. Norton. "The development of a dementia screening interview in two distinct languages." *International Journal of Methods in Psychiatric Research* (1993).

Hegarty, Mary, Daniel R. Montello, Anthony E. Richardson, Toru Ishikawa, and Kristin Lovelace. "Spatial abilities at different scales: Individual differences in aptitude-test performance and spatial-layout learning." *Intelligence* 34, no. 2 (2006): 151–176.

Hill, Nicole T. M., Loren Mowszowski, Sharon L. Naismith, Verity L. Chadwick, Michael Valenzuela, and Amit Lampit. "Computerized cognitive training in older adults with mild cognitive impairment or dementia: a systematic review and meta-analysis." *American Journal of Psychiatry* 174, no. 4 (2017): 329–340.

Hort, Jakub, Jan Laczó, Martin Vyhnálek, Martin Bojar, Jan Bureš, and Kamil Vlček. "Spatial navigation deficit in amnestic mild cognitive impairment." *Proceedings of the National Academy of Sciences* 104, no. 10 (2007): 4042–4047.

Hota, Sunil Kumar, Vijay Kumar Sharma, Kalpana Hota, Saroj Das, Priyanka Dhar, Bidhu Bhusan Mahapatra, Ravi Bihari Srivastava, and Shashi Bala Singh. "Multi-domain cognitive screening test for neuropsychological assessment for cognitive decline in acclimatized lowlanders staying at high altitude." *Indian Journal of Medical Research* 136, no. 3 (2012): 411–420.

Hsieh, Sharpley, Sarah McGrory, Felicity Leslie, Kate Dawson, Samrah Ahmed, Chris R. Butler, James B. Rowe, Eneida Mioshi, and John R. Hodges. "The Mini-Addenbrooke's Cognitive Examination: a new assessment tool for dementia." *Dementia and Geriatric Cognitive Disorders* 39, no. 1–2 (2015): 1–11.

Htut, Thwe Zar Chi, Vimonwan Hiengkaew, Chutima Jalayondeja, and Mantana Vongsirinavarat. "Effects of physical, virtual reality-based, and brain exercise on physical, cognition, and preference in older persons: a randomized controlled trial." *European Review of Aging and Physical Activity* 15, no. 1 (2018): 1–12.

Huang, Kuo-Ting. "Exergaming executive functions: An immersive virtual reality-based cognitive training for adults aged 50 and older." *Cyberpsychology, Behavior, and Social Networking* 23, no. 3 (2020): 143–149.

Hwang, Jungha, and Sunmin Lee. "The effect of virtual reality program on the cognitive function and balance of the people with mild cognitive impairment." *Journal of Physical Therapy Science* 29, no. 8 (2017): 1283–1286.

Iype, Thomas, B. K. Ajitha, P. Antony, N. B. Ajeeth, S. Job, and K. S. Shaji. "Usefulness of the Rowland universal dementia assessment scale in South India." *Journal of Neurology, Neurosurgery & Psychiatry* 77, no. 4 (2006): 513–514.

Johnson, Nancy, A. Barion, A. Rademaker, G. Rehkemper, and S. Weintraub. "The Activities of Daily Living Questionnaire: a validation study in patients with dementia." *Alzheimer Disease & Associated Disorders* 18, no. 4 (2004): 223–230.

Julayanont, Parunyou, and Ziad S. Nasreddine. "Montreal Cognitive Assessment (MoCA): concept and clinical review." In *Cognitive screening instruments*, pp. 139–195. Springer, Cham, 2017.

Kang, Jae Myeong, Young-Sung Cho, Soowon Park, Byung Ho Lee, Bo Kyung Sohn, Chi Hyun Choi, Jeong-Seok Choi et al. "Montreal cognitive assessment reflects cognitive reserve." *BMC Geriatrics* 18, no. 1 (2018): 1–8.

Kar, Bhoomika R., Shobini L. Rao, B. A. Chandramouli, and K. Thennarasu. "Growth patterns of neuropsychological functions in Indian children." *Frontiers in Psychology* 2 (2011): 240.

Karr, Justin E., Raquel B. Graham, Scott M. Hofer, and Graciela Muniz-Terrera. "When does cognitive decline begin? A systematic review of change point studies on accelerated decline in cognitive and neurological outcomes preceding mild cognitive impairment, dementia, and death." *Psychology and Aging* 33, no. 2 (2018): 195.

Kennedy, Robert S., Norman E. Lane, Kevin S. Berbaum, and Michael G. Lilienthal. "Simulator sickness questionnaire: An enhanced method for quantifying simulator sickness." *The International Journal of Aviation Psychology* 3, no. 3 (1993): 203–220.

Kober, Silvia Erika, Guilherme Wood, Daniela Hofer, Walter Kreuzig, Manfred Kiefer, and Christa Neuper. "Virtual reality in neurologic rehabilitation of spatial disorientation." *Journal of Neuroengineering and Rehabilitation* 10, no. 1 (2013): 1–13.

Krishnan, Syam, Sunitha Justus, Radhamani Meluveettil, Ramshekhar N. Menon, Sankara P. Sarma, and Asha Kishore. "Validity of Montreal Cognitive Assessment in non-english speaking patients with Parkinson's disease." *Neurology India* 63, no. 1 (2015): 63.

Lampit, Amit, Harry Hallock, and Michael Valenzuela. "Computerized cognitive training in cognitively healthy older adults: a systematic review and meta-analysis of effect modifiers." *PLoS Medicine* 11, no. 11 (2014): e1001756.

Lebedeva, Aleksandra K., Eric Westman, Tom Borza, Mona K. Beyer, Knut Engedal, Dag Aarsland, Geir Selbaek, and Asta K. Haberg. "MRI-based classification models in prediction of mild cognitive impairment and dementia in late-life depression." *Frontiers in Aging Neuroscience* (2017): 13.

Lee, Geun-Ho. "Effects of virtual reality exercise program on balance, emotion and quality of life in patients with cognitive decline." *The Journal of Korean Physical Therapy* 28, no. 6 (2016): 355–363.

Lee, Jun-Young, Sooyeon Kho, Hye Bin Yoo, Soowon Park, Jung-Seok Choi, Jun Soo Kwon, Kyung Ryeol Cha, and Hee-Yeon Jung. "Spatial memory impairments in amnestic mild cognitive impairment in a virtual radial arm maze." *Neuropsychiatric Disease and Treatment* 10 (2014): 653.

Lehman, Sarah, Jenna Graves, Carlene Mcaleer, Tania Giovannetti, and Chiu C. Tan. "A mobile augmented reality game to encourage hydration in the elderly." In *International Conference on Human Interface and the Management of Information*, pp. 98–107. Springer, Cham, 2018.

Liao, Ying-Yi, I-Hsuan Chen, Yi-Jia Lin, Yue Chen, and Wei-Chun Hsu. "Effects of virtual reality-based physical and cognitive training on executive function and dual-task gait performance in older adults with mild cognitive impairment: a randomized control trial." *Frontiers in Aging Neuroscience* 11 (2019): 162.

Man, David W. K., Jenny C. C. Chung, and Grace Y. Y. Lee. "Evaluation of a virtual reality-based memory training programme for Hong Kong Chinese older adults with questionable dementia: a pilot study." *International Journal of Geriatric Psychiatry* 27, no. 5 (2012): 513–520.

Manera, Valeria, Grégory Ben-Sadoun, Teun Aalbers, Hovannes Agopyan, Florence Askenazy, Michel Benoit, David Bensamoun et al. "Recommendations for the use of serious games in neurodegenerative disorders: 2016 Delphi Panel." *Frontiers in Psychology* 8 (2017): 1243.

Manera, Valeria, Pierre-David Petit, Alexandre Derreumaux, Ivan Orvieto, Matteo Romagnoli, Graham Lyttle, Renaud David, and Philippe H. Robert. "'Kitchen and cooking,' a serious game for mild cognitive impairment and Alzheimer's disease: a pilot study." *Frontiers in Aging Neuroscience* 7 (2015): 24.

Mathuranath, P. S., P. J. Nestor, G. E. Berrios, Wojtek Rakowicz, and J. R. Hodges. "A brief cognitive test battery to differentiate Alzheimer's disease and frontotemporal dementia." *Neurology* 55, no. 11 (2000): 1613–1620.

Mayeaux Jr, E. J., T. C. Davis, R. H. Jackson, D. Henry, P. Patton, L. Slay, and T. Sentell. "Literacy and self-reported educational levels in relation to Mini-mental State Examination scores." *Family Medicine* 27, no. 10 (1995): 658–662.

Mukundan, C. R., and V. N. Murthy. Lateralization and Localizing Cerebral Lesions by a Battery of Neuropsychological Tests. Paper Presented *at the Joint Conference of Neurology, Psychiatry, Clinical Psychology and Psychiatric Social Work Societies of India*, NIMHANS, Bangalore, India; 1979.

Nasreddine, Ziad S., Natalie A. Phillips, Valérie Bédirian, Simon Charbonneau, Victor Whitehead, Isabelle Collin, Jeffrey L. Cummings, and Howard Chertkow. "The Montreal Cognitive Assessment, MoCA: a brief screening tool for mild cognitive impairment." *Journal of the American Geriatrics Society* 53, no. 4 (2005): 695–699.

Nehra, A., D. Pershad, and V. Sreenivas. "Indian Aphasia battery: Tool for specific diagnosis of language disorder post stroke." *Journal of the Neurological Sciences* 333 (2013): e165.

Noone, Peter. "Addenbrooke's cognitive examination-III." *Occupational Medicine* 65, no. 5 (2015): 418–420.

O'Bryant, Sid E., Joy D. Humphreys, Glenn E. Smith, Robert J. Ivnik, Neill R. Graff-Radford, Ronald C. Petersen, and John A. Lucas. "Detecting dementia with the mini-mental state examination in highly educated individuals." *Archives of Neurology* 65, no. 7 (2008): 963–967.

Palsetia, Delnaz, G. Prasad Rao, Sarvada C. Tiwari, Pragya Lodha, and Avinash De Sousa. "The clock drawing test versus mini-mental status examination as a screening tool for dementia: a clinical comparison." *Indian Journal of Psychological Medicine* 40, no. 1 (2018): 1–10.

Park, Eunhee, Byoung-Ju Yun, Yu-Sun Min, Yang-Soo Lee, Sung-Jun Moon, Jae-Won Huh, Hyunsil Cha, Yongmin Chang, and Tae-Du Jung. "Effects of a mixed reality-based cognitive training system compared to a conventional computer-assisted cognitive training system on mild cognitive impairment: a pilot study." *Cognitive and Behavioral Neurology* 32, no. 3 (2019b): 172–178.

Park, Jin Kyung, Eun Hye Jeong, and Gyeong Ae Seomun. "The clock drawing test: a systematic review and meta-analysis of diagnostic accuracy." *Journal of Advanced Nursing* 74, no. 12 (2018): 2742–2754.

Park, Mi Jin, Dong Jun Kim, Unjoo Lee, Eun Jin Na, and Hong Jin Jeon. "A literature overview of virtual reality (VR) in treatment of psychiatric disorders: recent advances and limitations." *Frontiers in Psychiatry* 10 (2019a): 505.

Paula, Jonas Jardim de, Debora Marques de Miranda, Edgar Nunes de Moraes, and Leandro Fernandes Malloy-Diniz. "Mapeando as engrenagens: o que o Teste do Desenho do Relogio avalia no envelhecimento normal e patologico?" *Arquivos de Neuro-Psiquiatria* 71 (2013): 763–768.

Pershad, Dwarka, and Santosh K. Verma. *Hand-book of PGI battery of brain dysfunction (PGI-BBD)*. National Psychological Corporation, 1990.

Pershad, Dwarka, and N. N. Wig. "Reliability and validity of a new battery of memory tests (PGI memory scale)." *Indian Journal of Psychiatry* 20, no. 1 (1978): 76–80.

Plancher, Gaën, A. Tirard, V. Gyselinck, S. Nicolas, and P. Piolino. "Using virtual reality to characterize episodic memory profiles in amnestic mild cognitive impairment and Alzheimer's disease: influence of active and passive encoding." *Neuropsychologia* 50, no. 5 (2012): 592–602.

Prince, M., Daisy Acosta, Cleusa P. Ferri, Mariella Guerra, Yueqin Huang, K. S. Jacob, Juan J. Llibre Rodríguez et al. "A brief dementia screener suitable for use by non-specialists in resource poor settings—the cross-cultural derivation and validation of the brief Community Screening Instrument for Dementia." *International Journal of Geriatric Psychiatry* 26, no. 9 (2011): 899–907.

Rao, S. L., D. K. Subbakrishna, and K. Gopukumar. "NIMHANS neuropsychological battery manual." *Bangalore: National Institute of Mental Health and Neurosciences* (2004).

Rohrbach, Nina, Philipp Gulde, Alan Robert Armstrong, Linda Hartig, Anas Abdelrazeq, Stefan Schröder, Johanne Neuse, Timo Grimmer, Janine Diehl-Schmid, and Joachim Hermsdörfer. "An augmented reality approach for ADL support in Alzheimer's disease: a crossover trial." *Journal of Neuroengineering and Rehabilitation* 16, no. 1 (2019): 1–11.

Rossetti, Heidi C., Laura H. Lacritz, C. Munro Cullum, and Myron F. Weiner. "Normative data for the Montreal Cognitive Assessment (MoCA) in a population-based sample." *Neurology* 77, no. 13 (2011): 1272–1275.

Ryan, Joseph J., Laura A. Glass, Jared M. Bartels, and Anthony M. Paolo. "Base Rates of "10 to 11" Clocks in Alzheimer's and Parkinson's Disease." *International Journal of Neuroscience* 119, no. 9 (2009): 1261–1266.

Sakhare, Ashwin R., Vincent Yang, Joy Stradford, Ivan Tsang, Roshan Ravichandran, and Judy Pa. "Cycling and spatial navigation in an enriched, immersive 3D virtual park environment: a feasibility study in younger and older adults." *Frontiers in Aging Neuroscience* 11 (2019): 218.

Schwenk, Michael, Marwan Sabbagh, Ivy Lin, Pharah Morgan, Gurtej S. Grewal, Jane Mohler, David W. Coon, and Bijan Najafi. "Sensor-based balance training with motion feedback in people with mild cognitive impairment." *Journal of Rehabilitation Research and Development* 53, no. 6 (2016): 945.

Serino, Silvia, Francesca Morganti, Fabio Di Stefano, and Giuseppe Riva. "Detecting early egocentric and allocentric impairments deficits in Alzheimer's disease: An experimental study with virtual reality." *Frontiers in Aging Neuroscience* 7 (2015): 88.

Sikkes, S. A. M., E. S. M. De Lange-de Klerk, Y. A. L. Pijnenburg, and P. Scheltens. "A systematic review of Instrumental Activities of Daily Living scales in dementia: room for improvement." *Journal of Neurology, Neurosurgery & Psychiatry* 80, no. 1 (2009): 7–12.

Sosa, Ana Luisa, Emiliano Albanese, Martin Prince, Daisy Acosta, Cleusa P. Ferri, Mariella Guerra, Yueqin Huang et al. "Population normative data for the 10/66 Dementia Research Group cognitive test battery from Latin America, India and China: a cross-sectional survey." *BMC Neurology* 9, no. 1 (2009): 1–11.

Sunderland, Trey, James L. Hill, Alan M. Mellow, Brian A. Lawlor, Joshua Gundersheimer, Paul A. Newhouse, and Jordan H. Grafman. "Clock drawing in Alzheimer's disease: a novel measure of dementia severity." *Journal of the American Geriatrics Society* 37, no. 8 (1989): 725–729.

Swati, B., V. Sreenivas, T. Manjari, and N. Ashima. "Dementia assessment by rapid test (dart): an Indian screening tool for dementia." *The Journal of Alzheimer Disease & Parkinsonism* 5, no. 198 (2015): 2161–2460.

Tarnanas, Ioannis, Winfried Schlee, Magda Tsolaki, René Müri, Urs Mosimann, and Tobias Nef. "Ecological validity of virtual reality daily living activities screening for early dementia: longitudinal study." *JMIR Serious Games* 1, no. 1 (2013): e2778.

Teng, E., and H. Chui. "The modified mini-mental state examination (3MS)." *The Canadian Journal of Psychiatry* 41, no. 2 (1987): 114–121.

Tripathi, Ravikesh, Janakiprasad Kumar Kumar, Srikala Bharath, Palaniappan Marimuthu, and Mathew Varghese. "Clinical validity of NIMHANS neuropsychological battery for elderly: A preliminary report." *Indian Journal of Psychiatry* 55, no. 3 (2013): 279.

Valenzuela, Michael J., and Perminder Sachdev. "Brain reserve and dementia: a systematic review." *Psychological Medicine* 36, no. 4 (2006): 441–454.

Van Schaik, Paul, Anthony Martyr, Tim Blackman, and John Robinson. "Involving persons with dementia in the evaluation of outdoor environments." *Cyber Psychology & Behavior* 11, no. 4 (2008): 415–424.

Verghese, Joe, Mohan L. Noone, Beena Johnson, Anne F. Ambrose, Cuiling Wang, Herman Buschke, Vayyattu G. Pradeep, Kizhakkaniyakath Abdul Salam, Kunnukatil S. Shaji, and Pavagada S. Mathuranath. "Picture-based memory impairment screen for dementia." *Journal of the American Geriatrics Society* 60, no. 11 (2012): 2116–2120.

Weiss, Barry D., Richard Reed, Evan W. Kligman, and Abdul Abyad. "Literacy and performance on the mini-mental state examination." *Journal of the American Geriatrics Society* 43, no. 7 (1995): 807–810.

Weniger, Godehard, Mirjana Ruhleder, Claudia Lange, Stefanie Wolf, and Eva Irle. "Egocentric and allocentric memory as assessed by virtual reality in individuals with amnestic mild cognitive impairment." *Neuropsychologia* 49, no. 3 (2011): 518–527.

Williams, Barbara, Nicole L. Doherty, Andrew Bender, Holly Mattox, and Jesse R. Tibbs. "The effect of Nintendo Wii on balance: A pilot study supporting the use of the Wii in occupational therapy for the well elderly." *Occupational Therapy in Health Care* 25, no. 2–3 (2011): 131–139.

Wolf, Dennis, Daniel Besserer, Karolina Sejunaite, Matthias Riepe, and Enrico Rukzio. "care: An augmented reality support system for dementia patients." In *The 31st Annual ACM Symposium on User Interface Software and Technology Adjunct Proceedings*, pp. 42–44. 2018.

Yepthomi, Tokugha, Robert Paul, Snigdha Vallabhaneni, N. Kumarasamy, David F. Tate, Suniti Solomon, and Timothy Flanigan. "Neurocognitive consequences of HIV in southern India: a preliminary study of clade C virus." *Journal of the International Neuropsychological Society* 12, no. 3 (2006): 424–430.

Zhu, Fan, Bharat Panwar, Hiroko H. Dodge, Hongdong Li, Benjamin M. Hampstead, Roger L. Albin, Henry L. Paulson, and Yuanfang Guan. "COMPASS: A computational model to predict changes in MMSE scores 24-months after initial assessment of Alzheimer's disease." *Scientific Reports* 6, no. 1 (2016): 1–12.

Zucchella, Chiara, Elena Sinforiani, Stefano Tamburin, Angela Federico, Elisa Mantovani, Sara Bernini, Roberto Casale, and Michelangelo Bartolo. "The multidisciplinary approach to Alzheimer's disease and dementia. A narrative review of non-pharmacological treatment." *Frontiers in Neurology* 9 (2018): 1058.

Zygouris, Stelios, Dimitrios Giakoumis, Konstantinos Votis, Stefanos Doumpoulakis, Konstantinos Ntovas, Sofia Segkouli, Charalampos Karagiannidis, Dimitrios Tzovaras, and Magda Tsolaki. "Can a virtual reality cognitive training application fulfill a dual role? Using the virtual supermarket cognitive training application as a screening tool for mild cognitive impairment." *Journal of Alzheimer's Disease* 44, no. 4 (2015): 1333–1347.

Zygouris, Stelios, Konstantinos Ntovas, Dimitrios Giakoumis, Konstantinos Votis, Stefanos Doumpoulakis, Sofia Segkouli, Charalampos Karagiannidis, Dimitrios Tzovaras, and Magda Tsolaki. "A preliminary study on the feasibility of using a virtual reality cognitive training application for remote detection of mild cognitive impairment." *Journal of Alzheimer's Disease* 56, no. 2 (2017): 619–627.

# 4 Characterization of Biomedical Signals in Neurological Disorders

*Priya Dev and Abhishek Pathak*
Banaras Hindu University, Varanasi, India

## 4.1 INTRODUCTION

Diseases are medically defined as neurological disorders that affect the brain and nervous system throughout the human body, including the spinal cord. The brain, nerve roots, cranial nerves, spinal cord, peripheral nerves, autonomic nervous system, and points of neuromuscular connection and muscles are all involved in nervous disorders. Neurological disorders can be inherited or acquired, regardless of their origin, and cause damage to the nervous system. The severity of the damage determines the extent of impairment, from paralysis to muscle weakness and seizures to loss of sensation. As per a recent study of disease burden and trends in neurological disorders at the state level in India, non-communicable neurological diseases increased from 4.0% (95% confidence interval 3.2 to 5.0) in 1990 to 8.2% (6.6 to 10.2) in 2019 with disability-adjusted total life years (DALY) (Singh et al. 2021).

Biomedical signals aid the better observation of an organism's physiological activities, ranging from gene sequences to proteins, neural and heart rhythms, to images of tissues and organs. By processing these biomedical signals, important information is extracted and the biologist can discover new aspects of biology and doctors can watch for a specific disease. Computer assisted diagnosis (CADx) or computer assisted detection (CADe) is a computer system that assists clinicians in making quick judgements. Imaging analysis is critical work in the medical profession since imaging is the most fundamental means of diagnosing any disease as fast as possible. These tests assist doctors in confirming or excluding the prevalence of a neurological or additional medical condition. For example, diagnosing diseases related to the brain, such as epilepsy, degenerative disorders, certain seizure disorders, autism, sleep disorders, migraines, and brain tumors. The electroencephalogram (EEG) is a technique for recording the activity of brain cells across the skull in order to determine the functional states of the brain. This helps doctors in the diagnosis of neurological impairments such as tumours, degenerative diseases, blood clots, and locating a stroke. The main purpose of CAD systems is to identify abnormal signs as early as possible and which a human professional cannot detect. As a result, there is a growing demand to build CAD systems for neurologists to automatically perform precise assessments for the detection of various neurological diseases.

## 4.2 DIFFERENT TYPES OF BIOMEDICAL SIGNALS USED IN THE DIAGNOSIS OF NEUROLOGICAL DISORDERS

### 4.2.1 ELECTROCARDIOGRAM (ECG)

The ECG is the easiest and fastest test to assess how well the heart is working. The heart's electrical activity is measured using electrodes placed in specific locations on the chest, arms, and legs, which are then connected to the ECG machine and the results are printed immediately. The ECG records


DOI: 10.1201/9781003245346-4

the heart's natural rhythm, as well as the strength of the electrical impulses and their timing as they travel through the heart's many chambers. The ECG is a realistic record of the direction and amplitude of electrical agitation caused by the atria and ventricles depolarizing and repolarizing. Changes in an ECG report can be an indication of heart problems. In the ECG signal, a cardiac cycle consists of Provocation, Quality, Region (or Radiation), Severity (or Scale), and Timing (PQRST) waves. The respective characteristics of the wave peaks in the ECG output determine the clinical information based on the intervals and amplitudes of the peaks with duration. Automatic analysis of ECG characteristics with an extremely fast and accurate performance is extremely important, especially for examining long recordings (Mahmoodabadi et al. 2005).

The regular electrical depolarization and repolarization of the myocardium are linked to atrioventricular and ventricular contractions which are determined by the representation of the P, QRS, and T waves. The P wave represents the two atrial activations located in the upper chamber of the heart, while the QRS complex and the T wave represent the ventricular excitation in the lower chamber of the heart. With automatic ECG analysis, QRS detection is the main problem. If successful, it is followed by a thorough examination of the ECG signal. In the trace of the ECG signal, the horizontal trough for the P wave is called the baseline or isopotential line. This is followed by the P wave which represents the depolarization of the atrial musculature. The QRS complex follows the P wave representing joint repolarization and ventricular depolarization that occur almost simultaneously. This is followed by the T wave which represents ventricular repolarization, while the U wave, if present, is generally considered to be the result of posterior potentials in the ventricular muscle. The normal heart rate ranges between 60 and 100 beats per minute, but abnormalities include a slower heart rate (bradycardia), a higher heart rate (tachycardia), while an abnormal ECG signal represents arrhythmia (Saritha et al. 2008, Ranjan and Giri 2012).

Over the past decade, several studies and algorithms have been developed for automated ECG signal extraction and analysis. Different classification methods have been proposed and evaluated with many advanced techniques showing their advantages and disadvantages, such as digital signal analysis, artificial neural networks, fuzzy logic methods, Bayesian algorithms, genetics, hidden Markov models, self-organizing maps, and supporting vector machines for accurate and fast ECG feature extraction. There are several systems for classifying and analysing ECG signals.

#### 4.2.1.1 Parkinson's Disease (PD)

PD is a debilitating neurological ailment that progresses over time, usually with a more than 50% loss of substantia nigra neurons and an 80% reduction in striatal dopamine levels by the time PD presents clinically (Fearnley and Lees 1991, Ross et al. 2012). Years or even decades before the characteristic motor signs appear, the disease process may be active. Diagnostic methods for detecting early prodromal signs are required for the development and implementation of possible treatment drugs to delay disease progression. Autonomic pathology and cardiac sympathetic denervation in the early stages are among the non-motor signs of Parkinson's disease, which is regarded as having non-motor symptoms and being a systemic illness with broad anatomic involvement. Advanced ECG analysis can be used to extract more information and identify people who are at high risk of developing PD. Research has proposed that a conventional ten-second ECG can be used for prodromal PD as a biomarker that is universally accessible, non-invasive, and affordable. Using such an ECG and machine learning methods, early pathogenic cardiac autonomic innervation might be detected.

The relationship between clinical characteristics and electrocardiogram parameters in PD patients was explored in a study. In patients with PD, BMI was found to be positively linked with PR and QRS intervals. The QRS interval was associated with disease duration and the Hoehn and Yahr stages, while the QT interval and QTc were associated with age. Clinical characteristics and ECG values are likely to be tightly linked. Several ECG characteristics can indicate autonomic dysfunction or the course of a disease. In the treatment of PD patients, clinicians should pay more attention to ECG parameters. This research provided three major findings. First, BMI was found to have a favourable relationship with PR and QRS intervals. Second, the QRS interval was linked to the length of the sickness and the HY stage. Third, QTc was found to have a favourable relationship with age (Akbilgic et al. 2020, Mochizuki et al. 2017).

#### 4.2.1.2 Amylotrophic Lateral Sclerosis (ALS)

ALS is a deadly neurological illness characterized by the degradation of the first and second motor neurons. Recent research has revealed variability in the phenotype, clinical substrate, and genetic predisposition, implying that ALS should be treated as a syndrome rather than a single disease entity. As a result, the clinical manifestations and development of ALS might differ greatly. Although cognitive and behavioural changes are common in ALS, other non-motor clinical aspects, such as the autonomic nervous system (ANS), are often overlooked (Hardiman et al. 2011, Kiernan et al. 2011). The effect of ANS on ALS as part of a complicated degenerative process is gaining traction, and it is hypothesized that people with ALS acquire autonomic dysfunction, which can include cardiac involvement.

Various central nervous system problems, such as ST segment elevation, T wave inversion, and QT interval prolongation, are known to generate ECG abnormalities that mimic coronary syndromes. These findings in relation to subarachnoid or subdural hematomas have been well documented. It is generally recognized that ALS has a negative influence on the cardiovascular system. In patients with ALS, subclinical sympathetic hyperfunction and parasympathetic hypofunction have been demonstrated to cause cardiovascular disease (Pavlovic et al. 2010, Asai et al. 2007, Shimizu et al. 1994). There are only a few publications that describe the ECG's features in relation to this condition. A pseudo-ischemic pattern has been described in ALS, although a pseudo-myocardial infarction pattern has also been described (Li et al. 2000, Zhang et al. 2012). Additionally, increased troponin T levels have been recorded in patients with ALS who do not have underlying ischemic heart disease as a result of hypoxia respiratory failure or immune-mediated myocardial injury leading to ALS (Von Lueder et al. 2011).

The ECG revealed that the mean QT corrected for heart rate was considerably greater in individuals with ALS in favour of sympathetic disruption in motor neuron disease (Asai et al. 2007) in a study assessing alterations in the corrected QT interval (QTc) and QTc spread. Ion channel failure has been linked to cardiac illness, thus it's possible that ECG alterations in patients with ALS are due to ion channel dysfunction (Chockalingam and Wilde 2012). An ECG of an ALS patient shows negative T waves in the precordial leads, which mimic myocardial ischemia. Complementary studies ruled out systemic and cardiological causes of ECG abnormalities, implying a link between the pseudo-ischemic ECG and ALS. Although ANS dysfunction has been suggested, the mechanism behind this anomaly on the ECG has yet to be investigated.

ECG anomalies were found to cause main sympathetic-impaired autonomic regulation in ALS patients in other research (Pavlovic et al. 2010, Bella et al. 2015). The amygdala and hypothalamus have been implicated as major sympathetic structures in studies of transactive response (TAR) DNA-binding protein-43 (pTDP-43) disease in the brain and related neuronal loss (Brettschneider et al. 2013, Cykowski et al. 2014). Given that sympathetic hyperactivity has been linked to sudden cardiac death and stress-induced cardiomyopathy, this idea could explain why, after respiratory failure, sudden cardiac arrest is one of the leading causes of mortality in ALS. As a result, cardiovascular magnetic resonance imaging (CMR) appears to be more sensitive compared to cardiac parameters found in blood tests for detecting cardiac involvement in ALS.

### 4.2.2 Electroencephalogram (EEG)

Electroencephalography is the technique that reads the electrical potential of the brain and is measured using a special device called an electroencephalogram (EEG). This device contains electrodes, a conductive gel, amplifiers, and an analogue-to-digital converter. Electrodes or wires are used to conduct electrical activity starting at the scalp of the brain. Different types of electrodes are generally used for the EEG analysis. The reusable disc is one kind of electrode. With a little amount of conductive gel (AgCl) under the disc, these electrodes are placed on the scalp (Tallgren et al. 2005). The disc will consist of compositions of gold, tin, and silver. The cost of the electrode is low and the service life may depend on the metal used in the disc and the insulating back of the wire. These electrodes have the potential to fall out of the scalp, increasing the potential for artefacts (Taheri et al. 1994). The EEG cap is also available with reusable discs where conductive gel is injected onto the cap holes. Multi-channel recording is preferred, but a complex issue with this cap is that if one electrode fails, the entire cap has to be replaced, which is difficult (Stevens et al. 2007).

#### 4.2.2.1 EEG Signal Analysis and Its Phases

The raw EEG signals are obtained directly from the brain's scalp during the acquisition phase. The second stage is a pre-processing step that includes artefact removal (Ames 1971) and data filtering (Basar 1998). In signal capture and analysis, detecting and eliminating artefacts is a difficult task. Several variables might cause artefacts, including head motions during signal capture, physical flaws in the electrode/channel/probe, and head-to-device connection issues. These artefacts will also produce abnormally shaped frequency signals. The feature extraction stage of analysis divides the signal's features using Fourier transform (a signal processing technique), wavelets, principal component analysis, and significant features extracted (abnormal/normal) (Tong and Thankor 2009). The Fourier transform, which separates data into four frequency bands – delta (4 Hz), theta (48 Hz), alpha (813 Hz), and beta (1330 Hz) – is the most extensively used automated approach (Fonseca et al. 2006). For EEG signals with a greater noise ratio, the fast Fourier transform (FFT) approach is not recommended. To reduce spectral loss and improve frequency resolution, parametric spectrum estimation methods such as autoregression (AR) are applied. For non-stationary signals, such as the EEG signal (Jasper 1958), the parametric technique is ineffective. Another essential stage is classification, which uses extracted features to obtain target observations (Kaneko et al. 1996). In time domain analysis, the extraction and classification of functions are two essential concerns.

#### 4.2.2.2 Signals and Their Characterizations

The frequency, amplitude, shape, and location of the electrodes on the scalp are all used to classify EEG waveforms. The main unit used to determine normal or aberrant rhythms is frequency (Hz). The frequency of the signal determines the well-known classification of waveforms such as alpha, beta, theta, delta, and gamma. The shape, head distribution, and symmetry features of some waves can be identified (Salmelin and Hari 1994). At a given age, state of attention, and sleep, certain waveform patterns are natural. Frequency bands are used to categorize continuous brain rhythms or brain waves. Different brain wave frequencies are associated with various mental and behavioural states (Birbaumer et al. 1990, Kaufman 2001, Fell et al. 2010).

#### 4.2.2.3 Role of EEG in Diagnosis of Neurological Diseases

##### *4.2.2.3.1 Parkinson's Disease*

The commencement of PD freezing may be recognized with 75% accuracy, specificity, and sensitivity using the back propagation neural network (BPNN) classifier. EEG data in the raw form (the area under the receiver operating characteristic curve, AROC, = 0.59–0.86) is proven to be more robust than clean EEG data in classifying PD patients with a healthy individual (0.57–0.72). The raw EEG attributes for muscular artefacts and non-linear extraction and sorting of raw EEG are employed as biomarkers for PD. Analysis of power spectral density (PSD) and centroid frequency (CF) on the EEG using the BPNN classifier provides 27% of the performance and 80% of the sensitivity and precision, respectively. The novel approach, which combines the spectral, spatial, and temporal characteristics of surface EEG recordings, may be an effective method to predict freezing of gait in patients affected by PD and leaves room for future research when taking into account a superior classifier that can enhance the usefulness of this method (Kumar and Bhuvaneswari 2012).

#### 4.2.2.3.2 Alzheimer's Disease (AD)

To diagnose AD in healthy controls, brain signals should be recorded and analysed. The following literature review offers an overview of various approaches and classifiers that can be utilized to diagnose AD using EEG waves. AD patients had less complex EEG signals than healthy controls. The signals were evaluated for characteristics such as spectral centre of gravity (SC), zero crossing rate (ZCR), spectral decay (SR), spectral entropy (SE), and Higuchi fractal dimension (HFD). In patients with AD, these features are less complicated and inferior, containing significant information in the primary and temporal lobes. The coherence and frequency analysis of the quantitative electroencephalography (QEEG) were investigated in order to improve the accuracy of AD diagnosis. The absolute power values in the delta and theta bands will increase in AD patients, according to this investigation (Kumar and Bhuvaneswari 2012).

#### 4.2.2.3.3 Epilepsy

Epilepsy is one of the most common brain illnesses, affecting 65 million individuals globally (Thurman et al. 2011). Electroencephalography is the most effective epilepsy diagnosis tool (Noachtar and Rémi 2009). A total of 4444 investigations have been conducted with the goal of developing CAD for epilepsy. To construct an EEG-based CAD for epilepsy, a study proposed employing a multi-stage nonlinear pre-treatment filter in combination with an artificial neural network (ANN) (Nigam and Graupe 2004). The proposed technique has a 97.2% accuracy rate. Other research compared various entropy algorithms and hypothesized that entropy values be used to differentiate neurotypic and epileptic EEGs (Kannathal et al. 2005). For categorization, they used an adaptive neuroflurry inference method, which had a 92.2% accuracy. This was followed by using an adaptive fuzzy neural network for epilepsy diagnosis (Sadati et al. 2006). The sub-band energy of the discrete wavelet transform (DWT) was used to extract functions. Their proposed method, on the other hand, had an accuracy of 85.9%. Ocak (2009) suggested a method for feature extraction using DWT that employs an estimated Shannon entropy and achieves an accuracy of better than 96% when the DWT is used and 73% when it is not. Subasi and Gursoy (2010) investigated various analysis strategies for integrating EEG data with independent component analysis (ICA), linear discriminant analysis (LDA), and principal component analysis (PCA) to reduce the dimension of EEG data. Subasi (2007) employed the wavelet transform for feature extraction and classification with an expert model. The overall accuracy of the proposed approach was 94.5%. Chen (2014) recently introduced a complicated feature extraction method, using the double-tree wavelet transform, which obtained perfect classification accuracy using the closest neighbour classification (100%).

#### 4.2.2.3.4 Autism Spectrum Disorder (ASD)

Researchers are focusing on enhancing an EEG-based CAD technique for ASD (Patel et al. 2014). ASD has been diagnosed using CAD tools in several earlier investigations. Short-term Fourier transform (STFT) was utilized for extracting the properties of the EEG signal in the study reported by Sheikhani et al. (2008); the k-nearest neighbour (KNN) was employed as a classifier. This approach achieves an overall accuracy of up to 82.4%. The researchers developed the proposed strategy using more data for testing in a subsequent publication (Sheikhani et al. 2012), achieving an accuracy of 96.4%. The fractal dimension (FD) was described by Ahmadlou et al. (2010) as a way to quantify dynamic changes and complexity in the brains of people with ASD.

The classifier was based on a radial basis function. The accuracy of this procedure has been reported to be as high as 90%. The authors presented ASD diagnosis using a visibility graph technique (VG) (Ahmadlou et al. 2012b), fuzzy synchronization likelihood (Fuzzy SL), and better neural network classification in another study (Ahmadlou et al. 2012a). The accuracy of the two proposed approaches was 95.5%. To categorize signals from neurotypic and autistic individuals, Bosl et al. (2011) employed a minimal square error as a characteristic multi-class KNN, vector of EEG signals, support vector machine (SVM), and naive Bayesian as classification methods. The categorization accuracy was better than 80% for infants under the age of nine months, nearly 100% for males under the age of nine months, and between 70 and 90% for children aged 12–18 months. At six months of age, the overall accuracy of the assessment was highest for girls.

### 4.2.3 Electromyography (EMG)

The study of electrical impulses produced by muscles is known as EMG. The phrase "myoelectric activity" is used to characterize EMG. Electrical potentials are carried by muscle tissue in the same manner as nerves do, and these electrical messages are known as muscle action potentials. The information included in these muscular action potentials is recorded using surface EMG. There are two main issues that affect the fidelity of the EMG signal when it is detected and recorded; that is, the energy in EMG signals is divided by the energy in the noise signal. Electrical impulses that are not part of the targeted EMG signal are referred to as noise (Reaz et al. 2006).

The signal obtained from electrodes placed directly on the skin is a combination of all muscle fibre action potentials occurring underneath the skin's surface. Individual action potentials of muscle fibres can occasionally be acquired by inserting wire or needle electrodes into the muscle:

$$x(n) = \sum_{r=0}^{N=1} h(r)e(n-r) + w(n)$$

Where the modelled EMG signal is denoted by $x(n)$, the point processed EMG signal by $e(n)$, the motor unit action potential (MUAP) by $h(r)$, zero mean addictive white Gaussian noise by $w(n)$, and the number of motor unit firings is $N$ (Reaz et al. 2006).

#### 4.2.3.1 PD

Artificial intelligence approaches can be utilized as medical assistance to improve diagnostic accuracy. In order to assess neuromuscular dysfunction, electromyography (EMG) signals are used. An automatic approach for detecting neuromuscular dysfunction in PD using surface EMG (sEMG) signals was proposed. To distinguish healthy EMG signals (normal) from abnormal EMG signals, the proposed system employs the ANN method. Following the detection of EMG activity zones using the fine modified adaptive linear energy detector (FM-ALED) approach, the DWT was used to extract the features. ECOTECH's project dataset is used to conduct an experimental analysis, which focuses on the accuracy parameter (Acc). Furthermore, for the identification of healthy and Parkinsonian people, a multi-class neural networks classification method combining the voting rule and the wavelet cepstral coefficient (WCC) has been devised. Various investigations using surface EMG signals are used to assess the correctness of the diagnosis. The proposed methodology achieves 100% classification accuracy (Bengacemi et al. 2021).

#### 4.2.3.2 Amylotrophic Lateral Sclerosis (ALS)

In diagnostics, EMG signal parameters can be extremely valuable. The majority of EMG signal characteristics are derived using the time domain, frequency domain, and time–frequency domain. Time domain features such as spectrogram, root mean square, entropy, power, and kurtosis have been used to classify ALS and healthy signals. For categorization of ALS and healthy EMG signals, mel-frequency cepstral coefficient-based features were employed as input to a KNN classifier. To categorize the healthy and ALS signals, discrete wavelet transform coefficients were used. A KNN classifier was used for ALS classification and healthy signals of EMG using frequency-based time parameters such as mean frequency, average value of spectral peak, zero-crossing rate, and autocorrelation. To distinguish ALS and normal EMG signals, researchers evaluated the number of onset peak characteristics recovered from the short-time Fourier transform, as well as the power level of the spectrum and frequency shifting to higher areas. The least square SVM (LS-SVM) classification offers the advantages of modest complexity, a nonlinear decision region method, adaptive implementation, and converges to solutions with the lowest mean square error. The kernel function selected determines the LS-SVM classifier's capability. The complicated regression and pattern recognition issues are successfully solved as a result of this. The basic goal of this classification is to find a hyperplane that maximizes the separation margin between it and each class's closest data points. In the second intrinsic mode function (IMF) with a polynomial kernel function, the six functions combined with the LS-SVM classification to yield an accuracy of 95%. Clinicians may find the proposed strategy useful when making decisions about ALS disease. Other brain illnesses (essential tremors, Tourette's syndrome, multiple sclerosis, etc.) may be classified using these traits in the future (Mishra et al. 2016).

#### 4.2.3.3 Spinal Cord Injury (SCI)

EMG is extensively used because it is seen as a basic and straightforward method of assessing motor dysfunction and rehabilitation following an SCI. However, a couple of investigations state that while performing surface EMG (sEMG) examinations in clinical practice, there are a variety of parameters to consider (Pilkar et al. 2020, Merletti et al. 2021). For equipment, training, and maintenance, sEMG, for example, necessitates specific resources and infrastructure. Specialized training, continuing support, and simple sEMG interfaces are required for healthcare practitioners. In light of this, a consistent body of evidence was found showing that EMG is a valuable addition to current clinical studies, but that the information it can provide is unlikely to be completely explored. Engineers and software developers should build sEMG devices in the future that allow for a broader range of measurements at the caring point, rather than merely computations based on amplitude. When attempting surgical nerve transfer to restore upper limb function in SCI, for example, having easy-to-use sEMG information available prior to surgery can help avoid frequent mistakes in selecting possible donor and recipient muscles. In general, having a thorough grasp of the spontaneous recovery profile in sEMG can help guide therapy selection and development (Balbinot et al. 2021).

### 4.2.4 Heart Rate Variability (HRV)

HRV has been linked to stress, morbidity and mortality, athletic performance, and fatigue in a number of studies. HRV is principally used to examine the operation of the ANS, which is made up of the sympathetic nervous system (SNS) and the parasympathetic nervous system (PNS), and is a portion of the peripheral nervous system that controls the body's unconscious actions. The fight-or-flight response SNS is a part of the central nervous system that becomes active in response to stress, generating a spike in the heart rate, blood vessel constriction, and to maintain equilibrium in blood pressure or a healthy/stable state of the body. The PNS, also known as the rest and digest mechanism, relaxes the heart, slowing down the heart rate, lowering stress, and lowering blood pressure. SNS and PNS collaborate to maintain a balance, also known as sympathovagal equilibrium, that allows humans to be safe and healthy; a lack of balance indicates heart irregularities (Ishaque et al. 2021).

#### 4.2.4.1 Muscular Dystrophies

Cardiovascular involvement is commonly observed in patients with muscular dystrophy. Atrial and ventricular arrhythmias, as well as conduction abnormalities, are not uncommon in these patients. The deficiency of HRV in patients with muscular dystrophies has been described since the early 1990s. In addition, change in HRV was linked to disease progression. The same pattern was observed for time domain indices. These results were subsequently confirmed by other authors. Lanza et al. (2001) described lower HRV values in 60 patients with Duchenne muscular dystrophy (DMD) compared to control patients. The most significant differences between the studied patients and a control group were observed for pNN50 and high frequency power (HF) potency. Interestingly, no significant correlation was observed, except for HF power, between HRV indices and the left ventricular ejection fraction. Inoue et al. (2009) assessed HRV indices in 57 patients with DMD and related them to brain natriuretic peptide (BNP) levels and the shortening fraction of the left ventricle. They found HRV measurements even in patients with normal BNP and a shortening fraction of left ventricular ejection (LV), which may suggest that the alteration of HRV can be considered a preclinical marker of cardiovascular damage in this group.

#### 4.2.4.2 PD

Several dysfunctions of the autonomic nervous system accompany the classic symptoms of akinesia, stiffness, and tremor seen in PD. As with other neurological diseases, in patients with PD HRV is consistently reported to have decreased (Turkka et al. 1987, Ludin et al. 1987, van et al. 1993. Autonomic dysfunction in PD has been demonstrated by a variety of measurements, ranging from the bedside autonomic reflex test to long-term HRV analysis. As demonstrated by Kallio et al. (2000), the alteration of HRV is already present in untreated patients with mild clinical symptoms, indicating early involvement of the ANS in this group. In addition, classical autonomic reflex tests showed that autonomic dysfunction is more attenuated in patients with hypokinesia/stiffness as the first symptom compared to a subgroup with tremor at disease onset (Kallio et al. 2000). The same group then compared 4444 traditional HRV parameters, as well as 4444 selected nonlinear parameters analysed from 24-hour recordings, between 4444 untreated PD patients and a healthy control group of 4444 (Haapaniemi et al. 2001). A lower standard deviation of NN (normal R-peak)-intervals (SDNN), all spectral indices, and a slope of the power–law relationship were found in a Parkinson group. When HRV was correlated with total score and motor score, a significant inverse relationship of very low frequency (VLF) with low frequency (LF) power spectra was observed.

#### 4.2.4.3 Epilepsy

Data on HRV in untreated patients with approximately premature seizures are conflicting. Persson et al. (2007) compared 22 untreated epilepsy patients with healthy disposition and found no change in the HRV measurements evaluated from the 24-hour Holter follow-up. On the other hand, Evrengül et al. (2005) more clearly identified SDNN, reduced HF, and better LF values evaluated from tachycardia records in untreated epilepsy patients, suggesting increased sympathetic tone. Nevertheless, it is difficult to examine these effects because they were obtained from long and short duration recordings. In more advanced stages of the disease, especially in refractory epilepsy, significant changes in HRV have been reported consistently over decades (Drake et al. 1998, Tomson et al. 1998, Ansakorpi et al. 2002). The nonlinear HRV parameters, the power law slope, and the ApEn were significantly lower in patients with temporal epilepsy than in healthy subjects. Further worsening of HRV was observed in refractory patients compared to patients with well-controlled disease. EEG, and ECG during seizures, were assessed in the post-critical period in patients undergoing preoperative evaluation, and it was found that a decrease in HRV parameters occurred in the time domain immediately after seizures and during the 5–6 hours of observation that followed.

### 4.2.5 Magnetoencephalography (MEG)

The confusing intervening structures' effects that substantially hinder attempts to precisely determine the source of the signal drastically limit the variations in electrical potential associated with brain activity detected on the scalp by EEG. MEG, on the other hand, monitors the alterations in the magnetic field generated by the flow of an intracellular current, the production of which follows the "right-hand rule" of Ampère's law. Unlike EEG measurements, these are relatively unaffected by the dura, skull, and scalp. The technology thus provides a safe, non-invasive method of "listening" in to brain activity at rest and during simple tasks, which, although measuring hundreds of channels, is gentle and rapid for setting up from the subject's perspective. Mathematical modelling of these data allows for source identification while maintaining sampling frequencies of up to tens of thousands of times per second (Proudfoot et al. 2014).

The net contributions from post-synaptic potentials, dendritic exciters, and inhibitors, rather than the axonal action potentials (too brief) of pyramidal cells, generate the neuronal activity detected by MEG. Since the current through the apical dendrites (represented by a "dipole") generates a magnetic field that extends radially, MEG excels at detecting dipoles located tangentially to the skull. Fortunately, the majority of cortical micro-columns prefer this orientation due to the widely folded grooves of the human cortex. MEG, on the other hand, is less sensitive to deeper sources (such as the sub-cortical) because the magnetic field changes rapidly. The strength of the signals recorded by MEG is 1014 orders less than that of a conventional clinical magnetic resonance (MR) scanner with a magnetic field of 1.5 teslas. This has been compared to being at a rock concert and hearing a pin. The lowest quantifiable variations in the magnetic field are thought to be created by 50,000 pyramidal cells operating simultaneously on a cortical surface with a diameter of 0.9 mm. Since the modulation of self-generated oscillatory activity is well recognized as a major mechanism by which geographically distant network sections communicate, there is an instant requirement for a brain-scale imaging technique with great time sensitivity (Proudfoot et al. 2014).

#### 4.2.5.1 The Applications and Potential of MEG

MEG has a close association with invasive studies of brain activity and has found early therapeutic utility in discovering the etiology of epilepsy, notably for scheduling later procedures (Stufflebeam 2011). MEG had previously begun characterizing total brain activity during the resting state at the network level (Brookes et al. 2011) in addition to task performance at a later stage, and it is no longer restricted to the description of rather basic neurophysiology (Luckhoo et al. 2012). MEG now verifies these findings by removing the artefactually based explanations exclusively on correlated models of vascular activity, which were generated by fMRI (Smith et al. 2009). MEG can also be used to interrupt the temporal flow of communication between "nodes" in such networks, evaluate their functionality during task execution, and even explain their dysfunction. MEG additionally adds to the fMRI data by revealing the disease's ambiguous impact on the course of hemodynamic response function across time. During brain activation, blood oxygen-level-dependent (BOLD) sequences promote the capture of multimodal data (Singh 2012).

#### 4.2.5.2 Role of EEG in the Diagnosis of Neurological Diseases

##### *4.2.5.2.1 AD*

MEG is a strong technology for recording changing brain function activities. A regular and persistent slowdown of brain oscillations has been identified in AD using single channel analysis. In comparison to controls, AD patients have lower connectivity in functional connectivity (FC) studies. To get to any conclusions, further EC studies must be carried out. In comparison to healthy control (HC) participants, the connection of parietal and temporal areas has been identified with AD progression. The hippocampus has also been shown to be involved, but additional research is needed. Other electrophysiological metrics such as EEG, local field potential (LFP), fMRI, positron emission tomography (PET), and brain stimulation can be bridged with MEG. It paves the way for cross-validation of research findings across multiple modalities.

Furthermore, MEG can be used in conjunction with other modalities in determining the changes in neurotransmitters like glutamate, gamma-aminobutyric acid (GABA), and other neurotransmitters (Muthukumaraswamy 2014, Kujala et al. 2015). MEG has the potential to bring up new clinical research avenues in AD. Another factor to consider is that the AD population is different in terms of gender, age, demography, disease progression, and other factors, making it difficult to find research that is similar. Modality integration is also significant in experimental design for AD research. To obtain additional information, several modalities including EEG, fMRI, PET, and diffusion tensor imaging (DTI) have been combined with MEG. Another key study path to consider for AD research is the availability of data.

#### 4.2.5.2.2 *Traumatic Brain Injury (TBI)*

MEG, when used in conjunction with anatomical MRI, stands as a method of functional brain imaging that ensures a high degree of temporal and spatial resolution. MEG has demonstrated itself to be beneficial in identifying mild TBI as well as assessing functional network connectivity abnormalities produced by TBI that are not detectable using traditional anatomical imaging techniques. Combining MEG with additional techniques, such as EEG or DTI, can help researchers better understand how TBI affects connectivity. Researchers can gain a better understanding of how TBI impacts connection if MEG is used in combination with other techniques like EEG or DTI. Although MEG's application in TBI is currently limited to research, future studies may uncover a clinical purpose for it in TBI, as it has in epilepsy (Peitz et al. 2021).

#### 4.2.5.2.3 *Epilepsy*

Aside from the non-invasive aspect of the test, MEG provides intrinsic advantages for detecting language function. This contains milliseconds rather than seconds of temporal resolution, which is substantially higher than fMRI, which captures vascular changes during an eight-second time interval, yielding static pictures with critical and non-critical language localizations. When anomalies in the vasculature, such as arteriovenous malformations (AVMs), are present, fMRI has the potential to provide misplaced localizations. Each MEG image, on the other hand, measures brain neuronal activation over the whole length of the magnetic evoked response with millisecond time precision, allowing for the systematic study of sequential stages involved in language function. MEG has also been used to assess memory function in a number of smaller studies. It's not hard to imagine MEG replacing the intracarotid amobarbital test (IAP), also known as the WADA test for language and memory lateralization purposes, depending on the findings of future studies in this field (Ray and Bowyer 2010).

MEG is a valuable method with a wide range of known and potential uses. It could be used to supplement EEG for seizure focus localization because it has intrinsic advantages over the latter. When compared to other existing techniques, the combination of non-invasiveness and exceedingly high spatial and temporal resolution is unparalleled. MEG source localization is more accurate than EEG in terms of overall accuracy. Furthermore, because MEG is not contaminated by solely radial signals, it is a simpler source to model. Apart from epileptic focal localization, functional localization in the brain cortex is anticipated to be the technique's most important use in the future. MEG can be used to define far more complicated cognitive processes such as language and memory, in addition to relatively simple functions like sensation and vision, and hence has the potential to modify current paradigms for eloquent cortex localization (Ray and Bowyer 2010).

## 4.3 LIMITATIONS OF BIOMEDICAL SIGNALS

The limitations of all the biomedical signals discussed in this chapter are shown in Table 4.1.

### 4.3.1 Artefacts of ECG

- Incorrect electrode placement;
- Accidental left arm–right arm reversal;
- Differential diagnosis with dextrocardia;
- Right arm/left leg (RA/LL) electrode reversal;
- Truncal or non-standard limb lead placement;
- Accidental reversal of right leg and right arm electrodes;
- Accidental reversal of left arm/right leg;
- Arms and legs reversal or bilateral arm-leg reversal.

(Pérez-Riera et al. 2018)

**TABLE 4.1**
**Limitations of Biomedical Signals**

| Biomedical Signals | Limitations | References |
|---|---|---|
| ECG | • Presence of artefacts<br>• Performance measures<br>• Complexity of signal analysis algorithm<br>• Types of electrodes used<br>• ECG wave morphology<br>• P-wave and T-wave analysis | Khairuddin et al. (2017) |
| EEG | • The main disadvantage of EEG recording is poor spatial resolution.<br>• The EEG signal is not useful for pin-pointing the exact source of activity. In other words, they are not very exact.<br>• EEG waveform does not help researchers to distinguish between activities originating in different but closely adjacent locations. | Sangam et al. (2020) |
| EMG | • Limitations with recording dynamic muscle activity.<br>• It is used for superficial muscles only.<br>• No standard electrode placement.<br>• May affect movement patterns of subject.<br>• Cross-talk is a concern.<br>• Detection area may not be representative of the entire muscle. | Katzberg and Abraham (2021) |
| MEG | • Patients need to remain relatively still during a MEG examination<br>• Patients with a pacemaker or similar device may not be able to undergo a MEG study | Burgess (2020) |

### 4.3.2 Artefacts of EEG

- Environmental artefacts and experimental errors, arising from external factors, are classified as extrinsic artefacts;
- Physiological artefacts are EKG, eye movements, glossokinetic, pacemaker, pulse, sniffling, myogenic, and sway artefacts;
- Non-physiological artefacts are bed motions, room electronical equipment's attached to or around the patient, loose and high impedance electrodes, and 60 Hz artefacts;
- Ocular artefacts, muscle artefacts, cardiac artefacts, and extrinsic artefacts.

(Sazgar and Young 2019, Jiang et al. 2019)

### 4.3.3 Artefacts of EMG

- There are several sources of low-frequency noise, both intrinsic and extrinsic, that can contaminate the sEMG signal;
- Power line noise and cable motion artefacts are two examples of extrinsic noise sources;
- The skin–electrode interface (electrochemical noise) and the electronic amplification system (thermal noise) are the two intrinsic noise sources;
- The movement artefact is an electrochemical noise that occurs when a force impulse flows through the muscle and skin creating a movement in the sensor at the skin–electrode interface.

(De Luca et al. 2010)

### 4.3.4 Artefacts of MEG

- Interference coming in from the outside of the shielded room;
- Inside the shielded chamber, there are other individuals and devices;

- Sources inside-the-patient, including physiological and non-physiological;
- Inside-the-head activity that is unrelated to the signal of interest;
- Noise from sensors and recording electronics that are intrinsic to the system;
- Artefacts from other recording equipment, such as evoked response stimulators;
- The patient is not properly positioned;
- Head posture changes during the recording;
- Mistaken co-registration;
- Input of faulty signals during post-processing;
- Fitting mistakes.

(Burgess 2020)

## 4.4 FUTURE APPROACHES

The Internet of Things (IoT) is altering the health-care industry as one of the most essential interconnected technologies. According to the literature, the IoT can enable a variety of medical and health-care applications. For example, remote health monitoring and delivery, exercise programmes, chronic diseases, geriatric care, treatment compliance, and drug administration at home could all benefit from the IoT. Additionally, medical gadgets, such as ECGs, sensors, and other diagnostic and imaging devices, can also be connected via the IoT. IoT-based device networks are expected to improve disease diagnosis and prevention, as well as reduce medical costs, increase quality of life, and improve patients' experiences with these devices. Finally, the IoT has the potential to pave the way for a more logical and pragmatic approach to building and creating ECG devices that can not only meet present demands but also change how health care is monitored and delivered in the future.

In comparison to older methods, machine learning as an emerging technology provides principled, automatic, and objective algorithms for high-dimensional and intricate data, demonstrating its superiority in EEG signal processing. Regardless of the benefits of machine learning (e.g. low bias and high sensitivity to pattern identification), reliable classifiers, particular feature extraction, well-selected data, and computing costs must all be considered. For example, channel selection under specific situations can reduce feature extraction and pattern recognition computation loading, which is viable for online computation, especially for some wearable or implantable devices in real-world applications. Another option is to use cloud computing, which is enabled by 5G technology, to achieve real-time EEG recording exchange. Deep learning is a trendy technology in image processing, but it is only now making an appearance in EEG processing, demonstrating its superiority in EEG pattern detection.

Most likely, with the advent of different communication modules like Bluetooth, Wi-Fi, Near Field Communication (NFC), and Wireless Body Area Networks (WBAN), healthcare wearable devices (HWDs) may now visualize and share data in real time. These HWDs aid in the quantification of a wide range of metrics and biopotentials. ECG which measures heart function, EMG which monitors muscle activity in response to nerve stimulation, EEG which monitors brain activity and the electro-oculogram (EOG) which records eye movements, are all examples of biopotentials. These HWDs are widely employed as non-invasive medical devices, especially at the point-of-care (POC). Additionally, since wearable devices are non-invasive, they have simplified treatment procedures and reduce the risk of infection, which was formerly connected with blood.

HWDs have completely transformed the health-care industry. They have proven to be effective in monitoring a variety of physiological parameters, as previously mentioned. They have been found to have a wide range of applications for monitoring; consequently, further work is needed to make them appropriate for diagnostic use. This is due to the fact that most diagnostic techniques require the use of samples such as blood, urine, and saliva, which HWDs have trouble integrating. Furthermore, AI algorithms can be used to track the behaviour of several factors for prognosis, such as the supervised learning regression method. Similarly, the wearer's security is vital, and because HWDs carry protected health information (PHI), the wearer's privacy must be protected. Secure communication techniques in HWDs are required for this reason in order to ensure the confidentiality and privacy of wearers. HWDs have also been found to be useful in the monitoring of physiological ailments such as cardiovascular disease, muscle disorders, blood, and glucose levels. However, limited uses of HWDs for psychiatric diseases such as PD, AD, and other psychological disorders are available. As a result, the expanded use of HWDs for psychological illnesses could be useful in the near future.

## 4.5 SUMMARY

This chapter has focussed on various biomedical signals used for the diagnosis of neurological disorders. In the teaching and research domains of biomedical engineering, various techniques in the processing of biomedical signals and images are widely used. The advancement of the physiological understanding of biomedical signals has led to the development of novel clinical approaches. The integration of electrophysiological signals with imaging modalities is a vital strategy in the field of neuroscience. This chapter has presented quite a few extensively employed algorithms based on the combination of electrophysiological signals and functional imaging. Because of the usefulness of this technique in this context, the case studies included a commentary on ECG, EEG, EMG, MEG, and HRV signals. In the future, the performance of sophisticated algorithms and techniques that combine electrophysiological signal and functional imaging could be compared.

## REFERENCES

Ahmadlou, Mehran, Hojjat Adeli, and Amir Adeli. "Fractality and a wavelet-chaos-neural network methodology for EEG-based diagnosis of autistic spectrum disorder." *Journal of Clinical Neurophysiology* 27, no. 5 (2010): 328–333.

Ahmadlou, Mehran, Hojjat Adeli, and Amir Adeli. "Fuzzy synchronization likelihood-wavelet methodology for diagnosis of autism spectrum disorder." *Journal of Neuroscience Methods* 211, no. 2 (2012a): 203–209.

Ahmadlou, Mehran, Hojjat Adeli, and Amir Adeli. "Improved visibility graph fractality with application for the diagnosis of autism spectrum disorder." *Physica A: Statistical Mechanics and Its Applications* 391, no. 20 (2012b): 4720–4726.

Ai-Hsien, Li, Kwan-Lih Hsu, Chiau-Suong Liau, Yung-Zu Tseng, and Lee Yuan-Teh. "Amyotrophic Lateral Sclerosis with a 'Pseudo-Infarction' Pattern on the Electrocardiograph." *Cardiology* 93, no. 1–2 (2000): 133.

Akbilgic, Oguz, Rishikesan Kamaleswaran, Akram Mohammed, G. Webster Ross, Kamal Masaki, Helen Petrovitch, Caroline M. Tanner, Robert L. Davis, and Samuel M. Goldman. "Electrocardiographic changes predate Parkinson's disease onset." *Scientific Reports* 10, no. 1 (2020): 1–6.

Ames, F. R. "'Self-induction' in photosensitive epilepsy." *Brain* 94(4) (1971): 781–798.

Ansakorpi, Hanna, J. T. Korpelainen, H. V. Huikuri, U. Tolonen, V. V. Myllylä, and J. I. T. Isojärvi. "Heart rate dynamics in refractory and well controlled temporal lobe epilepsy." *Journal of Neurology, Neurosurgery & Psychiatry* 72, no. 1 (2002): 26–30.

Asai, Hirohide, Makito Hirano, Fukashi Udaka, Keiji Shimada, Masaya Oda, Tamotsu Kubori, Kazuto Nishinaka et al. "Sympathetic disturbances increase risk of sudden cardiac arrest in sporadic ALS." *Journal of the Neurological Sciences* 254, no. 1–2 (2007): 78–83.

Balbinot, Gustavo, Guijin Li, Matheus Joner Wiest, Maureen Pakosh, Julio Cesar Furlan, Sukhvinder Kalsi-Ryan, and Jose Zariffa. "Properties of the surface electromyogram following traumatic spinal cord injury: a scoping review." *Journal of Neuroengineering and Rehabilitation* 18, no. 1 (2021): 1–23.

Basar, E. *Brain Function and Oscillations: Integrative brain function. Neurophysiology and cognitive processes*. Springer; (1998).

Bella, S. D., Benoit, C. E., Farrugia, N., Schwartze, M., and Kotz, S. A. "Effects of musically cued gait training in Parkinson's disease: Beyond a motor benefit." *Annals of the New York Academy of Sciences* 1337 (2015): 77–85. doi: 10.1111/nyas.12651.

Bengacemi, Hichem, Abdenour Hacine-Gharbi, Philippe Ravier, Karim Abed-Meraim, and Olivier Buttelli. "Surface EMG Signal Classification for Parkinson's Disease using WCC Descriptor and ANN Classifier." In *ICPRAM*, pp. 287–294. 2021.

Birbaumer, Niels, Thomas Elbert, Anthony G. Canavan, and Brigitte Rockstroh. "Slow potentials of the cerebral cortex and behavior." *Physiological Reviews* 70, no. 1 (1990): 1–41.

Bosl, William, Adrienne Tierney, Helen Tager-Flusberg, and Charles Nelson. "EEG complexity as a biomarker for autism spectrum disorder risk." *BMC Medicine* 9, no. 1 (2011): 1–16.

Brettschneider, J., Del Tredici, K., Toledo, J. B., Robinson, J. L., Irwin, D. J., Grossman, M. et al. Stages of pTDP-43 pathology in amyotrophic lateral sclerosis. *Annals of Neurology* 74, no. 1 (2013): 20–38

Brookes, Matthew J., Mark Woolrich, Henry Luckhoo, Darren Price, Joanne R. Hale, Mary C. Stephenson, Gareth R. Barnes, Stephen M. Smith, and Peter G. Morris. "Investigating the electrophysiological basis of resting state networks using magnetoencephalography." *Proceedings of the National Academy of Sciences* 108, no. 40 (2011): 16783–16788.

Burgess, Richard C. "Recognizing and correcting MEG artifacts." *Journal of Clinical Neurophysiology* 37, no. 6 (2020): 508–517.

Caller, Tracie A., James W. Doolin, James F. Haney, Amanda J. Murby, Katherine G. West, Hannah E. Farrar, Andrea Ball, Brent T. Harris, and Elijah W. Stommel. "A cluster of amyotrophic lateral sclerosis in New Hampshire: a possible role for toxic cyanobacteria blooms." *Amyotrophic Lateral Sclerosis* 10, no. sup2 (2009): 101–108.

Chen, Guangyi. "Automatic EEG seizure detection using dual-tree complex wavelet-Fourier features." *Expert Systems with Applications* 41, no. 5 (2014): 2391–2394.

Chockalingam, Priya, and Arthur Wilde. "The multifaceted cardiac sodium channel and its clinical implications." *Heart* 98, no. 17 (2012): 1318–1324.

Cykowski, Matthew D., Hidehiro Takei, Paul E. Schulz, Stanley H. Appel, and Suzanne Z. Powell. "TDP-43 pathology in the basal forebrain and hypothalamus of patients with amyotrophic lateral sclerosis." *Acta Neuropathologica Communications* 2, no. 1 (2014): 1–11.

Dalla Vecchia, Laura, Beatrice De Maria, Kalliopi Marinou, Riccardo Sideri, Anna Lucini, Alberto Porta, and Gabriele Mora. "Cardiovascular neural regulation is impaired in amyotrophic lateral sclerosis patients. A study by spectral and complexity analysis of cardiovascular oscillations." *Physiological Measurement* 36, no. 4 (2015): 659.

De Luca, Carlo J., L. Donald Gilmore, Mikhail Kuznetsov, and Serge H. Roy. "Filtering the surface EMG signal: Movement artifact and baseline noise contamination." *Journal of Biomechanics* 43, no. 8 (2010): 1573–1579.

Drake Jr, Miles E., Jodie M. Andrews, and Christina M. Castleberry. "Electrophysiologic assessment of autonomic function in epilepsy." *Seizure* 7, no. 2 (1998): 91–96.

Evrengül, Harun, Halil Tanriverdi, Dursun Dursunoglu, Asuman Kaftan, Omur Kuru, Unal Unlu, and Mustafa Kilic. "Time and frequency domain analyses of heart rate variability in patients with epilepsy." *Epilepsy Research* 63, no. 2–3 (2005): 131–139.

Fearnley, Julian M., and Andrew J. Lees. "Ageing and Parkinson's disease: substantia nigra regional selectivity." *Brain* 114, no. 5 (1991): 2283–2301.

Fell, Juergen, Nikolai Axmacher, and Sven Haupt. "From alpha to gamma: electrophysiological correlates of meditation-related states of consciousness." *Medical Hypotheses* 75, no. 2 (2010): 218–224.

Fonseca, Lineu C., Glória M. A. S. Tedrus, Marcelo G. Chiodi, Jaciara Näf Cerqueira, and Josiane M. F. Tonelotto. "Quantitative EEG in children with learning disabilities: analysis of band power." *Arquivos de neuro-psiquiatria* 64 (2006): 376–381.

Haapaniemi, T. H., Ville Pursiainen, J. T. Korpelainen, H. V. Huikuri, K. A. Sotaniemi, and V. V. Myllylä. "Ambulatory ECG and analysis of heart rate variability in Parkinson's disease." *Journal of Neurology, Neurosurgery & Psychiatry* 70, no. 3 (2001): 305–310.

Hardiman, Orla, Leonard H. Van Den Berg, and Matthew C. Kiernan. "Clinical diagnosis and management of amyotrophic lateral sclerosis." *Nature Reviews Neurology* 7, no. 11 (2011): 639–649.

Inoue, Miki, Kazuhiro Mori, Yasunobu Hayabuchi, Katsunori Tatara, and Shoji Kagami. "Autonomic function in patients with Duchenne muscular dystrophy." *Pediatrics International* 51, no. 1 (2009): 33–40.

Ishaque, Syem, Naimul Khan, and Sri Krishnan. "Trends in heart-rate variability signal analysis." *Frontiers in Digital Health* 3 (2021): 639444.

Jasper, Herbert H. "The ten-twenty electrode system of the International Federation." *Electroencephalography and Clinical Neurophysiology* 10 (1958): 370–375.

Jiang, Xiao, Gui-Bin Bian, and Zean Tian. "Removal of artifacts from EEG signals: a review." *Sensors* 19, no. 5 (2019): 987.

Kallio, M., T. Haapaniemi, J. Turkka, K. Suominen, U. Tolonen, K. Sotaniemi, V-P. Heikkilä, and V. Myllylä. "Heart rate variability in patients with untreated Parkinson's disease." *European Journal of Neurology* 7, no. 6 (2000): 667–672.

Kaneko, W. M., E. L. Phillips, E. P. Riley, and C. L. Ehlers. "EEG findings in fetal alcohol syndrome and Down syndrome children." *Electroencephalography and Clinical Neurophysiology* 98, no. 1 (1996): 20–28.

Kannathal, N., Min Lim Choo, U. Rajendra Acharya, and P. K. Sadasivan. "Entropies for detection of epilepsy in EEG." *Computer Methods and Programs in Biomedicine* 80, no. 3 (2005): 187–194.

Katzberg, H.D., and Abraham, A. "Electrodiagnostic assessment of neuromuscular junction disorders." *Neurologic Clinics* 39, no. 4 (2021): 1051–1070. doi: 10.1016/j.ncl.2021.06.013.

Kaufman, Marc J., ed. *Brain imaging in substance abuse: research, clinical, and forensic applications*. Totowa, NJ: Humana Press, 2001.

Khairuddin, A. M., Ku Nurul Fazira Ku Azir and P. E. Kan. "Limitations and future of electrocardiography devices: A review and the perspective from the Internet of Things." *2017 International Conference on Research and Innovation in Information Systems (ICRIIS)* (2017): 1–7.

Kiernan, M. C., S. Vucic, B. C. Cheah, M. R. Turner, A. Eisen, O. Hardiman, J. R. Burrell, and M. C. Zoing. "Amyotrophic lateral sclerosis." *The Lancet* 377, no. 9769 (2011): 942–955.

Kujala, Jan, Julien Jung, Sandrine Bouvard, Françoise Lecaignard, Amélie Lothe, Romain Bouet, Carolina Ciumas, Philippe Ryvlin, and Karim Jerbi. "Gamma oscillations in V1 are correlated with GABAA receptor density: A multi-modal MEG and Flumazenil-PET study." *Scientific Reports* 5, no. 1 (2015): 1–12.

Kumar, J. Satheesh, and P. Bhuvaneswari. "Analysis of Electroencephalography (EEG) signals and its categorization–a study." *Procedia Engineering* 38 (2012): 2525–2536.

Lanza, Gaetano Antonio, Antonio Dello Russo, Vincenzo Giglio, Lucia De Luca, Loredana Messano, Cesare Santini, Enzo Ricci et al. "Impairment of cardiac autonomic function in patients with Duchenne muscular dystrophy: relationship to myocardial and respiratory function." *American Heart Journal* 141, no. 5 (2001): 808–812.

Li, J., Wang, X. Q., Watson, M. B., and Assmann, S. M. "Regulation of abscisic acid-induced stomatal closure and anion channels by guard cell AAPK kinase." *Science* 287, no. 5451 (2000): 300–303. doi: 10.1126/science.287.5451.300.

Luckhoo, Henry, Joanne R. Hale, Mark G. Stokes, Anna Christina Nobre, Peter G. Morris, Matthew J. Brookes, and Mark William Woolrich. "Inferring task-related networks using independent component analysis in magnetoencephalography." *Neuroimage* 62, no. 1 (2012): 530–541.

Ludin, Sabina M., Ursula H. Steiger, and Hans-Peter Ludin. "Autonomic disturbances and cardiovascular reflexes in idiopathic Parkinson's disease." *Journal of Neurology* 235, no. 1 (1987): 10–15.

Mahmoodabadi, S. Z., Alireza Ahmadian, and M. D. Abolhasani. "ECG feature extraction using Daubechies wavelets." In *Proceedings of the fifth IASTED International conference on Visualization, Imaging and Image Processing*, pp. 343–348. 2005.

Merletti, Roberto, Isabella Campanini, William Z. Rymer, and Catherine Disselhorst-Klug. "Surface electromyography: barriers limiting widespread use of sEMG in clinical assessment and neurorehabilitation." *Frontiers in Neurology* 12 (2021): 642257.

Mishra, Vipin K., Varun Bajaj, Anil Kumar, and Girish Kumar Singh. "Analysis of ALS and normal EMG signals based on empirical mode decomposition." *IET Science, Measurement & Technology* 10, no. 8 (2016): 963–971.

Mochizuki, Hitoshi, Nobuyuki Ishii, Kazutaka Shiomi, and Masamitsu Nakazato. "Clinical features and electrocardiogram parameters in Parkinson's disease." *Neurology International* 9, no. 4 (2017): 7356.

Muthukumaraswamy, Suresh D. "The use of magnetoencephalography in the study of psychopharmacology (pharmaco-MEG)." *Journal of Psychopharmacology* 28, no. 9 (2014): 815–829.

Nigam, Vivek Prakash, and Daniel Graupe. "A neural-network-based detection of epilepsy." *Neurological Research* 26, no. 1 (2004): 55–60.

Noachtar, Soheyl, and Jan Rémi. "The role of EEG in epilepsy: a critical review." *Epilepsy & Behavior* 15, no. 1 (2009): 22–33.

Ocak, Hasan. "Automatic detection of epileptic seizures in EEG using discrete wavelet transform and approximate entropy." *Expert Systems with Applications* 36, no. 2 (2009): 2027–2036.

Patel, Vinood B., Victor R. Preedy, and Colin R. Martin, eds. *Comprehensive guide to autism*. Springer New York, 2014.

Pavlovic, S., Stevic, Z., Milovanovic, B., Milicic, B., Rakocevic-Stojanovic, V., Lavrnic, D., and Apostolski, S. "Impairment of cardiac autonomic control in patients with amyotrophic lateral sclerosis." *Amyotrophic Lateral Sclerosis* 11, no. 3 (2010): 272–276. doi: 10.3109/17482960903390855.

Peitz, Geoffrey W., Elisabeth A. Wilde, and Ramesh Grandhi. "Magnetoencephalography in the detection and characterization of brain abnormalities associated with traumatic brain injury: A comprehensive review." *Medical Sciences* 9, no. 1 (2021): 7.

Pérez-Riera, Andrés Ricardo, Raimundo Barbosa-Barros, Rodrigo Daminello-Raimundo, and Luiz Carlos de Abreu. "Main artifacts in electrocardiography." *Annals of Noninvasive Electrocardiology* 23, no. 2 (2018): e12494.

Persson, Håkan, Mats Ericson, and T. Tomson. "Heart rate variability in patients with untreated epilepsy." *Seizure* 16, no. 6 (2007): 504–508.

Pilkar, Rakesh, Kamyar Momeni, Arvind Ramanujam, Manikandan Ravi, Erica Garbarini, and Gail F. Forrest. "Use of surface EMG in clinical rehabilitation of individuals with SCI: barriers and future considerations." *Frontiers in Neurology* 11 (2020): 578559.

Proudfoot, Malcolm, Mark W. Woolrich, Anna C. Nobre, and Martin R. Turner. "Magnetoencephalography." *Practical Neurology* 14, no. 5 (2014): 336–343.

Raman, Sahana Sundar, A. S. Lakshmi, Prerana Ananda Murthy, and Mohammed Faizan. "Electroencephalogram (EEG), its processing and feature extraction." *International Journal of Engineering and Technical Research* 9 (2020): 1030–1034.

Ranjan, Rajiv, and V. K. Giri. "A unified approach of ECG signal analysis." *International Journal of Soft Computing and Engineering* 2, no. 3 (2012).

Ray, Amit, and Susan M. Bowyer. "Clinical applications of magnetoencephalography in epilepsy." *Annals of Indian Academy of Neurology* 13, no. 1 (2010): 14–22.

Reaz, Mamun Bin Ibne, M. Sazzad Hussain, and Faisal Mohd-Yasin. "Techniques of EMG signal analysis: detection, processing, classification and applications." *Biological Procedures Online* 8, no. 1 (2006): 11–35.

Ross, G. Webster, Robert D. Abbott, Helen Petrovitch, Caroline M. Tanner, and Lon R. White. "Pre-motor features of Parkinson's disease: the Honolulu-Asia Aging Study experience." *Parkinsonism & Related Disorders* 18 (2012): S199–S202.

Sadati, Nasser, Hamid Reza Mohseni, and Arash Maghsoudi. "Epileptic seizure detection using neural fuzzy networks." In *2006 IEEE international conference on fuzzy systems*, pp. 596–600. IEEE, 2006.

Salmelin, Riitta, and Riitta Hari. "Spatiotemporal characteristics of sensorimotor neuromagnetic rhythms related to thumb movement." *Neuroscience* 60, no. 2 (1994): 537–550.

Sangam, V.G., M. Sushrutha Bharadwaj, Sundar Raman, Sahana, Lakshmi, Ananda Murthy Prerana, and Mohammed Faizan. "Electroencephalogram (EEG), its processing and feature extraction." *International Journal of Engineering Research & Technology (IJERT)*, 09, no. 06 (2020).

Saritha, C., V. Sukanya, and Y. Narasimha Murthy. "ECG signal analysis using wavelet transforms." *Bulgarian Journal of Physics* 35, no. 1 (2008): 68–77.

Sazgar, Mona, and Michael G. Young. *Absolute epilepsy and EEG rotation review: Essentials for trainees*. Springer, 2019.

Sheikhani, Ali, Hamid Behnam, Mohammad Reza Mohammadi, Maryam Noroozian, and Pari Golabi. "Connectivity analysis of quantitative Electroencephalogram background activity in Autism disorders with short time Fourier transform and Coherence values." In *2008 Congress on Image and Signal Processing*, vol. 1, pp. 207–212. IEEE, 2008.

Sheikhani, Ali, Hamid Behnam, Mohammad Reza Mohammadi, Maryam Noroozian, and Mohammad Mohammadi. "Detection of abnormalities for diagnosing of children with autism disorders using of quantitative electroencephalography analysis." *Journal of Medical Systems* 36, no. 2 (2012): 957–963.

Shimizu, Toshio, Hideaki Hayashi, Shuichi Kato, Michiyuki Hayashi, Hitoshi Tanabe, and Masaya Oda. "Circulatory collapse and sudden death in respirator-dependent amyotrophic lateral sclerosis." *Journal of the Neurological Sciences* 124, no. 1 (1994): 45–55.

Singh, Gagandeep, Meenakshi Sharma, G. Anil Kumar, N. Girish Rao, Kameshwar Prasad, Prashant Mathur, Jeyaraj D. Pandian et al. "The burden of neurological disorders across the states of India: the Global Burden of Disease Study 1990–2019." *The Lancet Global Health* 9, no. 8 (2021): e1129–e1144.

Singh, Krish D. "Which "neural activity" do you mean? fMRI, MEG, oscillations and neurotransmitters." *Neuroimage* 62, no. 2 (2012): 1121–1130.

Smith, Stephen M., Peter T. Fox, Karla L. Miller, David C. Glahn, P. Mickle Fox, Clare E. Mackay, Nicola Filippini et al. "Correspondence of the brain's functional architecture during activation and rest." *Proceedings of the National Academy of Sciences* 106, no. 31 (2009): 13040–13045.

Stevens, Todd K., John R. Ives, L. Martyn Klassen, and Robert Bartha. "MR compatibility of EEG scalp electrodes at 4 tesla." *Journal of Magnetic Resonance Imaging: An Official Journal of the International Society for Magnetic Resonance in Medicine* 25, no. 4 (2007): 872–877.

Stufflebeam, Steven M. "Clinical magnetoencephalography for neurosurgery." *Neurosurgery Clinics* 22, no. 2 (2011): 153–167.

Subasi, Abdulhamit. "EEG signal classification using wavelet feature extraction and a mixture of expert model." *Expert Systems with Applications* 32, no. 4 (2007): 1084–1093.

Subasi, Abdulhamit, and M. Ismail Gursoy. "EEG signal classification using PCA, ICA, LDA and support vector machines." *Expert Systems with Applications* 37, no. 12 (2010): 8659–8666.

Taheri, Babak A., Robert T. Knight, and Rosemary L. Smith. "A dry electrode for EEG recording." *Electroencephalography and Clinical Neurophysiology* 90, no. 5 (1994): 376–383.
Tallgren, Pekka, Sampsa Vanhatalo, Kai Kaila, and Juha Voipio. "Evaluation of commercially available electrodes and gels for recording of slow EEG potentials." *Clinical Neurophysiology* 116, no. 4 (2005): 799–806.
Thurman, D. J., E. Beghi, C. E. Begley, A. T. Berg, J. R. Buchhalter, D. Ding, D. C. Hesdorffer et al. "ILAE Commission on Epidemiology. Standards for epidemiologic studies and surveillance of epilepsy." *Epilepsia* 52, no. suppl 7 (2011): 2–26.
Tomson, Torbjörn, Mats Ericson, Christina Ihrman, and Lars Erik Lindblad. "Heart rate variability in patients with epilepsy." *Epilepsy Research* 30, no. 1 (1998): 77–83.
Tong, Shanbao, and Nitish V. Thankor. *Quantitative EEG analysis methods and clinical applications*. Artech House, 2009.
Turkka, Jukka T., Uolevi Tolonen, and Vilho V. Myllylä. "Cardiovascular reflexes in Parkinson's disease." *European Neurology* 26, no. 2 (1987): 104–112.
van Dijk, J. Gert, J. Haan, Koos Zwinderman, Berry Kremer, B. J. Van Hilten, and R. A. Roos. "Autonomic nervous system dysfunction in Parkinson's disease: relationships with age, medication, duration, and severity." *Journal of Neurology, Neurosurgery & Psychiatry* 56, no. 10 (1993): 1090–1095.
Von Lueder, Thomas G., Morten Nissen Melsom, Dan Atar, and Stefan Agewall. "Amyotrophic lateral sclerosis (ALS), a novel rare cause of elevated plasma troponin T levels." *Clinical Laboratory* 57, no. 7–8 (2011): 615–618.
Zhang, Jian, Shi-Wei Yang, Zheng Wang, Guang-Ru Wei, and Yu-Jie Zhou. "Pseudo-ischaemic ECG in a patient with amyotrophic lateral sclerosis surviving for a decade." *Case Reports* 2012 (2012): bcr0120125543.

# 5 An Overview of Distinct Electronic Devices and Circuits

*B. V. Srividya and Sasi Smitha*
Dayanand Sagar College of Engineering, Bengaluru, India

## 5.1 INTRODUCTION

Cognitive problems often begin gradually, but as they worsen, they significantly lower the affected person's quality of life. Understanding the various forms of cognitive illnesses, their symptoms, and the therapies that are available is essential [1].

Epilepsy is a condition marked by abnormal brain activity that can result in seizures, as well as periods of strange behaviour, emotions, and occasionally unconsciousness. There are a number of potential seizure signs. Certain epileptics only stare blankly for a brief period of time during a seizure, while others repeatedly twitch their arms or legs [2]. Typically, at least two separate seizures that happen at least 24 hours apart are needed to make an epilepsy diagnosis. Most epilepsy sufferers can control their seizures with medication, though rarely surgery is necessary. Others finally achieve a seizure cessation, while some patients require continued treatment to manage their seizures. Some young people with epilepsy may eventually outgrow their condition.

A variety of seizures are brought on by the long-term neurological condition of epilepsy, some of which are characterised by uncontrollable repetitive convulsions that have a substantial impact on patients' everyday lives. The part of the device that the patient should wear has been given particular thought, and details are provided. This study will focus on how epileptic detection is implemented, analyses the results, and identifies the objectives of the monitoring tool [3].

Parkinson's disease (PD) is a neurological condition that happens when the brain's dopamine levels are too low. The degree of incapacity grows over time as the sickness gets worse. About 1% of persons over 60 in industrialised countries have PD, a neurological movement disorder. Levodopa can be used to treat the three main motor symptoms of the disease: tremors (particularly when at rest), rigidity, and slowness of movement (bradykinesia). The severity of these motor symptoms worsens over time, making daily tasks challenging and lowering the quality of life. Dopaminergic medications can help with some of these symptoms, but as the illness progresses and affects more body parts, their benefits tend to wear off more quickly [4].

Machine learning algorithms could automate the diagnosis of Parkinson's symptoms and the tracking of the disease's progression by utilising data streams from soft wearable sensors [5]. These algorithms would be trained to recognise symptoms with the aid of annotated data provided by clinical specialists. This study focuses on the importance of the required number of sensors and the relevant data in order to successfully deploy these sensor models outside of clinical trials.

With current research into different illness conditions, deep brain stimulation (DBS) [6] has developed into an approved and effective treatment for movement, obsessive–compulsive, and epilepsy disorders that are resistant to pharmacological treatments.

DOI: 10.1201/9781003245346-5

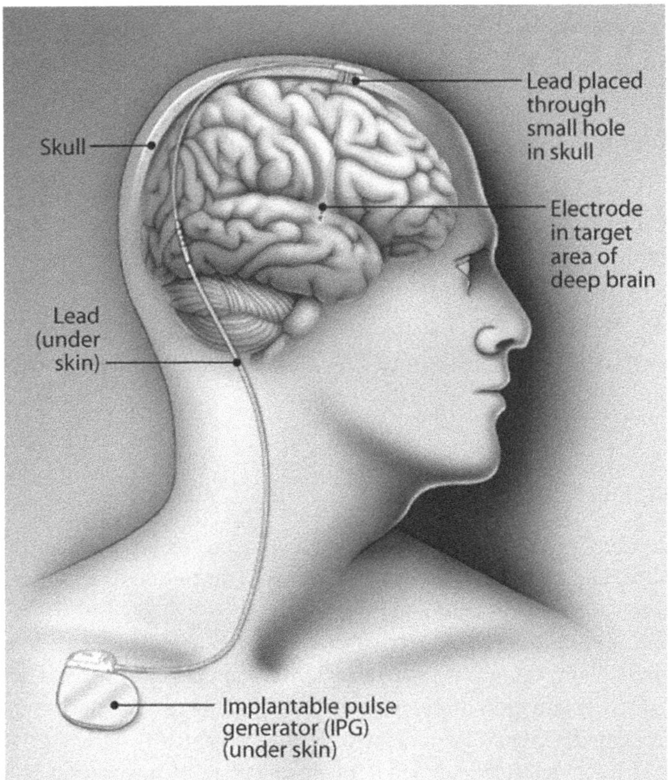


**FIGURE 5.1** Placement of deep brain stimulators [7].

These deep brain stimulators use:

1. Leads (thin insulated wires) that are implanted in the brain and end in electrodes;
2. An implantable pulse generator (IPG);
3. An extension cable linking these two parts;
4. A device that can be turned on and off and adjusts the signals used by the device.

In DBS, electrodes are positioned in a number of brain regions as can be seen in Figure 5.1 [7]. These electrodes provide electrical impulses that regulate erroneous impulses. The electrical impulses may also have an impact on the cells of the brain and various chemicals secreted. An electronic circuitry that is placed beneath the skin in the upper chest region is the main part of the deep brain stimulator, similar to a pacemaker. A wire that travels beneath the skin connects this gadget to the electrodes in the brain.

## 5.2 ELECTRODES IN DEEP BRAIN STIMULATORS

Medical electrodes typically consist of a lead (for electrical current conduction), a metal electrode, and, for surface electrodes [8], an electrode-conducting gelatin or adhesive. The electrodes are able to pick up on minute electrical charges generated by the activity of brain cells. The charges are boosted, and the monitoring equipment displays them as a graph.

Ionic potentials are transformed into electronic potentials via electrodes. The anatomical location of the bioelectric event to be detected determines the type of electrode utilised for the measurements. It is preferable to transform ionic conduction into electronic conduction in order to process the signal in electronic circuits (Figure 5.2).

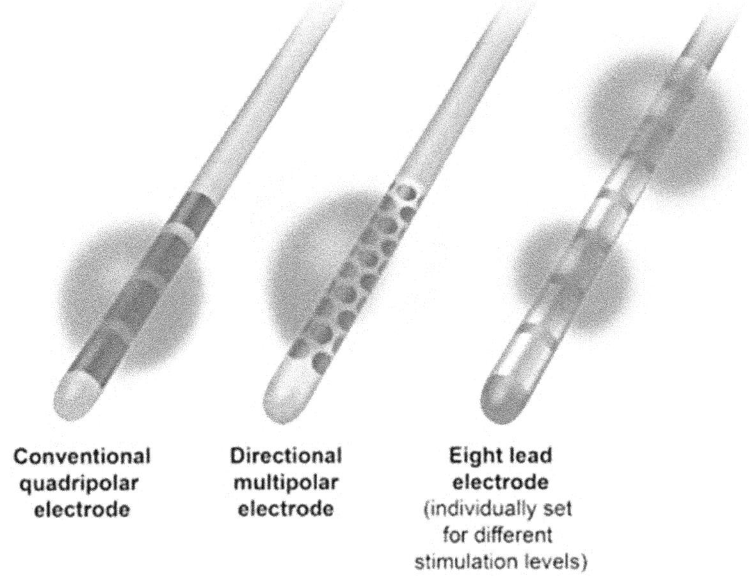


**FIGURE 5.2** Conventional deep brain stimulator electrodes [8].

Electrodes are conductors used to make contact with a non-metallic component. An anode and a cathode are the two electrodes that make up a diode. In the upcoming sections, the various electronic circuits and devices are discussed.

## 5.3 AN IMPLANTABLE PULSE GENERATOR (IPG)

An electrical source called an IPG [9] sends current through a lead and extension wires to an electrode, across the electrode–tissue interface, and back through the tissue to the return electrode in the IPG case. Both a current source and a voltage source can be used by an IPG.

The block diagram shown in Figure 5.3 depicts the usage of various electronic circuits like the power supply, anode and cathode electrodes, and the field effect transistor (FET). The details of these electronic circuits and devices will be elaborated in the subsequent sections.

The lead is connected to the IPG via an extension cable, which is an insulated wire that is inserted under the skin of the head, neck, and shoulder. The third component of the IPG, known as the

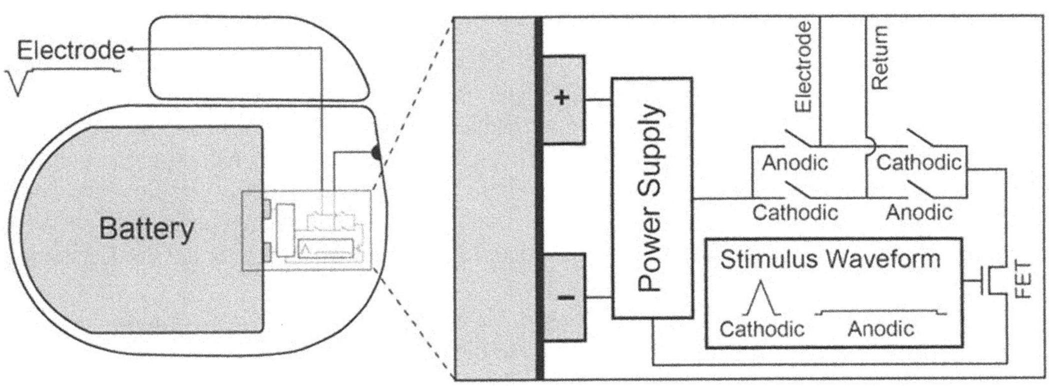


**FIGURE 5.3** An implantable pulse generator in a deep brain stimulator [9].

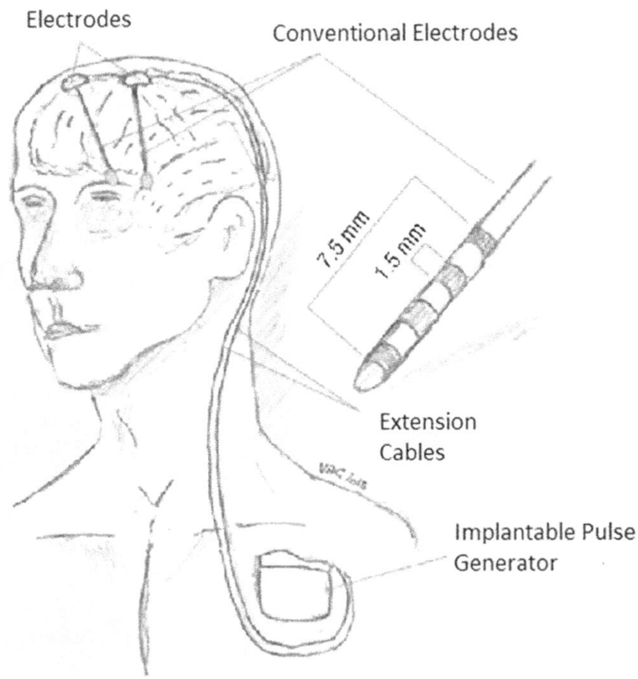


**FIGURE 5.4** Schematic of a deep brain stimulator [10].

"battery", is often inserted under the skin close to the collarbone. In some circumstances, it might be placed beneath the skin over the abdomen or lower in the chest. These extension cables, as shown in Figure 5.4, are usually made up of a non-magnetic alloy housed in ethylene tetrafluoroethylene and insulated with polycarbonate polyurethane.

When DBS is used, electrodes are placed in several areas of the brain. The electrical impulses of these electrodes regulate the irregular impulses. Alternatively, the electrical impulses might have an impact on the cells of the brain and various chemicals secreted. The level of DBS is controlled by an electronic device that looks like a pacemaker and is positioned just beneath the skin in the upper chest. An under-the-skin connection connects this gadget to the electrodes in the brain.

## 5.4 VARIOUS ELECTRONIC DEVICES

### 5.4.1 PN Junction Diode

The metallurgical separation at the intersection of the P and N regions of a semiconductor crystal is known as the PN junction as can be seen in Figure 5.5. The symbolic representation of the PN junction diode is shown in Figure 5.6. Two semiconductor areas with opposing doping types make up a PN junction. While the area on the right is N-type with a donor density Nd, the area on the left is P-type with an acceptor density Na. Since it is believed that the dopants are shallow, the donor density and electron density in the N-type area are roughly equal. An instantaneous flow of electrons from the N to the P side happens when an N-type and P-type semiconductor is involved, leaving a blank zone between the two [11].

Consider a PN diode with bias voltage applied, Va. Applying a positive voltage to the anode in relation to the cathode is what is meant by a forward bias.

When "+" is attached to the anode side and "–" to the cathode side of a semiconductor, the "+" and "–" charges bind together at the P and N junction and cancel each other out, though electrons are still free to travel from the cathode to the anode, allowing electricity to flow as shown in Figure 5.7.

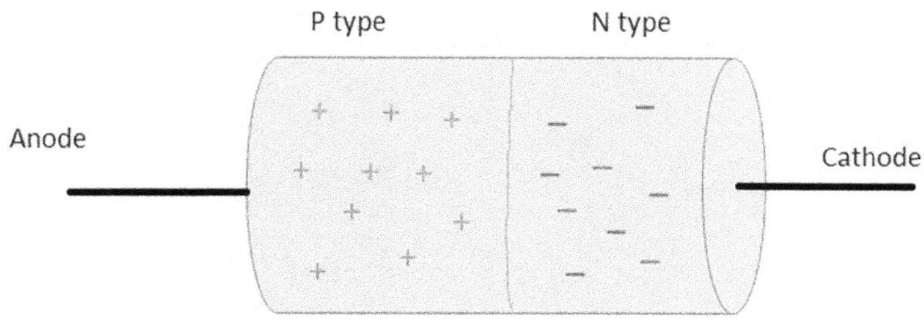


**FIGURE 5.5** PN junction diode.

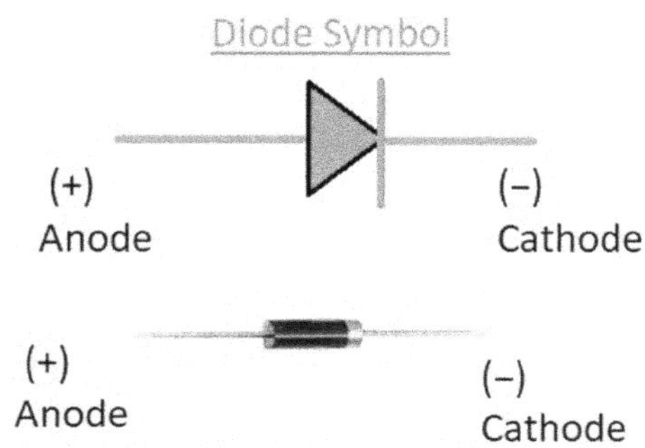


**FIGURE 5.6** Schematic of diode symbol.

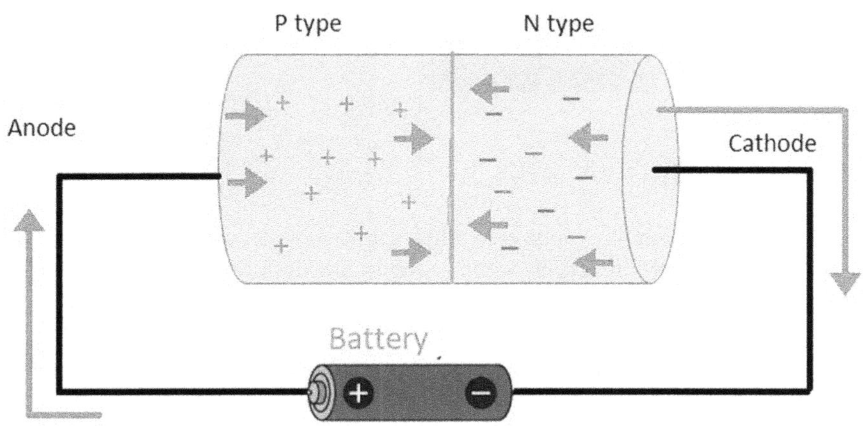


**FIGURE 5.7** Forward bias in a PN junction diode.

In this case, the junction barrier potential is the inverse of the applied voltage. In turn, this results in a decrease in the junction's effective potential barrier and width, which further favours the flow of most carriers through the junction. Additionally, for the barrier to be totally removed, less voltage is required.

The majority of charge carriers must pass through a forward biased PN junction. The depletion of the layer's width thus gets smaller. The quantity of holes and electrons mingle with one another after the connection has been crossed.

A negative voltage delivered to the cathode is equivalent to a reverse bias.

A PN junction produces a blank zone of electricity when "–" is linked to the anode side of a PN diode and "+" is connected to the cathode side. As a result, the semiconductor's electrons are drawn to the anode side, thus the circuit has no electrical current as shown in Figure 5.8.

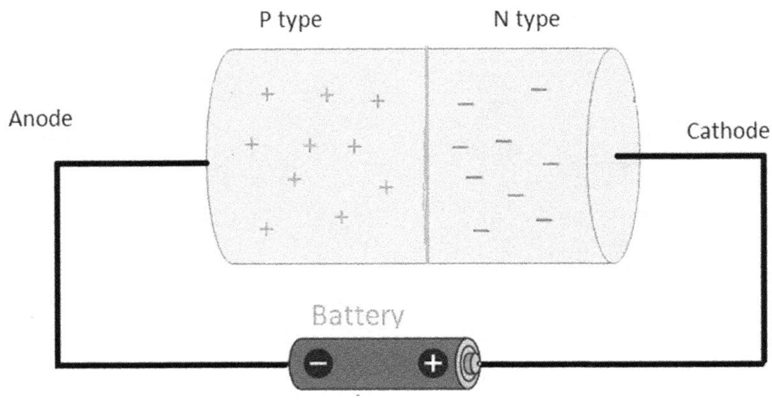


**FIGURE 5.8** Reverse bias using a PN junction diode.

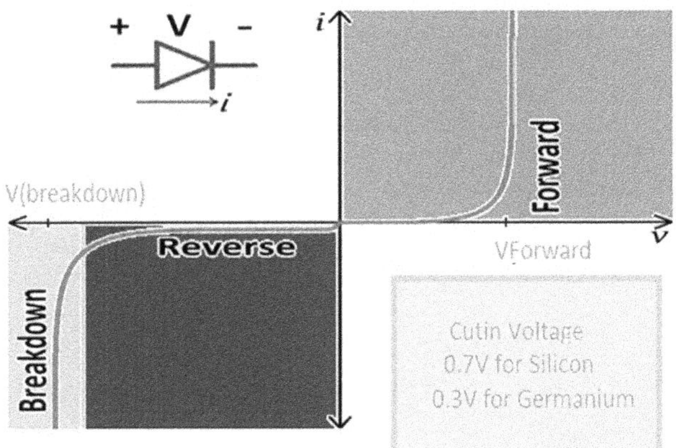


**FIGURE 5.9** VI characteristics of a diode [12].

The most frequent function of a diode is to allow the flow of electric current to be unidirectional (known as the diode's forward direction) while preventing it from flowing in the opposite direction (the reverse direction). The diode can therefore be viewed as an electrical control valve.

A diode offers extremely little resistance to the flow of current in a unidirection but very strong resistance to the other reverse direction. The diode is a unidirectional device as a result, as shown in Figure 5.9.

### 5.4.2 Bipolar Junction Transistors (BJTs)

One of the fundamental components of all contemporary electronic systems is the transistor. This is a device which is referred to as tri-terminal, and the input current determines the output current, voltage, and power. It serves as the main constituent of the amplifier in communication systems. A circuit called an amplifier is used to boost the power of an AC signal.

There are essentially two categories of transistors: an FET and a BJT. The transistor's ability to strengthen a weak signal is a crucial characteristic. This quality is known as amplification. Digital computers, satellites, mobile phones, communication systems, as well as control systems, medical equipment, and other devices, all require transistors.

There are two PN junctions inside of a transistor. As seen in Figure 5.10, the junction is created by sandwiching either P-type or N-type semiconductor layers between two pairs of opposing kinds [11, 13].

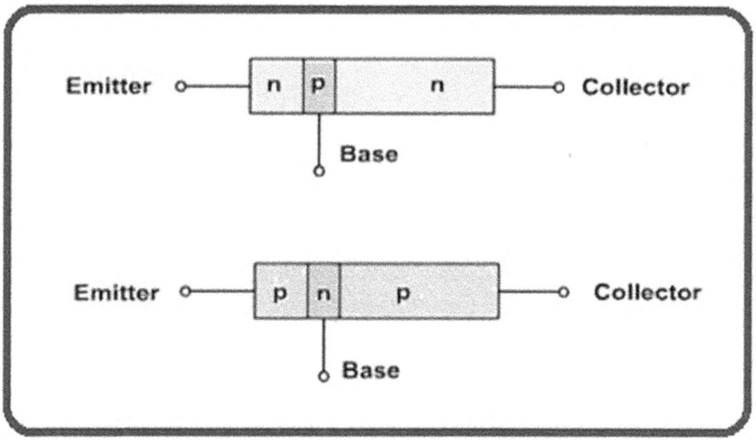


**FIGURE 5.10** A PNP and NPN transistor.

The emitter, base, and collector are the three regions that make up a transistor. An emitter is an area on one side that provides the other two regions with charge carriers (e.g., electrons and holes). The emitter is a highly doped area. The next area is the base which is the central area in the transistor between two PN junctions. The transistor's base is a weakly doped region and is thinner than the emitter. A transistor's other side, or the side opposite the emitter, is where the charge carriers are collected, commonly termed "the collector". A transistor's base and emitter are always smaller than its collector. The collector is slightly more heavily doped than the emitter but less heavily doped than the base.

The emitter of the transistor symbol has an arrowhead pointing from the P-area to the N-region. The arrowhead shows the transistor's typical current flow in that direction. In NPN and PNP transistors, the arrowheads at the emitter point in the opposite directions as seen in Figure 5.11. A complement to the NPN transistor is the PNP transistor. Free electrons make up the majority of carriers in NPN transistors, whereas holes do so in PNP transistors. Unbiased or open-circuited transistors are those that have the emitter, base, and collector terminals unconnected.

The emitter-base and collector-base junctions of the NPN transistor are forward biased and reverse biased, respectively, in the forward active bias mode. Only when V is higher than the barrier potential of 0.7 volts for silicon and 0.3 volts for germanium transistors is the emitter-base junction forward biased. The N-type emitter's free electrons flow in the direction of the base area due to the forward bias at the emitter-base junction. This constitutes the emitter current.

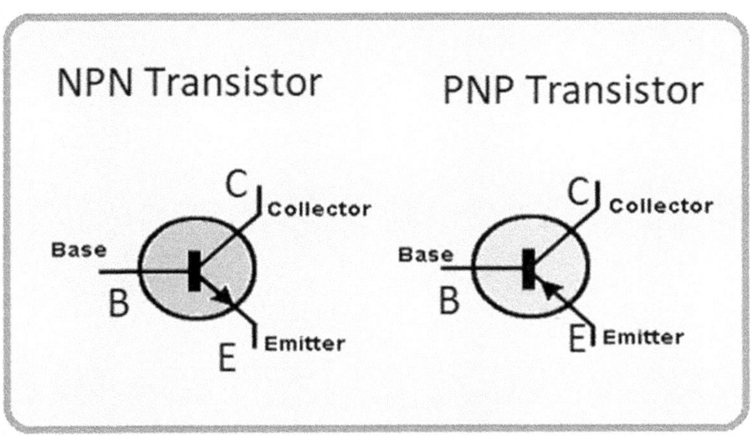


**FIGURE 5.11** Schematic representation of an NPN and PNP transistor.

The flow of electrons is opposite to the flow of the conventional current direction. Once in the base region, electrons have a tendency to join with the holes. These liberated electrons become a base current when they join holes in the base.

Most of the unpaired electrons do not combine with the base's holes. This is because there are not enough holes available for recombination for the electrons due to the base width being made incredibly tiny. Therefore, the majority of the electrons will diffuse to the collector region, which results in a collector current. Because it is formed by electrons injected from the emitter region, the collector current is also known as the injected current. The thermally produced carriers add another element to the collector current. The reverse saturation current, which is what this is, is a very small current.

For a transistor to function, there are three different configurations, as discussed below [14].

## 5.5 STANDARD BASE CONFIGURATION

This design is sometimes referred to as a grounded base. The emitter serves as the input terminal in this setup, the collector serves as the output terminal, and the base serves as the common terminal (Figure 5.12).

A diode offers extremely little resistance to the flow of current in one direction and very strong resistance to the other direction. The diode is a unidirectional device as a result.

## 5.6 THE TYPICAL EMITTER DESIGN: THE COMMON EMITTER (CE)

Additionally known as a grounded emitter setup, the base serves as the input terminal, the collector serves as the output terminal, and the emitter serves as the common terminal.

The position of the emitter between the collector and base is a typical emitter configuration. As shown in Figure 5.13, the emitter current ($I_B$) fluctuates as a function of the base-emitter voltage (VBE), while the collector-emitter voltage (VCE) remains constant (see also Figure 5.14).

## 5.7 A CONFIGURATION OF TYPICAL COLLECTORS: THE COMMON COLLECTOR (CC)

Additionally known as the grounded collector setup, the base serves as the input terminal, or as the output terminal, and the collector serves as the common terminal.

The collector terminal is considered to be shared in a common collector configuration. As a result, the output is produced from the emitter and collector terminals while the input is placed between the base and collector terminals. Because the output emitter voltage always tracks the base input voltage, the common collector design is frequently referred to as an emitter follower or voltage follower, as shown in Figure 5.15.

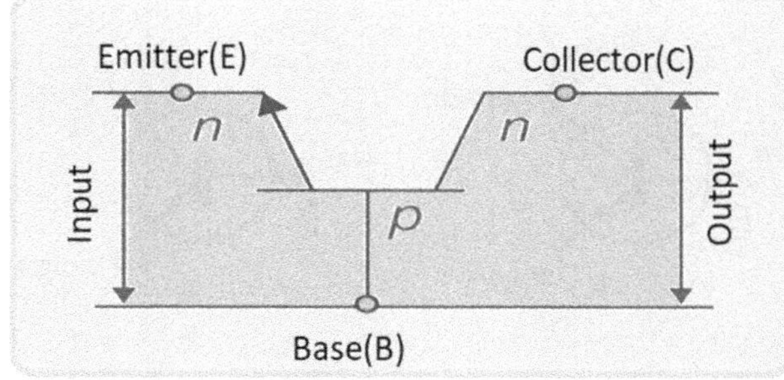


**FIGURE 5.12** Common base configuration.

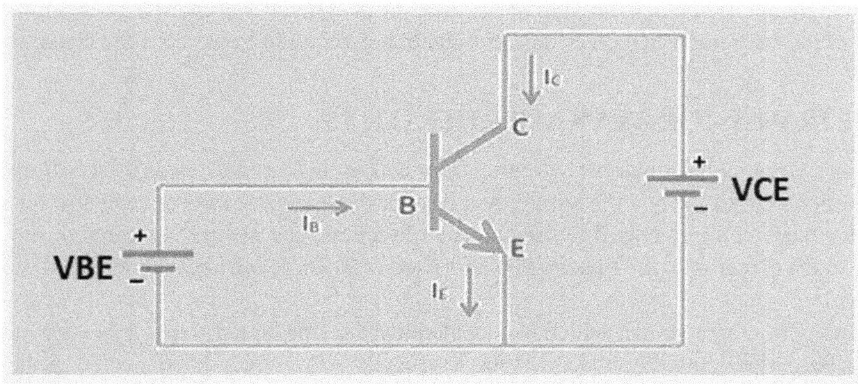


**FIGURE 5.13** Common emitter configuration.

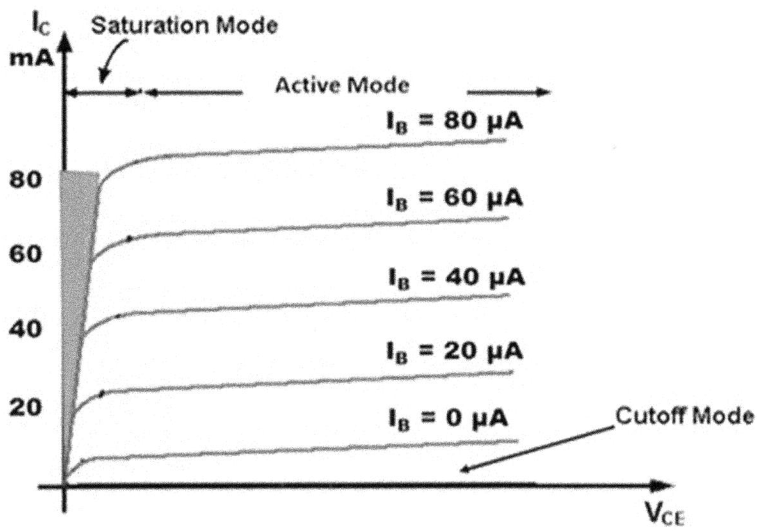


**FIGURE 5.14** VI characteristics of the transistor in the common emitter mode.

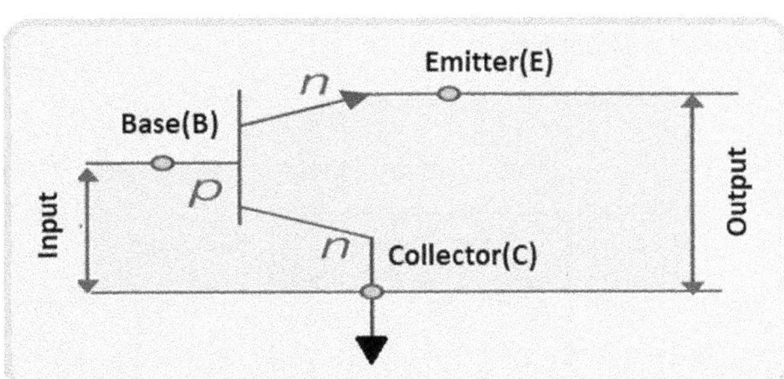


**FIGURE 5.15** Common collector configuration.

As seen in the internal block diagram of the deep brain stimulator (Figure 5.3), an implicit amplifier is one of the very important electronic circuits that is required to increase the signal strength.

## 5.8 THE TRANSISTOR AS AN AMPLIFIER [11, 15]

By boosting a weak signal's intensity, the transistor acts as an amplifier. Figure 5.16 shows the transistor amplifier's circuit. While the emitter and base of the transistor are connected in forward bias, the collector base region is biased in the opposite direction. The positive terminal of the supply is connected to the P-region of the transistor in a forward bias, while the negative terminal is connected to the N-region.

By applying the input signal, which is considered weak (the signal strength is very low), across the emitter base, the output is obtained at the load resistor $R_C$, which is connected in the collector circuit. Both the input signal and the DC voltage VEB are applied to the input circuit in order to produce the amplification. The DC voltage VEB, also known as a bias voltage, keeps the emitter-base junction in the forward biased condition regardless of the polarity of the input signal.

When a weaker signal is delivered, even a minute change in signal voltage causes a variance in emitter current because of the input circuit's incredibly low resistance (which implies that a small variation of 0.1 V of the signal generates a variation of 1 mA in the emitter current). As a result of how the transmitter works, the change in collector current is almost identical.

A load resistor $R_C$ with a high value is connected to the collector circuit. There is a significant voltage drop across such a high resistance when collector current passes through it. As a result, a weak signal of 0.1 V applied to the input circuit manifests in the collector circuit in an amplified form producing 10 V as shown in the amplification waveform of Figure 5.17.

$$\text{Voltage amplifier gain: } Av = \frac{OutputVoltage}{InputVoltage} = \frac{Vout}{Vin}$$

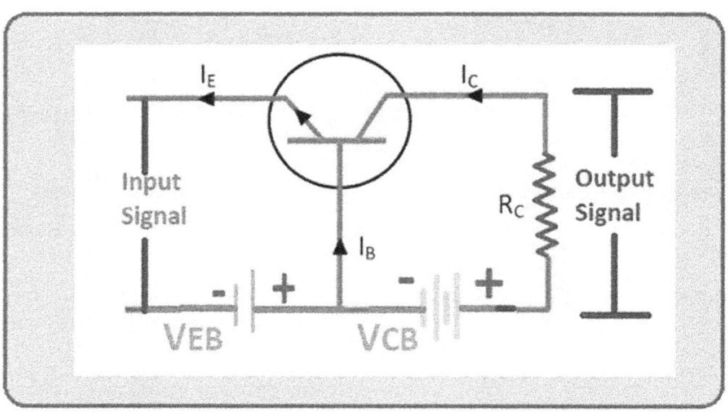


**FIGURE 5.16** The transistor as an amplifier.

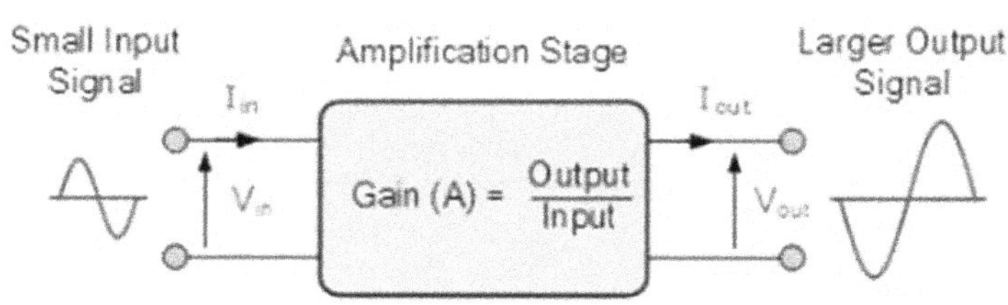


**FIGURE 5.17** Schematic of the amplification.

$$\text{Current amplifier gain: } A_I = \frac{OutputCurrent}{InputCurrent} = \frac{Iout}{Iin}$$

$$PowerGain\left(A_P\right) = Av \times A_I$$

The following section deals with the various types of power amplifier, their working, and their efficiency. The main aim of elaborating amplifiers is due to the fact that they are one of the basic building blocks of the deep brain stimulator.

## 5.9 CLASSES OF AMPLIFIERS

Audio power amplifiers are categorised according to their operating modes and circuit layouts. Different classes of operation, such as class "A", class "B", class "C", and class "AB", are used to identify amplifiers. These various amplifier classes range from having a non-linear output with a high efficiency to having an output that is nearly linear but has a poor efficiency.

- Class D amplifiers: A non-linear switching amplifier or pulse width modulated (PWM) amplifier is essentially what a class D audio amplifier is. Since current is exclusively pulled through the on transistor, there is never a time during a cycle when the voltage and current waveforms overlap. This allows class-D amplifiers to theoretically achieve 100% efficiency.
- Class F amplifiers: Using harmonic resonators in the output network, Class-F amplifiers can boost output and efficiency by converting the output waveform into a square wave. Class-F amplifiers are capable of high efficiency of more than 90% when infinite harmonic tuning is used [16, 17].
- Class G amplifiers: These amplifiers provide enhancements over the conventional class AB amplifier design. Class G uses a number of power supply rails of various voltages and switches between them automatically when the input signal changes. This constant switching lowers the average power consumption and, as a result, the power loss through wasted heat [16, 18].
- Class I amplifiers: These amplifiers are made up of two complementary sets of parallel push–pull output switching devices that sample the same input waveform. One device switches the positive half of the waveform while the other switches the negative half, similar to a class B amplifier. When a signal reaches the zero crossing point or when there is no input signal applied, the switching devices are simultaneously turned ON and OFF, with a 50% PWM duty cycle cancelling out any high frequency impulses. The duty cycle of the negative switching device is decreased to generate the opposite effect, whilst the duty cycle of the positive switching device is increased to produce the positive half of the output signal. When a class I amplifier runs at switching frequencies of more than 250 kHz, it is referred to as an "interleaved pulse width modulated amplifier" because the different switching signal currents are said to be interleaved at the output [19].
- Class S amplifiers: These power amplifiers are non-linear switching mode amplifiers that function similarly to class D amplifiers. Analogue input signals are converted by a delta-sigma modulator into digital square wave pulses, which are then amplified by a class S amplifier to increase output power and then demodulated by a band pass filter. Since the digital signal of this switching amplifier is always fully "ON" or "OFF", efficiency levels of 100% are possible [20].
- Class T amplifiers: This class of amplifier is a distinct type of digital switching amplifier architecture. Class T amplifiers are beginning to become more well-liked as an audio

amplifier design since digital signal processing (DSP) chips and multi-channel surround sound amplifiers are readily available. Class T amplifiers boost their efficiency by transforming analogue signals into digital PWM signals before amplification. Class T amplifier designs combine the low distortion signal levels of a class AB amplifier with the power efficiency of a class D amplifier [19].

The primary distinction between the BJT and the junction field effect transistor (JFET) is that a BJT is a device in which the base current regulates the output current. The input potential which is applied to a JFET, on the other hand, controls the device's output current. In contrast to JFETs, which have high input impedance, BJTs have low to medium input impedance.

The FET is unique among the primitive devices used in the pulse generator of the deep brain stimulator, as shown in Figure 5.3.

## 5.10 FIELD EFFECT TRANSISTOR

### 5.10.1 Junction Field Effect Transistor (JFET) [21, 22]

The JFET shown in Figure 5.18 is a unipolar device in which the electric field at a reverse biased PN-junction controls the flow of current between its two electrodes. The FET utilises the voltage that is supplied to its input terminal, known as the gate, so as to regulate. The output current is proportional to the input voltage due to the current flowing through them. The FET is a "voltage" operated device since it depends on an electric field produced by the input gate voltage for operation. The low power consumption and dissipation of FETs, combined with their ability to be more miniaturised than their counterpart, that is, BJT transistors, make them ideal for being utilised in integrated circuits such as the complementary metal oxide semiconductor family of digital logic processors.

The V-I characteristics of an N-channel JFET are shown in Figure 5.19. The gate voltage (VGS) in this N-channel JFET arrangement regulates the flow of current between the source and drain.

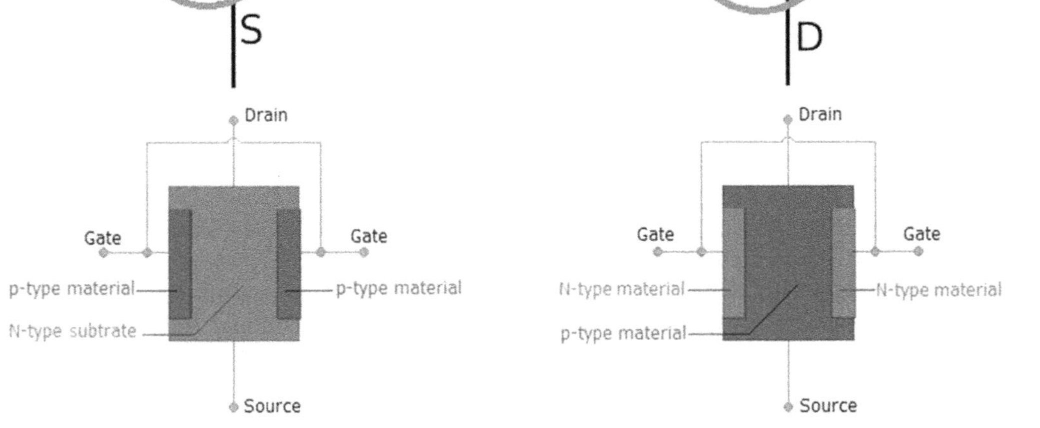


**FIGURE 5.18** Junction Field Effect Transistor.

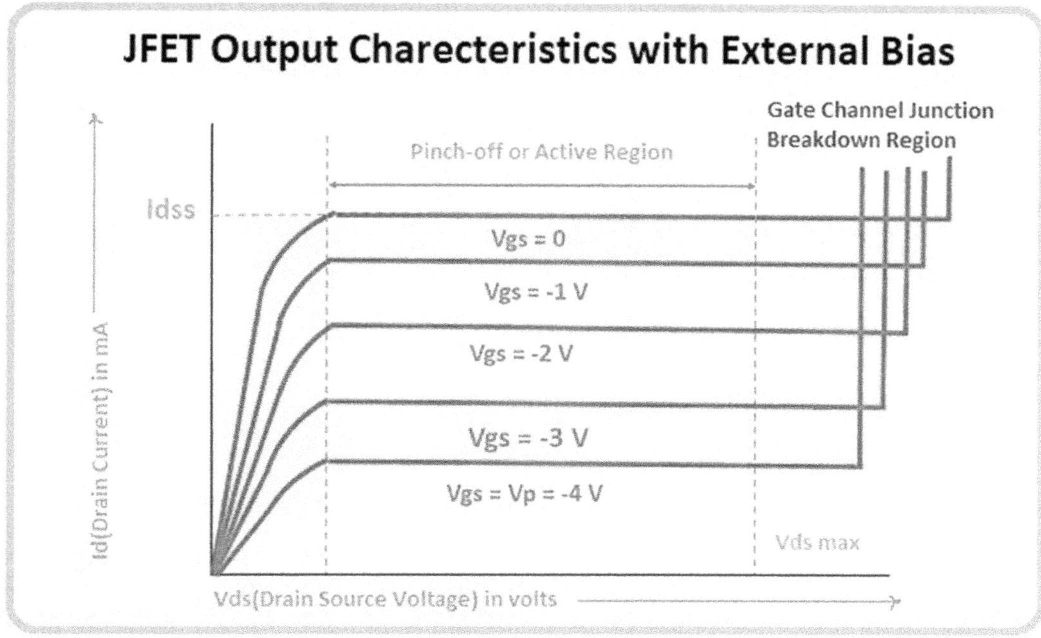


**FIGURE 5.19** VI characteristics of a JFET [24].

Since the JFET is termed a voltage-controlled device and zero current flows through the gate, the drain current ($I_D$) and the source current ($I_S$),that is, $I_D$ and $I_S$, are equal.

The voltages VGS and VDS in these V-I characteristics stand for the applied voltage between the gate and the source and the applied voltage between the drain and the source, respectively [23].

The characteristics of the JFET [24] in various regions are described as follows. The characteristics at various phases of operation rely on the input voltages:

- *Ohmic area*: The JFET acts as a voltage-controlled resistor in the extremely small depletion zone of the channel if VGS = 0.
- *Cut-off region*: The pinched-off region is another name for this area. The JFET moves into this region when the gate voltage is noticeably negative. The channel then seals off and stops carrying current.
- *Saturation region*: The gate voltage controls how the channel performs in the saturation or active region.
- *Breakdown region*: If the drain to source voltage (VDS) is high enough, the JFET channel breaks down, causing an unregulated maximum current to flow through the device.

With a few exceptions, the curves of the V-I characteristics of P-channel JFET transistors are similar to those of N-channel JFET transistors. For example, the drain current drops when the gate to source voltage (VGS) increases in a positive direction.

When the pinch-off voltage VP is equal to the applied voltage VGS, then no drain current ID flows throughout the channel. It is possible to determine the drain current ID flowing through the channel in a JFET when the gate voltage VGS applied is between 0 and VP. The drain current $I_D$ is

$$I_D = I_{DSS}\left(1-\left({}^{V_{GS}}\!/\!_{V_P}\right)\right)^2$$

The input impedance of the FET (Rin) is extremely high (thousands of Ohms), but that of the bipolar transistor (BJT) is relatively low, giving it a significant advantage over the BJT. They are particularly sensitive to input voltage signals because of their extremely high input impedance, but this sensitivity comes at a cost because static electricity may quickly harm them.

The insulated-gate field effect transistor (IGFET), also known as the ordinary metal oxide semiconductor field effect transistor or MOSFET for short, and the JFET are the two primary varieties of FETs.

MOSFET offers many advantages when compared to JFET:

- The leakage current is incredibly low;
- It has an extremely high input impedance of around $10^{14}$ ohm;
- Less power is used by MOSFET;
- It is utilised in very high RF, high noise applications;
- Compared to JFET, it has an extremely rapid switching speed.

### 5.10.2 The Metal Oxide Semiconductor Field Effect Transistor (MOSFET)

The drain, gate, source, and body terminals of a MOSFET [25] are its four terminals. The source terminal and the body terminal are frequently shorted together to create three terminals. Between the gate and the drain-source channel of a MOSFET is an insulating layer made of metal oxide, which raises the input impedance and electrically separates the gate from the channel. Additionally, it lessens leakage current. JFETs do not have this insulating layer, hence they do not have such a high input impedance or low leakage current.

The P-substrate substance, which is properly referred to as the substrate, is what causes the body to develop in N-channel MOSFETs. The creation of the terminals known as source and drain depends on the N-type material. Here, the N-type impurities are strongly doped whereas the P substrate impurities are lightly doped. Both enhancement mode and depletion mode are available for use with these MOSFETs as shown in Figure 5.20.

The enhancement type of N Channel MOSFET and its symbol is shown in Figures 5.21 and 5.22 respectively. The depletion type of N Channel MOSFET and its symbol is shown in Figures 5.23 and 5.24 respectively.

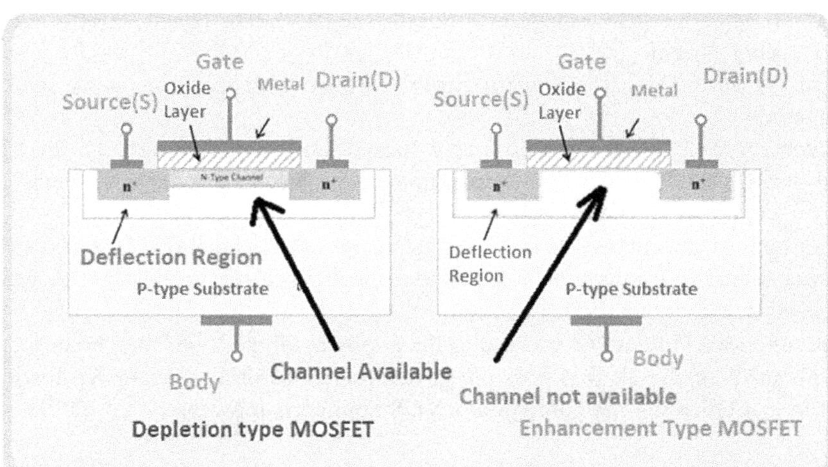


**FIGURE 5.20** Schematic highlighting the difference between the enhancement type and depletion type of MOSFET.

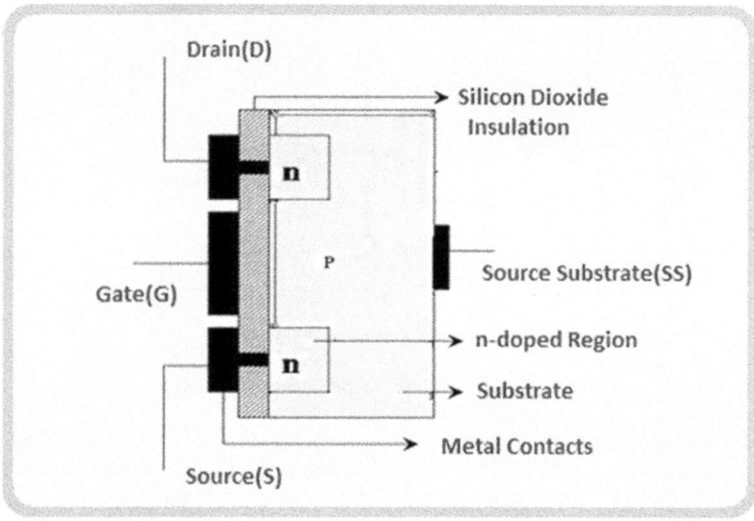


FIGURE 5.21 N channel enhancement MOSFET.

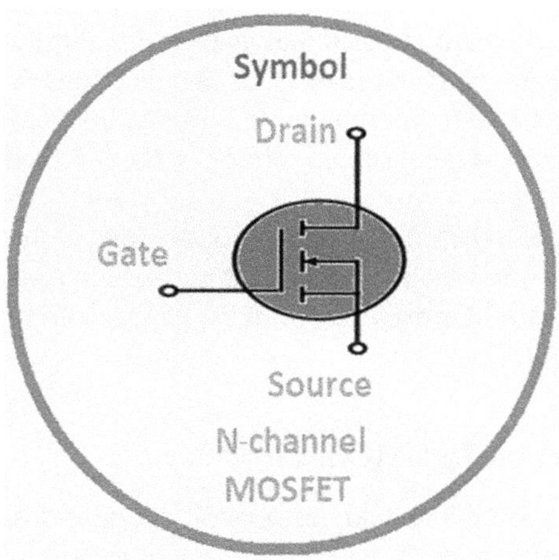


FIGURE 5.22 Symbolic representation of N-channel MOSFET.

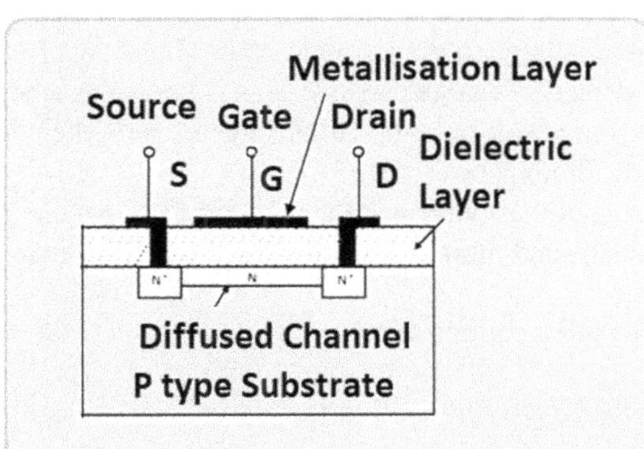


FIGURE 5.23 N-channel depletion MOSFET.

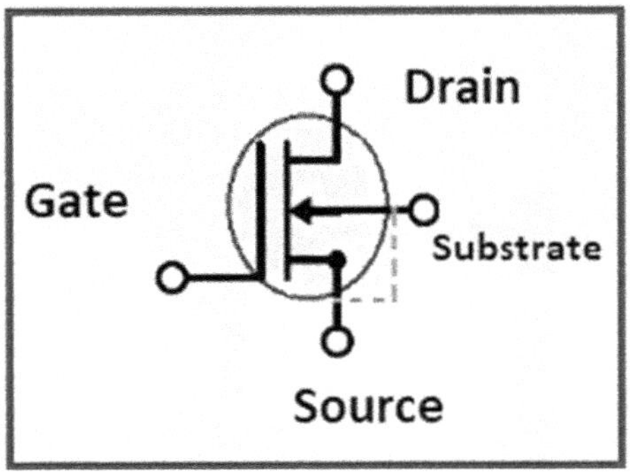


**FIGURE 5.24** Symbolic representation of N-channel depletion type MOSFET.

It was possible to develop a MOSFET where the majority of the charge carriers, or electrons, are in charge of conduction. When this MOSFET is activated to be in the ON state, the device experiences the highest level of current flow. N-channel MOSFET is the name given to this kind of MOSFET. The terminal source and the device body that results from a P-type are coupled to a common ground. The terminal gate receives a voltage with a positive polarity. It corresponds to a capacitor effect because of this positivism. Thus, in the P substrate, the free electron minority carriers are drawn to and migrate toward the terminal gate. As a result, a layer of exposed ions forms below the dielectric layer, where the pairings of holes and electrons take place. The minority carriers, the electrons, are able to prevent recombination with the holes as the applied positive voltage progressively increases and crosses the minimal threshold; they also create the channel between the two P-type materials [26].

The transistor's current flows when the positive voltage value at the drain is applied further. The channel is created as a result of the electron concentrations, which rely on the applied potential. The application of voltage at the gate improves current flow. As a result, it is referred to as an enhancement type N-channel MOSFET.

### 5.10.3 N-Channel Depletion Type MOSFET

The enhanced MOSFET has a similar design; however, it operates differently from it.

The N-type impurities make up the area between the terminals of the drain and the terminal source. The region's current flow is caused by a difference in potential between the terminal source and drain. At the gate, a voltage value with a negative polarity is applied. The electrons that are present in it are attracted to the dielectric layer and settle there. Depletion of the charge carriers thus takes place, which lowers the conductance as a whole. In this case, the current value decreases even after applying the same voltage to the terminal drain. The flow of current at the drain can be managed by adjusting the depletion charge carriers. This is known as a depletion MOSFET for this reason. Here, the terminal source still has a potential value of zero, the gate has a negative polarity, and the potential value at the drain is positive [27].

Compared to the terminals of the source and the gate, the difference in potential values is greater at the drain and gate terminals, and more so at the drain than the source – the depletion width will be visible (Figure 5.25).

MOSFET operates in the three regions of:

*Cut off region*: The MOSFET will be OFF in the cut-off zone since there won't be any current flowing through it. When they are needed to act as electronic switches, MOSFETs are chosen because they behave in this region like an open switch.

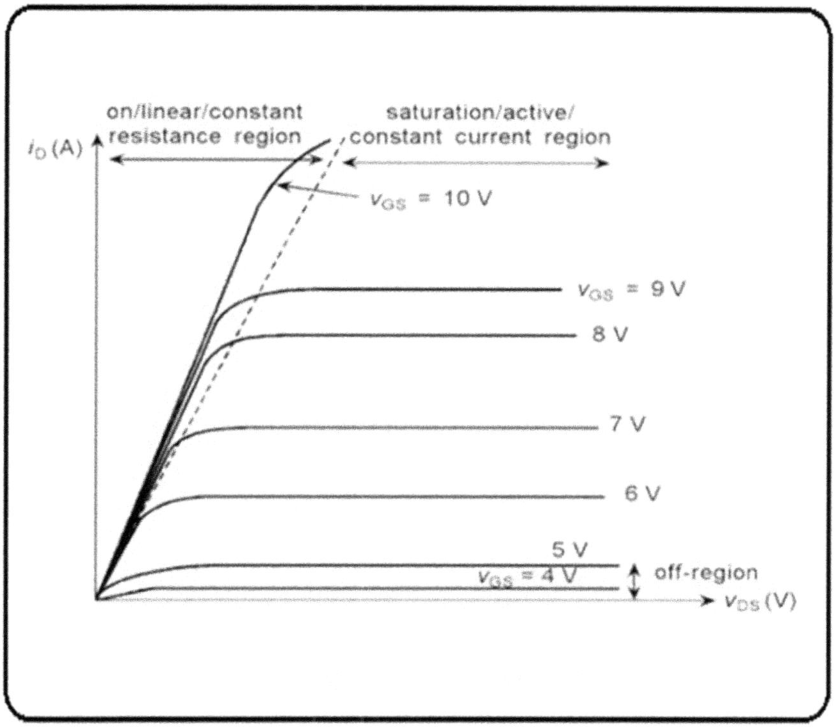


**FIGURE 5.25** Representation of VI characteristics of MOSFET.

*Ohmic or linear region*: A zone known as an ohmic or linear region is one in which the current IDS rises as the value of VDS rises. MOSFETs can be utilised as amplifiers if they are designed to function in this range.

*Saturation region*: The MOSFETs' IDS remains constant during the saturation area even as VDS increases, which happens once VDS surpasses the pinch-off voltage VP. When this occurs, the device behaves as a closed switch through which an IDS value saturated with information flows. As a result, whenever MOSFETs are needed to carry out switching operations, this operational area is picked [28].

## 5.11 CONCLUSION

The primary goal of this survey has been to investigate the many electronic circuit designs that could be used to build a device that gives tailored stimulation to specific brain regions for people with tremors, drug-resistant epilepsy, or PD. The various types of electronic equipment that are used to implement biomedical electronic solutions and that enhance the quality of life for persons who experience such conditions have been covered in this chapter. DBS, a technique used to treat epileptic seizures, is similar to cardiac pacemaking in that it generates and delivers high frequency electric pulses into the sub-thalmic nucleus or globus pallidus internus regions of the brain through extension wires and electrodes. Machine learning techniques can be used to automatically identify PD symptoms and follow the evolution of the condition by utilising data streams from soft wearable sensors. The numerous electronic circuits and parts used in these sensors must be carefully considered.

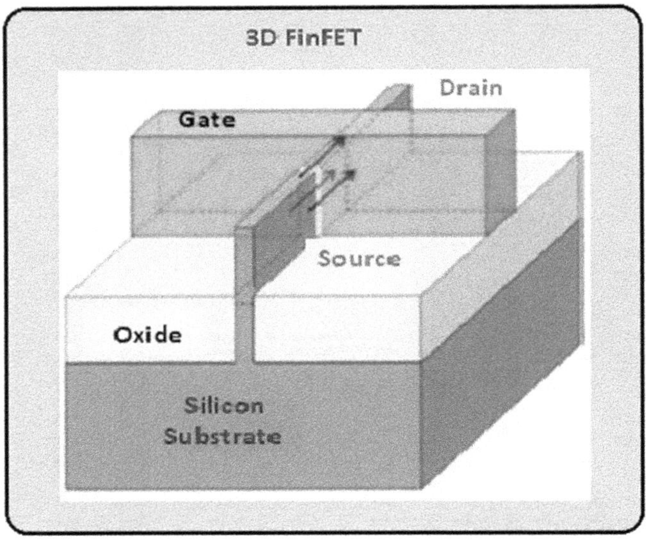


**FIGURE 5.26** Schematic of FinFET [29].

### 5.11.1 Fin Field Effect Transistor (FinFET)

MOSFET is a planar transistor, whereas FinFETs are three-dimensional transistors.

A vertical fin-shaped structure known as a FinFET serves as the drain and source of the device. The source and drain are encircled by a gate. With this design, the gate is sufficiently long and the channel of carriers between the drain and source is better electrostatically controlled. Metal, oxide, and semiconductors all play a role in the fundamental construction of MOSFETs, which are planar devices. A planar N-channel MOSFET is made by diffusing heavily doped N regions onto a P-substrate body. Over this planar structure, silicone dioxide is created as a layer. Metallic terminals are etched onto the insulating layer of silicon dioxide. The metallic terminals that are in touch with the N areas below create the drain and source. The gate terminal is the metallic layer on silicon dioxide that is not in contact with the N regions (Figure 5.26).

When compared to MOSFETS, FinFETs have significant advantages thanks to their three-dimensional structure [30]. These attributes include, among others:

- A single chip can have a considerable number of transistors. Due to its higher scalability than MOSFETs for a given footprint size, FinFET technology is appropriate for the production of integrated circuits.
- Transistors reduce in size along with chips. This compactness decreases the gate's control over the channel carriers and brings the drain and source closer together. In MOSFETs, this kind of short-channel impact can lead to significant problems. FinFETs exhibit superior short-channel performance due to the presence of fins.
- Planar MOSFETs frequently employ channel doping to enhance short-channel behaviour. Channel doping in FinFETs is optional due to the wrap-around gate covering the thin body. Therefore, FinFETs don't have any dopant-induced fluctuations.
- In order to reduce leakage current and, in turn, leakage power, the gate's length is important. In FinFETs, the gate is long enough to wrap around the drain-source channel, preventing leakage current when the gate is not activated. However, as the gate is shrunk in MOSFETs, leakage current occurs.
- In switching devices, leakage power results from leakage current and voltage. FinFETs consume less electricity than MOSFETs because they have low leakage current devices.

- A planar MOSFET's drive strength depends on the channel width, whereas a FinFET transistor's drive strength can be increased by merging more and longer fins.
- Faster switching times in FinFETs can be a result of a larger drive current. In contrast to planar MOSFETs, three-dimensional FinFETs can be regarded as high-speed electronics.
- FinFET technology makes multi-gate devices simple to manufacture. Multi-gate fabrication in MOSFETs is laborious due to planar architecture.
- Compared to planar MOSFETs, FinFETs have a better sub-threshold slope and a larger voltage gain.

## REFERENCES


1. https://www.psychguides.com/ An American Addiction Centres Resource.
2. M.E. Berryhill, D. Peterson, K. Jones, R. Tanoue, "Cognitive Disorders", in *Encyclopaedia of human behaviour*, 2nd Edition, 2012.
3. L.D. Ravdin, *Cognitive disorders*, International Encyclopaedia of Public Health, 2008.
4. Mild Cognitive Impairment (MCI), https://www.mayoclinic.org/diseases-conditions/mild-cognitive-impairment/symptoms-causes/syc-20354578
5. F. Elizabeth Godkin, Erin Turner, "Feasibility of a continuous, multi-sensor remote health monitoring approach in persons living with neurodegenerative disease", *Journal of Neurology*, October 2021.
6. Shweta Gupta, Shashi Kumar Singh, "Neurostimulators Used in Brain for Parkinson's disease and Epilepsy Using Bionics", *International Journal of Scientific Research Engineering & Technology (IJSRET)*, 1(5), 049–052, August 2012, ISSN 2278 – 0882.
7. https://www.defeatingepilepsy.org/treatment-for-epilepsy/deep-brain-stimulation/
8. Patrick Hickey, Mark A. Stacy, "Deep Brain Stimulation: A Paradigm Shifting Approach to Treat Parkinson's Disease", *Frontiers in Neuroscience*, https://doi.org/10.3389/fnins.2016.00173, April 2016.
9. Thomas J. Foutz, D. Michael Ackermann Jr., Kevin L. Kilgore, Cameron C. McIntyre, "Energy Efficient Neural Stimulation: Coupling Circuit Design and Membrane Biophysics", *PLOS One*, https://doi.org/10.1371/journal.pone.0051901, December 2012.
10. Volker A. Coenen, Florian Amtage, Jens Volkmann, Thomas E. Schlaepfer, "Deep Brain Stimulation in Neurological and Psychiatric Disorders," *Deutsches Ärzteblatt International* 112(31–32): 519–526. https://doi.org/10.3238/arztebl.2015.0519, August 2015.
11. Robert L. Boylestad, Louis Nashelsky, *Electronic devices and circuit theory*, Pearson Education, Edition 10.
12. https://learn.sparkfun.com/tutorials/diodes/real-diode-characteristics
13. https://www.sathyabama.ac.in/sites/default/files/course-material/2020-10/UNIT-2_5.pdf
14. https://www.physics-and-radio-electronics.com/electronic-devices-and-circuits/transistors/bipolar junctiontransistor/commonemitterconfiguration.html
15. https://physicscourses.colorado.edu/phys3330/phys3330_fa13/Documents/Manual/Exp_7_Fall13.pdf
16. https://www.electronics-tutorials.ws/amplifier/amplifier-classes.html
17. Andrei Grebennikov, Nathan O. Sokal, "Class F Power Amplifier", *Switch Mode RF Power Amplifiers* 2007, pp. 95–149.
18. Kunhee Cho, Ranjit Gharpurey "An Efficient Class-G Stage for Switching RF Power Amplifier Applications", September 2018, *IEEE Transactions on Circuits and Systems II: Express Briefs*, https://doi.org/10.1109/TCSII.2018.2870277
19. https://www.electroschematics.com/audio-amplifiers-from-class-a-to-t
20. John Dooley, Ronan Farrell, *A practical class S power amplifier for high frequency transmitters*, January 2008.
21. Kirti, "Basic study of Junction Field Effect Transistor (JFET)", *International Journal of Science and Research (IJSR)* 3(9), 2319–7064, September 2014.
22. Abbas Panahi, "Open-Gate Junction Field Effect Transistor (OG-JFET) for Life Science Applications: Design, Implementation, and Characterization", *IEEE Sensors Journal*, 21(23), October 2021.
23. Hideharu Matsuura, Kenji Akatani, Michihisa Ueda, "A New N-Channel Junction Field-Effect Transistor Embedded in the i Layer of a Pin Diode", *Japanese Journal of Applied Physics* 38(9AB), September 1999, https://doi.org/10.1143/JJAP.38.L1015
24. https://electronicscoach.com/characteristics-of-jfet.html

25. C. H. Wann, K. Noda, T. Tanaka, M. Yoshida, Chenming Hu "A Comparative Study of Advanced MOSFET Concepts", *IEEE Transactions on Electron Devices* 43(10), October 1996.
26. Samares Kar, "MOSFET: Basics, Characteristics, and Characterization", *Springer Series in Advanced Microelectronics* 43, 47–152, https://doi.org/10.1007/978-3-642-36535-5_2, July 2013.
27. https://www.watelectronics.com/basics-of-n-channel-mosfet-working-and-characteristics
28. Vasily Orlov, A. S. Bakerenkov, Vladislav Felitsyn, Gennady Zebrev "Compact Modeling of MOSFET I-V Characteristics and Simulation of Dose-Dependent Drain Currents", *IEEE Transactions on Nuclear Science*, https://doi.org/10.1109/TNS.2017.2712284, February 2017.
29. Vaishali Thakur, Pallavi Pahadiya, "A Review on MOSFET and its limitations: New era of transistor 'FinFET Technology'", *Pramana Research Journal*, 10(5), 2020, ISSN NO: 2249-2976
30. https://resources.system-analysis.cadence.com/blog/msa2021-using-finfets-vs-mosfets-for-ic-design

# 6 Exploration and Application of Cognitive Illness Predictors, such as Parkinson's and Epilepsy

*B. V. Srividya and Sasi Smitha*
Dayanand Sagar College of Engineering, Bengaluru, India

*Meenakshi Bannerjee*
O.P. Jindal Global University, Sonepat, Haryana, India

## 6.1 COGNITIVE DISORDERS

Cognitive disorders frequently start off slowly but progress until they dramatically reduce the quality of life for the person who has them. It's crucial to comprehend the numerous types of cognitive diseases, their signs and symptoms, and the available treatments [1].

Neurocognitive diseases include cognitive impairments. Any condition that significantly hinders a person's ability to think clearly to the point where they cannot function normally in society without therapy is referred to as a cognitive illness. Among the widespread cognitive diseases are:

1. Developmental diseases;
2. Dementia;
3. Motor skill deficiencies;
4. Amnesia;
5. Cognitive impairment brought on by substance abuse.

Similar to the majority of mental illnesses, a range of factors can contribute to cognitive impairments. Others are caused by a hereditary predisposition, and still others are caused by unbalanced hormone levels in the womb. Common environmental causes of cognitive issues include inadequate nourishment and interaction during crucial periods of cognitive development, notably during infancy [2].

Substance misuse and physical harm are two additional prominent causes of cognitive disorders. Cognitive dysfunction can come from those neurophysiological changes when a part of the brain that controls cognitive function is harmed, whether by excessive drug or alcohol use, physical trauma, or any combination of these [3].

Various cognitive predictive maintenance tools need to be used for the early detection of a variety of cognitive diseases, such as Alzheimer's disease, bipolar disorder, epilepsy, Parkinson's disease, and depression [4]. These tools are essential today because there are no reliable medical tests that can detect these diseases in their earliest stages.

According to [5], two types of eHealth platforms have been created for the real-time identification and/or diagnosis of illnesses: wearable devices (WDs) and/or body sensor networks (BSNs). WDs are often provided for data collecting, measuring biological variables, or user input, with local processing done via mobile cloud computing (MCC) or cloud computing (CC) services. Model learning and computationally expensive activities, as well as sampling data from sensors, are often

DOI: 10.1201/9781003245346-6

handled by CC services, which also offer a presentation layer that includes user alarms for patients or medical professionals, patients' relations being informed, and even visualisations and data analytics for forthcoming investigations [5].

Future technologies like the industrial Internet of Things, artificial intelligence, machine learning, data sciences, big data, and different communication protocols could be examined and developed for use in the early detection of a variety of cognitive illnesses, which would be beneficial to society. It would also be beneficial to compare newly designed equipment using future technologies with technologies or devices currently accessible for cognitive illnesses.

This chapter focuses on the design, analysis, and use of various cognitive predictive maintenance tools for the early detection of a variety of cognitive diseases, such as epilepsy or Parkinson's disease.

## 6.2 EPILEPSY

Seizure monitoring is essential for managing epilepsy and assessing therapy outcomes. Currently, clinical seizure surveillance may miss seizures, so long-term peripheral monitoring may be required. In this work, wearable biosensors are used to evaluate how well machine learning (ML) algorithms created specifically for the detection of seizures perform across a wide range of epileptic episodes [6].

An aberrant brain activity that can cause seizures or periods of bizarre behaviour, feelings, and occasionally loss of consciousness is what is known as epilepsy. There are several possible seizure symptoms. Some epileptics simply stare mindlessly for a brief period of time during a seizure, while others repeatedly twitch their limbs or legs. A diagnosis of epilepsy typically requires at least two unrelated seizures that occur at least 24 hours apart. For most epilepsy patients, treatment with drugs or occasionally surgery can control seizures. While some people need ongoing medication to manage their seizures, others finally experience a cessation of them. With time, some epileptic youngsters may outgrow their affliction.

Seizures can disrupt any process your brain controls because epilepsy is brought on by aberrant brain activity. Among the seizure warning signs and symptoms are:

1. Confusion momentarily;
2. The action of staring;
3. Stiff muscles;
4. Jerking characterised by involuntary arm and leg movements;
5. Loss of perception or consciousness occurs;
6. Psychological signs like dread and anxiety.

The symptoms change according to the type of seizure. The symptoms will typically be consistent from episode to episode because an individual with epilepsy tends to have the same kind of seizure every time.

Based on how and where the aberrant brain activity starts, seizures are typically divided into two categories [7]:

1. Focal seizures;
2. Generalized seizures.

## 6.3 FOCAL SEIZURES

Seizures are referred to as focal seizures when they seem to be caused by abnormal activity in just one part of the brain. There are two types of these seizures:

1. *Seizures in a single area without losing consciousness.* These seizures, which were once known as simple partial seizures, don't result in unconsciousness. They may modify feelings or affect how objects appear, feel, sound, or smell. Along with involuntary jerking

of one body part, such the arm or leg, some seizures can also cause spontaneous sensory symptoms including tingling, vertigo, and flashing lights.
2. *Focal seizures accompanied with altered awareness.* These seizures, which were once known as complex partial seizures, include a shift or loss of consciousness or awareness. This kind of seizure could make you feel like you're dreaming. An individual experiencing a focal seizure with diminished consciousness may stare out into space, not react to their surroundings normally, or engage in repeated actions like pacing in circles or rubbing their hands together.

Focal seizures can mimic other neurological conditions such migraine, narcolepsy, or mental illness in their symptoms. To differentiate epilepsy from other illnesses, comprehensive evaluation and testing are required.

## 6.4 GENERALIZED SEIZURES

Generalized seizures are defined as seizures that seem to affect every part of the brain and can come in six different forms:

1. *Seizures when absent.* Children are often the ones that experience absence seizures, also known as petit mal seizures. They often last between five and ten seconds and are characterised by blank stares and with or without modest physical motions like lip smacking or eye blinking. There may be a brief loss of awareness during these clustered seizures, which can happen up to 100 times per day.
2. *Tonic seizure.* Tonic seizures result in tense muscles and can have an impact on consciousness. A patient's back, arms, and legs may become weakened by these seizures, which can result in a loss of balance.
3. *Atonic seizures.* Also known as drop seizures, these are associated with the loss of muscular coordination. Because the legs are usually affected, the patient commonly collapses or drops to the knees as a consequence.
4. *Clonic seizures.* Muscle jerking, repetition, or rhythmic movements are signs of clonic seizures. These seizures often involve the face, arms, and neck.
5. *Myoclonic seizures.* The upper torso, arms, and legs are typically affected by myoclonic seizures, which often present as quick, short jerks or twitches.
6. *Tonic-clonic seizures.* These, often known as grand mal seizures, are the most severe type of epileptic seizure. They may also cause the body to jerk, twitch, or shake, as well as an abrupt loss of consciousness. They can occasionally result in tongue biting or loss of bladder control.

A thorough evaluation and testing is needed to predict seizures early. In order to make an early diagnosis of epilepsy, the registered patients admitted to the epilepsy monitoring unit are required to be fitted with a wearable sensor on either their wrists or ankles. Body temperature, blood volume pulse, electrodermal activity, photoplethysmography (BVP), and accelerometry (ACC) are all measured by the sensor. These results are then confirmed by a board-certified epileptologist as a benchmark comparison for the electroencephalographic (EEG) seizure onset and offset.

Wearable sensors have been suggested as a way to get around these restrictions by automatically evaluating the signs of cognitive illnesses like epilepsy and Parkinson's disease.

The design, analysis, and application of various cognitive predictive maintenance tools for the early identification and prognosis of a variety of cognitive disorders, such as Parkinson's disease and epilepsy, are the main topics of this chapter.

## 6.5 AN INTERNET OF THINGS INFRASTRUCTURE FOR SCREENING AND MANAGING EPILEPSY

Heart rate variability (HRV), which is strongly associated with seizures and shows autonomous nervous system disturbance, can offer practical clinical data that can be used to identify seizures. It is necessary to possess a detection system that can deliver clear data, be simple to use, and be capable of early intervention, giving the patient the chance to avoid seizures and the side effects that go along with them.

This research explores generalized tonic-clonic seizures and common absence seizures, two distinct and common types of epilepsy crises. In these two situations, WDs with a triaxial accelerometer (ACM) and/or heart rate (HR) [8, 9] sensors can effectively detect seizures.

The ergonomic features of this system need to be examined because each patient is supposed to be subjected to variables including EEGs, electrocardiograms (ECGs), and the usage of ACMs and body temperature sensors.

### 6.5.1 Electroencephalograms (EEGs)

This is a method for analysing and logging the electrical activity that skeletal muscles create. A non-invasive brain imaging technique called an EEG [11] uses scalp electrodes to monitor voltage fluctuations brought on by the intense electrical activity of neurons.

### 6.5.2 Electromyography (EMG)

When a muscle is at rest and does not exhibit a recordable electrical potential, an electromyogram is created using EMG [11]. When muscle cells are electrically or neurologically active, an EMG detects the electrical potential that is produced by these cells. As the force of contraction increases, so does the potential's amplitude.

### 6.5.3 Electrocardiograms (ECGs)

In individuals with temporal lobe epilepsy (TLE), electrocardiography [12] provides the extra benefit of automatically detecting seizures, though it would be inappropriate to use the wired hospital system as a long-term seizure detection system at home.

### 6.5.4 Triaxial Accelerometer (ACM)

An instrument known as an ACM [13] monitors g-forces, or acceleration forces, in all three dimensions. This implies that movements will be recognised along with their directions, based on the frame of reference.

However, without a gyroscope, the orientation of the sensor cannot be explicitly known, even if it is simple to approximate for a stationary sensor by computing the gravitational acceleration vector.

A model for seizure prediction must be generalisable to new and previously unexplored ACM data as well as able to learn from the ACM data on seizures. The model must be capable of quickly identifying seizures that are occurring or about to begin. In this instance, the model ought to be able to ignore how the WD is oriented.

### 6.5.5 Body Temperature Sensor

A child who is between the ages of six months and five years old experiences febrile seizures when their body temperature is higher than 38 °C (100.4 °F). Children between the ages of 12 and

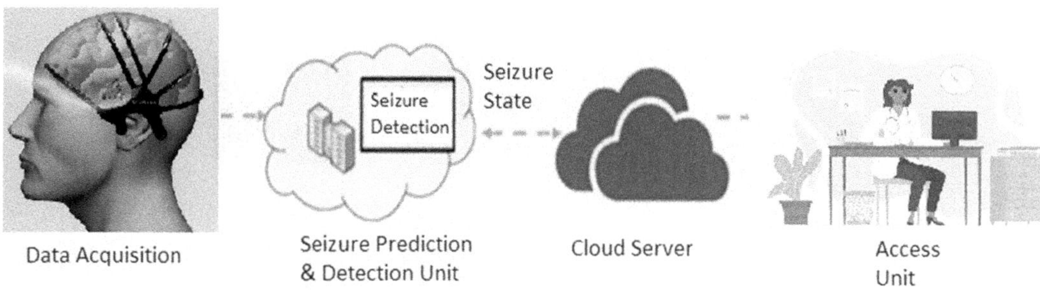


**FIGURE 6.1** Screening and managing Epilepsy.

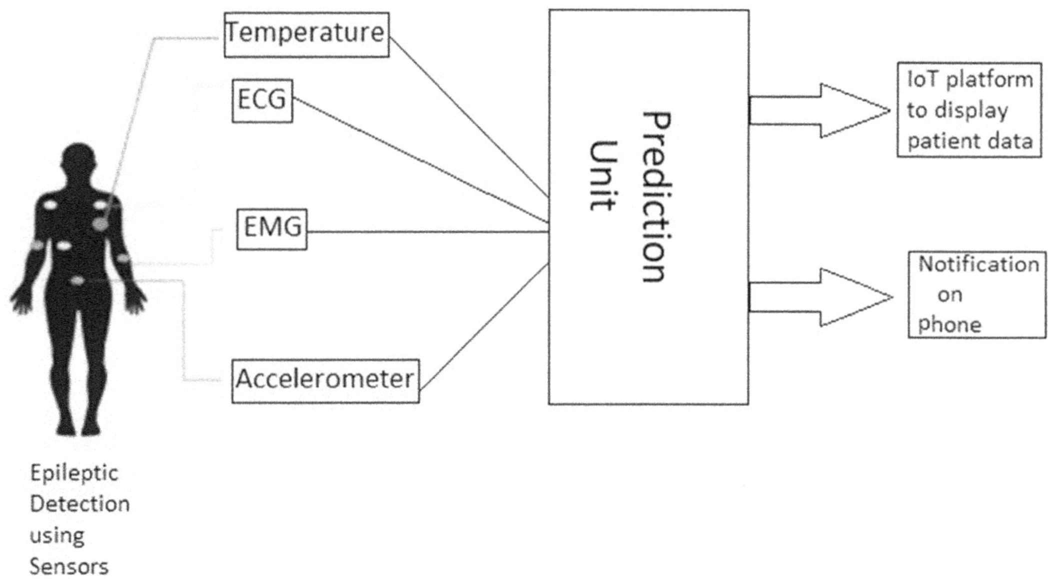


**FIGURE 6.2** Prediction of epilepsy using various wearable sensors.

18 months are most commonly affected by these seizures. A child does not necessarily have epilepsy just because they have a febrile seizure; epilepsy is characterised by two or more seizures that don't involve fever.

The survey in [14] found that 74% of patients with generalised tonic-clonic seizures exhibit the same symptoms and behaviours. These include loss of consciousness, which can cause the body to fall and be detected by the accelerometer sensor; muscle spasms, which can be intercepted by the EMG sensor; and rising heart rate, which can be detected by the ECG sensor [14].

As shown in Figure 6.1, the data from the various sensors are collected and processed periodically for predicting any possibility of occurrence of seizures. The data collected is stored in the cloud server and used to analyse the events that trigger the occurrence of seizures. The possibility of an occurrence is communicated to the carer in advance for the provision of acute treatment.

The prediction algorithm that was used to assess the necessary dataset of sick patients' parameters has enabled classification into several types of seizures, including body temperature, heart rate, muscle spasms, and falls. These are utilised as input to identify the type of seizure as an output, which is then graphically shown on the dashboard of an IoT platform (Think-Speak), where anomalous circumstances have been used to send an SMS message to notify the attendant or medical personnel of the issue.

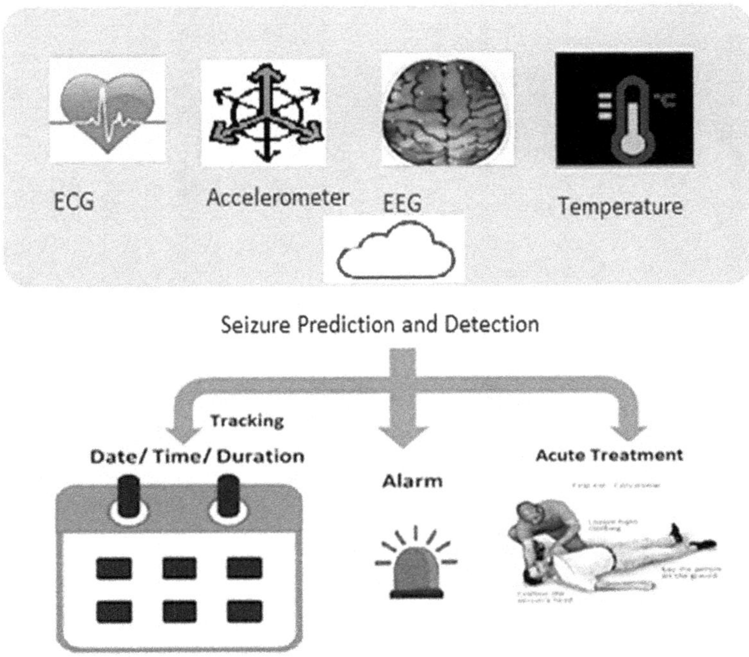


**FIGURE 6.3** Wearable sensor infrastructure for epilepsy prediction and detection [14].

## 6.6 EPILEPSY DETECTION AND PREDICTION USING EEG

Neurological research employs EEG signals to forecast epileptic seizures. Using an international standard recording device with 10–20 electrodes, EEG signals are captured. In this study, the health records of normal and sick individuals from varying age groups were taken from free online datasets (Figure 6.4).

The model provided by this work the execution of a combination operation of filtering and signal pre-processing. The network model is trained using this filtered data before being used to generate an estimate [15].

### 6.6.1 Filter

According to the survey conducted, filtering is carried out in three stages: Laplacian, spatial, and average filtering. The second derivatives of an image, which calculate the rate at which the first

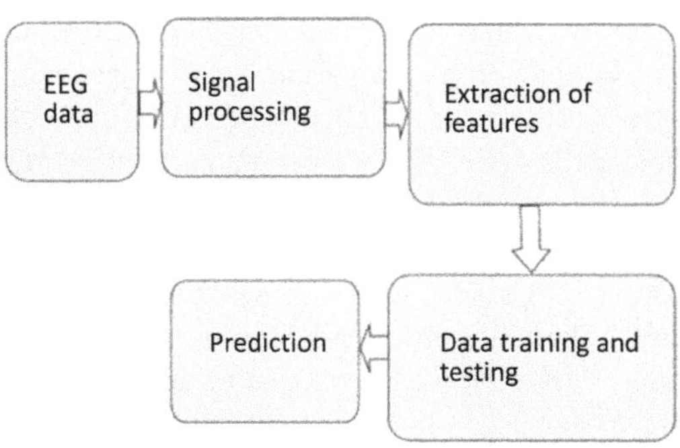


**FIGURE 6.4** Work flow.

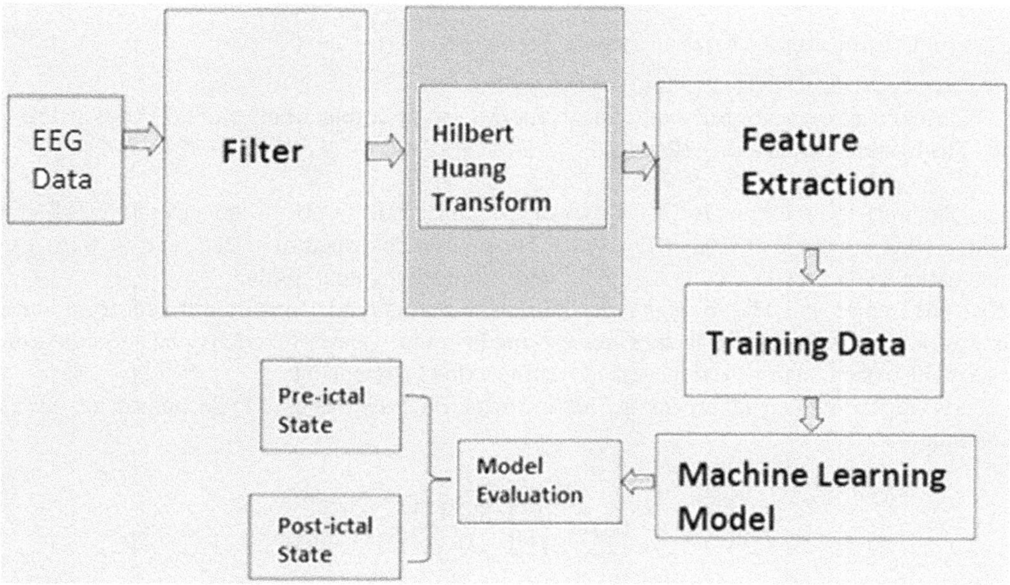


**FIGURE 6.5** Prediction steps.

derivatives change, are computed using a Laplacian filter, a type of edge detector. This establishes whether a change in adjacent pixel values results from an edge or continuous progression.

Through the process of "spatial filtering", specific spatial frequencies that make up an item can be removed to change the qualities of an optical image. In order to "smooth" photographs, average (or mean) filtering lessens the intensity fluctuation between adjacent pixels. The average filter operates by proceeding pixel-by-pixel through the image and replacing each value with the average of its own neighbouring pixels as well as its own.

### 6.6.2 Transformation

Image empirical or scientific mode decomposition (IEMD) is an extension of the Hilbert–Huang transform's (HHT) empirical mode decomposition concept into two dimensions for usage with images. By virtue of its unique capacity to locally separate superposed spatial frequencies, IEMD offers a tool for picture processing.

Empirical mode decomposition (EMD), often known as the intrinsic function mode, is a technique for breaking down signals into various simple oscillatory modes (intermaxillary fixation – IMF). As a result, the signal $x(t)$ can be represented by the residue and the sum of these IMF components:

$$x(t) = \sum_{m=1}^{M} D_m(t) + r_M(t)$$

where $r_M(t)$ is the residual and $M$ is the total number of IMFs. Two prerequisites must be met by the IMFs of a signal. First off, there is a maximum of one discrepancy between the total number of extrema and zero-crossings. Furthermore, the average value of the envelope defined by the local maxima and minima is zero or extremely close to zero at all sites. The EMD algorithm is shown by these steps:

1. From the signal of $x(t)$, extract local maxima and local minima
2. Connect all minima and all maxima to get two envelopes, $e\min(t)$ and $e\max(t)$

3. Compute the average between them as $m(t) = \frac{[e\min(t) + e\max(t)]}{2}$
4. Extract the detail from $x(t)$ as $d(t) = x(t) - m(t)$
5. Verify the aforementioned requirements for IMFs to determine whether or not $d(t)$ is an IMF
6. The residual $d(t)$ is to be reiterated.

Upon obtaining the preliminary IMF $D1(t)$ of the signal, and to obtain the successive IMFs, the residual $r(t)$ is generated as $r(t) = x(t) - D1(t)$. The process described from step (1) to step (6) needs to be continued until IMFs can no longer be obtained from the final residue.

The HHT employs EMD for signal decomposition and is fundamentally different from Fourier and wavelet transforms since it does not use predetermined basis functions and the conformity between the basic functions and the signal itself to extract components.

Each component in signal processing has its own HHT, which is used to decompose an intrinsic mode function:

$$yi(t) = \frac{1}{\Pi} \int_{-\infty}^{\infty} \frac{D_m j(\tau)}{t - \tau} d\tau$$

With the Hilbert transform, the analytic signal is defined as:

$$z(t) = x(t) + iy(t) = a(t)e^{i\theta(t)}$$

where

$$a(t) = \sqrt{x^2 + y^2}$$

and

$$\theta(t) = \arctan(y/x)$$

After performing the Hibert transform on each component, the original data can be expressed as the real part in the following form:

$$x(t) = \Re\left\{\sum_{i=1}^{n} a_j(t) \exp\left[i \int w_j(t) dt\right]\right\}$$

With the Hilbert spectrum defined, the marginal spectrum can be defined as:

$$h(w) = \int_{0}^{T} H(w,t) dt$$

### 6.6.3 Feature Extraction

Based on the survey carried out, wavelet transformation offers the best results for feature extraction. A time-frequency tool that is particularly effective for non-stationary signal analysis is the discrete wavelet transform (DWT). By scaling and shifting the mother function into wavelets, or by

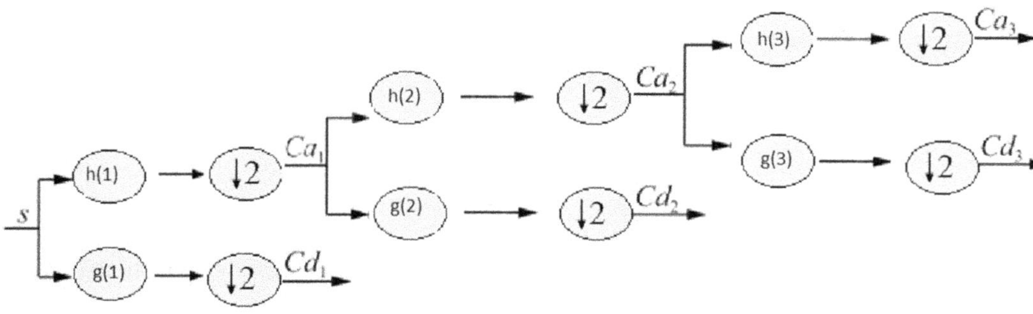


**FIGURE 6.6** Decomposition tree [15].

dividing a signal into two sub-bands with names like “approximation coefficients A” and “detailed coefficients D”, the DWT process enables the presentation of an input signal in sets of functions known as wavelets. Approximations and details can be separated out from the low frequency component. The frequency resolution is doubled and the temporal resolution is cut in half after each decomposition.

$$Dj(i) = \sum_k s(k).h(2.i - k)$$

$$A_j(i) = \sum_k s(k).l(2.i - k)$$

The line length feature parameter is retrieved from each frequency signal band and then DWT is applied. The EEG signal is categorised using an artificial neural network (ANN), which also helps to identify specific issues.

### 6.6.4 Prediction

It may be noted from the literature that a classifier such as random forest (RF) [16] produces results for seizure detection with a high degree of accuracy. The (RF) algorithm decides the outcome based on the predictions made by the decision trees. By averaging out the outcomes from various trees, predictions are provided. As there are more trees, the accuracy of the outcome improves. An RF technique overcomes the drawbacks of the decision tree technique: it raises accuracy and decreases dataset over-fitting.

The RF algorithm’s features are:

- It offers a useful way for handling missing data and is more accurate than the decision tree algorithm;
- It can produce an accurate prediction without hyper-parameter adjusting;
- It resolves the decision trees’ over-fitting issue;
- In each RF tree, a subset of characteristics is randomly selected at the node’s splitting point.

Using decision trees and RF, ML is effectively coupled. The RF identification approach works quickly and is appropriate for high-dimensional data. However, a significant amount of hyper-parameters are produced throughout the operation, and the model parameters need to be adjusted in order to achieve a higher accuracy when identifying the epileptic EEG signal. The selection of manual settings is typically reliant on experience because there are currently not many ways for optimising the RF method’s parameters.

A decision tree's Gini impurity function gauges how successfully it was split. In essence, it aids our ability to choose the finest splitter so that we may construct a straightforward decision tree. From 0 to 0.5 is the range of Gini impurity:

$$GINI(k) = 1 - \sum_{i=1}^{K} Pi$$

where $Pi$ is the probability of the $i^{th}$ category. The number of features corresponding to the sample training set are $\{n1, n2, \ldots nk\}$ $n = n1 + n2 + n3$, and the split Gini index is:

$$GINI(M^*) = \frac{n1}{n} GINI(M1) + \frac{n2}{n} GINI(M2) + \frac{n3}{n} GINI(M3)$$

Clustered decision trees $\{Tb\}_1^m$ are all used. The recognition results from the decision trees of size "m" for an input sample are size "m", and the RF acquires all of the recognition voting results. On the new node, forecasting is done, and the most recognisable amount of votes is the output $\left\{\hat{C}b(x)\right\}_1^m$.

The effectiveness of ML is when used with certain tools for computation to predict epileptic seizures using EEG inputs. However, in order to remove noise and distortions, EEG signals must be pre-processed and filtered as shown in Figure 6.5. The problem, referred to as a true positive, involves feature extraction and affects both time and the accuracy of predictions.

The model makes the assumption that epileptic seizures occur sufficiently in advance of their commencement and offers a higher true positive rate. Following pre-processing, a prediction model is trained using the time and frequency domain information that were retrieved. The pre-ictal state, which starts a few minutes before the start of the seizure, is examined by the planned model at its onset: 92% of seizures are detected using these procedures. Apart from EEG, the heart sensors and the temperature measurement can be utilised for the detection of pre-ictal seizures.

## 6.7 SEIZURE DETECTION AND PREDICTION USING HEART RATE SENSORS AND TEMPERATURE SENSORS

Further reducing computational complexity is the application of raw data such as body temperature and heartbeat signals. Sophisticated ML/deep learning techniques are used to estimate the model that derives the pertinent information from the temperature, heartbeat, and haemoglobin value through an ML method, as shown in Figure 6.7. This proposed method uses support vector machines (SVMs) and a convolutional neural network (CNN), which are said to produce the best outcomes for epileptic prediction. Edge calculation service makes the generated model independent and shows it

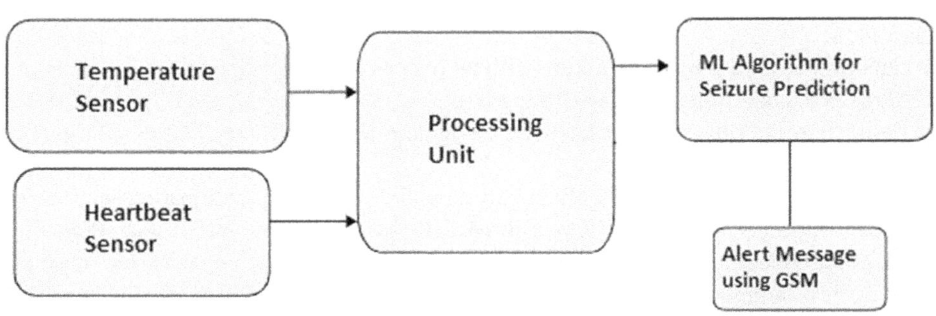


**FIGURE 6.7** Seizure prediction using a temperature sensor and heartbeat sensor.

to be useful in effective seizure prediction approaches. The outcomes may help epilepsy patients in the real world. Results have a 99% accuracy rate. The system anticipates some medication or prescribed quantity of medicines based on a health issue and sends an alarm message using the Global System for Mobile Communication (GSM) if an unusual scenario is observed. Also, the patient's position can be tracked, and when the patient falls, panics, or has abnormal health, a warning is sent as a notification.

In this investigation, epilepsy is detected using an ECG signal, which is produced by continuously measuring the electrical activity of the heart using electrodes implanted on the skin. An identification system based on the common spatial pattern (CSP) feature extraction technique is provided. Each patient's single- and multi-lead ECG signals are separated into non-overlapping segments, and various segment lengths are examined. Each signal segment's features are taken out by projecting them onto a CSP projection matrix [17, 18]. An SVM classifier built using a radial basis function kernel and trained using the retrieved features is then used in the identification stage.

In this research, the ECG signals from normal participants and those associated with neurological disorders are distinguished using the CSP technique. The following is a summary of the mathematical formulation from step 1 to 8 for the CSP approach.

1. Let $X_{in} \in R^{N\times S}$, be the $i$th segment of an ECG signal belonging to the $n$th patient. Here $N$ is the number of leads of the device and $S$ is the number of samples.
2. The covariance matrix in its normalised form for the $n$th patient is determined using

$$C_n = \left(\frac{1}{M}\right)\sum_{i=1}^{M}\frac{X_{in}X_{in}^T}{Trace\left(X_{in}X_{in}^T\right)},$$

   Here $M$ is the number of segments and $T$ is the transpose operation of the matrix.
3. The covariance matrix is obtained from all the patients:

$$C_0 = \left(\frac{1}{M(L\_1)}\right)\sum_{j=1}^{L}\sum_{i=1}^{M}\frac{X_{ij}X_{ij}^T}{Trace\left(X_{ij}X_{ij}^T\right)},$$

   where $L$ is the number of patients.
4. Compute the complex covariance matrix as

$$C_c = C_n + C_0$$

5. Perform the singular value decomposition (SVD) on the matrix $C_C$ to obtain the eigenvalues $\psi$ and eigenvectors $F_c$:

$$C_c = F_c\psi F_c^T$$

6. The QRS complexes are smartly emphasised, and the disturbances in the ECG signal are suppressed by using an improved whitening filter [19]. Perform a white transform on the covariance matrix $C_n$ and $C_0$ using the whitening matrix $P = \psi^{-1}F_c^T$ to obtain the matrices $D_n$ and $D_0$

$$D_n = PC_nP^T$$
$$D_0 = PC_0P^T$$

7. The matrices $D_K$ and $D_0$ are such that

$$D_n = U\Lambda_n U^T$$
$$D_0 = U\Lambda_0 U^T$$

These matrices have common eigenvectors, where $U$ and $\Lambda$ represent the eigenvectors and the diagonal matrix of eigenvalues respectively.

8. Finally the common spatial pattern matrix $W_n$ of size $N \times N$ is constructed as

$$W_n = \left(U^T P\right)^T$$

Here the spatial filter is every individual row of $W_n$ and the spatial pattern is every individual column of $W_n^{-1}$.

The training and testing feature vectors are extracted by projecting each segment $\chi$ of the ECG data sample by generating [20] $B_n = W_n\chi^T$ where $\chi$ is the segment from the $n$th patient under consideration. Therefore the feature vector $f_n$ pertaining to a given segment $\chi$ is defined as the log of the variance of each row of the matrix $B_n$.

The classifier for the $n$th subject will take as input the feature vector that was extracted from an ECG segment. The binary "1" for the target $n$th subject and "0" otherwise are the results of the classifier. The training dataset has a very imbalanced number of occurrences of each class as a result of using a one-versus-all classification method (i.e., the number of negative instances is much larger than that of positive instances). An approach of oversampling the positive cases is used to achieve a balance between the positive and negative instances.

## 6.8 AUTOMATED DETECTION OF SEIZURES USING AN ELECTROMYOGRAPHY (EMG) DEVICE

It is possible to detect seizures using EMG. When individuals with epilepsy are left unattended, bilateral (generalised) tonic-clonic seizures (TCSs) increase the risk of sudden unexpected death [21]. TCSs frequently go unreported while a person is sleeping, which can lead to poor treatment choices. Automated identification of these severe epileptic convulsions is required, and wearable technology can help. Specific to TCSs, quantitative surface EMG changes exhibit a dynamic evolution of the low and high-frequency signal components [22]. Seizure biomarkers are algorithms that aim to increase high-frequency EMG signals. They can be used to both identify seizures and tell them apart from convulsive non-epileptic seizures. There are numerous adhesive wearable sensors that can be applied to the arm as well as wearable biosensors in the armband form. Activities on the muscle can be utilised as a stand-in for convulsive seizure activity because this is a good place to measure EMG. The system detects changes in EMG to identify convulsions and is applied to the patient's bicep using an adhesive patch. This device can warn caregivers and features a cloud-based data platform. Further the ML algorithms can be incorporated after rigorous training and the testing phase to predict the possibility of the next occurrence of the convulsions and thus issue an alert to the caregiver [23, 24]. The mechanism of muscle activation during epileptic seizures has been found to differ from the normal one. In addition, TCSs have a distinct tonic phase from the tonic seizures in terms of persistent muscular activation: TCSs are caused by a considerable rise in signal frequency, whereas the tonic phase of TCSs is characterised by increased signal amplitude [25, 26].

Apart from the usage of wearable sensors, which requires maintenance, it is crucial to track behaviour at more complicated levels and that includes activity patterns, mobility range, sleep quality and

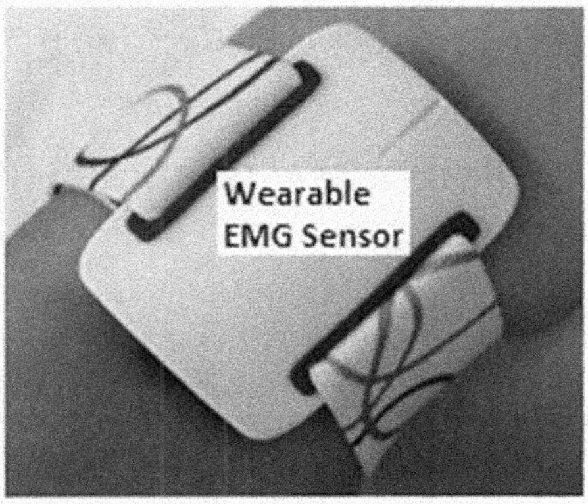


**FIGURE 6.8** Schematic of EMG sensors to detect seizures.

duration, and behavioural indications of mood, in addition to sensing fundamental bio-signals using wearable technology, for instance, based on studies of speech affect, social connection, or movement speed. Analysis of behavioural changes over days or weeks is thus necessary, as studies on prodromes and seizure triggering events suggest they may be related to seizure risk. Beyond passive monitoring, wearable technology can be used to actively ask the user questions to assess changes in mood and cognitive performance. In order to capture high level dynamic brain states, assessments can incorporate pop-up surveys at predetermined intervals as well as particular test batteries applied to general cognitive functions like attention or working memory [27] (see Figure 6.8).

## 6.9 PARKINSON'S DISEASE

Parkinson's disease (PD) is a neurological disorder that develops when dopamine levels in the brain are too low. As the illness worsens over time, the degree of disability increases. PD affects about 1% of adults over 60 in industrialised nations. Tremors (especially when at rest), rigidity, and slowness of movement are three primary motor symptoms of the disease that can be treated with levodopa (bradykinesia). These motor symptoms progressively get worse, making daily life difficult and degrading the quality of life [28]. Some of these symptoms can be treated with dopaminergic drugs, but as the disease worsens and spreads to additional areas of the body, their effects tend to fade more quickly. Some people also encounter frequent symptom changes (the "OFF/ON" condition) or uncontrollable transitions (dyskinesia) as a pharmaceutical adverse impact, which necessitates individualised dosage modifications.

When determining the rate of PD progression for a particular person, it is essential to monitor changes in motor symptoms and the reaction to treatment with time in order to develop individualised treatment plans. A skilled clinician will ask the patient to do a sequence of conventional motor tasks while visually evaluating the quality of their movements and assign a symptom score. This is the current gold standard of treatment for evaluating PD symptoms. The Movement Disorder Society Unified Parkinson Disease's Rating Scale is the most often used scale to carry out such evaluations. Patients may also be instructed to record their symptoms in a diary. However, due to their respective low accuracy and poor temporal precision, these approaches have limitations. It has been suggested that one method to get over these restrictions is to automate the diagnosis of PD symptoms using wearable, inertial, accelerometers and electromyography sensors. It has been demonstrated in several studies that information pertaining to wearable accessories like sensors and ML algorithms can be used to identify motor complaints. ML algorithms like neural networks and SVMs are being extensively utilised because of their capability to learn a classification model from the information and generalise to unforeseen scenarios, in contrast to the processing of signals, which were utilised for designing specific features manually and to identify symptoms. These models can be trained using movement data gathered from a variety of people while they carry out predetermined tasks in a clinic [29].

## 6.10 THE INTERNET OF THINGS INFRASTRUCTURE FOR PARKINSON'S DISEASE DETECTION

Typically, accelerometers, gyroscopes, or magnetometers make up the majority of wearable technology utilised in PD research. These devices can detect PD motion symptoms in real time and establish multiple data models by using certain motion programs. This makes it possible for clinicians to precisely assess the mobility state of patients in real time. In this investigation, the efficiency of collecting wearable sensor data for tremor and bradykinesia in the upper extremities was examined [30].

### 6.10.1 Bradykinesia

Bradykinesia, which refers to sluggishness of movement and pace, may manifest as gradual pauses or halts as motions proceed. It is one of the primary signs of PD.

### 6.10.2 Tremors

Uncontrollable shaking is a symptom of the neurological condition of tremor, which most frequently affects the hands and arms. Although the illness is rarely life-threatening, it can be very incapacitating. Parkinson's tremors frequently begin on one side of the body – often in the hands – and spread to the opposite side. The motions have a tendency to be stronger (high amplitude) and less frequent. The lower back is where the gyroscope is worn, as shown in Figure 6.9. The algorithm utilised in this system has been proved to estimate the risk of falling in PD patients based on variables such as smoothness of gait, consistency of gait patterns, and gait variability. It can identify slip-ups during activities of daily life [31].

A shuffling, restricted arm swing and a multi-step rotating gait are characteristics of PD. The potential for developing freezing and balance issues raises the danger of falling and has an unpredictably inconsistent response to the therapy. Wearable sensors have been widely employed in movement analysis because of their predictable movements and capacity to be tracked by a single sensor positioned with three-dimensional analysis. According to studies, jerk measurements recorded from the trunk are useful and accurate for detecting imbalance and standing difficulties in PD patients. The harmonic ratio, which is based on computations from three axes of motion, serves as a measure of the stability or fluctuation of walking from stride to stride. It has become a sensitive parameter for identifying patients with freezing as well as separating PD patients from controls.

To get adequate information on the transitions between the "OFF" and "ON" drug states, the data collecting technique frequently entails recordings from numerous patients wearing multiple sensors and enduring repeated clinical examinations over a large number of hours.

A tremor is distinguished by frequency and amplitude using tremor analysis. Accelerometers or gyroscopes can be used to distinguish the displacement of a tremor along an angular or linear axis, which has been shown to generate the greatest degree of handicap. A useful, measurable way for differentiating different tremor subtypes is provided by the addition of EMG to the investigation, which can further elucidate on the muscle groups recruited or synchronised during tremor formation [32].

This research's main objective is to compare the relative merits of several techniques for expanding the amount of training information while creating ML models for PD symptom identification during typical everyday activities. It was possible to capture movement using flexible wearable sensors that were fastened to the arms, hands, and thighs during the partial implementation, as shown

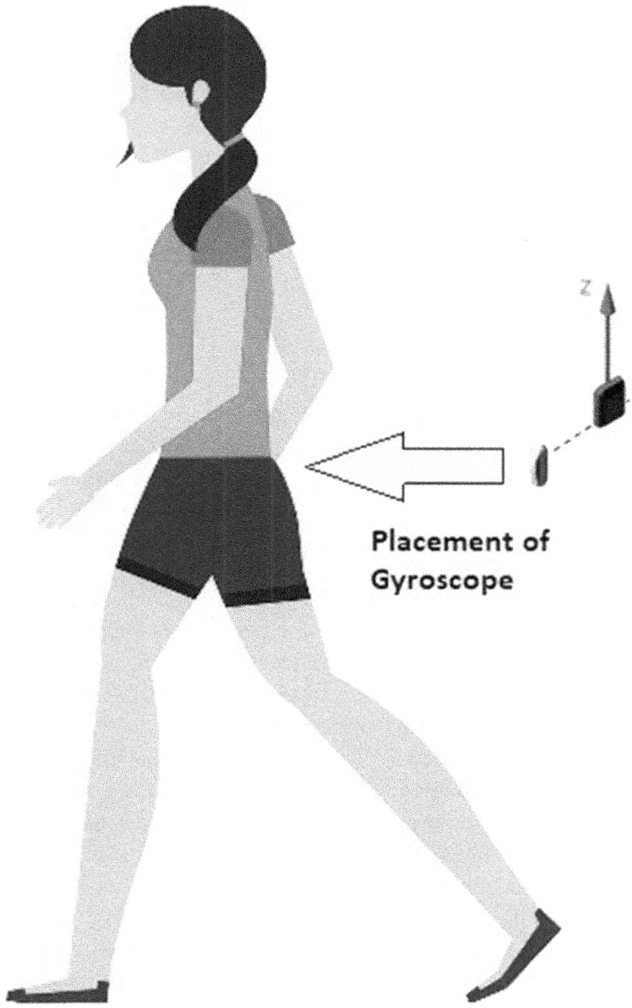


**FIGURE 6.9** Gyroscope sensor to detect PD.

in Figure 6.10. Then, using these findings, an ML classifier was trained to identify the presence of tremor or bradykinesia in the upper extremities, while people with PD underwent a number of routine everyday tasks and tasks used in clinical evaluations [33].

## 6.11 MACHINE LEARNING ALGORITHMS FOR PREDICTING PARKINSON'S DISEASE

CNN and random forest (RF) classifiers were fed data from a single sensor or a group of sensors to produce trained statistical ensembles. Because sensors are located on both sides of the body, these values were assessed using the data that was provided [33].

The implementation entailed training two RF classifiers, one for tremor detection and the other for determining whether an information segment had bradykinesia. Therefore, based on the symptom present, clinical scores for each segment were given a value of 0 to 5, with 5 being the highest. Each classifier took as input a vector of all the features, which were computed using the gyroscope

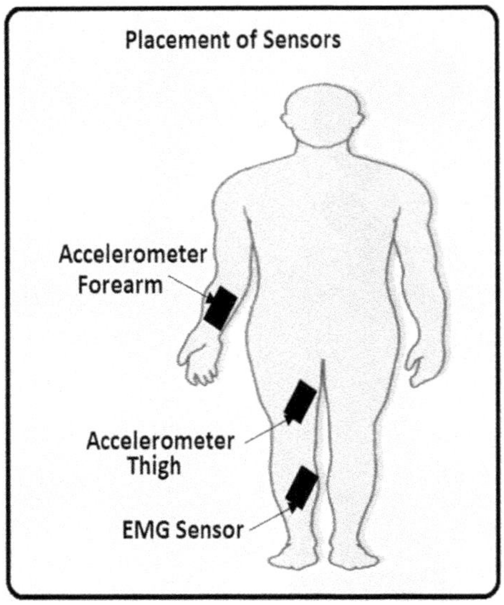


**FIGURE 6.10** Wearable devices for detecting PD.

and accelerometer information from each clip. These parameters successfully captured movement characteristics linked to speed and frequency in earlier PD research. The RF classifier's low number of adjustable hyper-parameters and capacity to minimise over-fitting are two reasons to utilise it. To minimise inaccuracy, the number of trees was set at an ideal level [34].

Two classification models using deep CNNs have been trained in this research project. CNN-based models do not require the creation of a set of features to encode an information segment because they can learn how to recognise symptoms from beginning to end from the raw sensor data. The weights across the network layers are encoded with features learned from the raw data that describe the correlation between sensor data and symptoms.

Each CNN had two convolutional layers, each having a kernel size of 32 or 16 samples and a rectified linear unit count of 16 or 32, succeeded by a max-pooling layer with a pool size of 4 or 6 units, respectively. The final two layers consist of two dense layers with a total of 32 neurons, each with the ability to activate ReLU. The likelihood that the input clip will display a symptom (bradykinesia/tremor) was output by the output layer using a softmax function for classification, with as many neurons as classes.

This research work was carried out in an institute which collaborated with the health sector. Initially the data available in open source was considered for implementation, training, and testing the model [34].

## 6.12 CONCLUSION

It is possible to automatically detect epileptic seizures of a wide range of seizure types using ML and wearable data. Initial findings demonstrate superior seizure identification above chance across a variety of seizure types. Future advancements may take into account alternative data balance, pre- and post-processing, fusion, and ensemble learning techniques, as well as clinical epileptic characteristics such as seizure length or syndrome. Therefore, despite the fact that current results point to viability, additional improvements in the future may enhance detection efficiency. Increased patient demand can put a burden on any neurology practice, forcing those with neurological issues to travel outside of a wide catchment area for care and leaving neurologists pressured for time and space to conduct examinations and treat patients. This is particularly true for epilepsy treatment, where there is a severe lack of neurologists or other epilepsy specialists, which severely restricts the number of patients who can be seen. With fewer medical resources overall and especially fewer neurologists, this burden increases on a worldwide scale. The health care sector is undergoing constant transformation as it strives to fulfil rising patient demand and complex treatment needs while also moving toward quality metrics and evidence-based treatment. In this setting, telemedicine has gained support from both patients and practitioners across several medical specialities. Nursing care, administrative support, certification, and sustainability are just a few prerequisites for successful epilepsy clinics or centres. It is crucial to make a plan for treating epilepsy that can be tailored to each patient's needs. Telemedicine also needs specific technology and information technology assistance in addition to these concerns. Computers, laptops with web cameras, smartphones, and connection to internet-based services are considered basic technological necessities. The ideal way to capture and record telemedicine encounters is also seen to require integration with the electronic health record system. Then, it will be simple and well supported to transfer data such as seizure logs, seizure action plans, and reports from investigations across web-based services. With the development of technology, concerns over privacy and the security of health information have emerged. Data encryption is a service that can be found on the network, which helps in this regard. Wearable motion sensors are rapidly expanding, and their use in PD symptom assessment offers novel clinical insights into the nature and traits of motor impairment. However, the unbiased, objective data offered by wearables not only has the potential to improve clinical care, but also creates the possibility of delivering a more customised therapeutic strategy to a disease that exhibits phenotypic and genotypic variability. The most often performed surgical treatment for Parkinson's is deep brain stimulation (DBS). Thin metal wires that provide electrical pulses to the brain, to assist with the control of some movement symptoms, are implanted by a surgeon. One can imagine sensor data acting as a feed-forward mechanism to fine-tune and modulate the degree of therapeutic gain, especially with closed-loop DBS and new drug delivery pump systems for PD. These real-time measures can also be used to stratify patients into different treatment modalities and build predictive models, allowing for a more effective management of their motor impairment.

## REFERENCES


1. https://www.psychguides.com/ An American Addiction Centres Resource
2. M.E. Berryhill, D. Peterson, K. Jones, R. Tanoue "Cognitive Disorders", in *Encyclopaedia of human behaviour*, 2nd Edition, 2012.
3. L.D. Ravdin, "*Cognitive disorders*", International Encyclopaedia of Public Health, 2008.
4. Mild Cognitive Impairment (MCI) https://www.mayoclinic.org/diseases-conditions/mild-cognitive-impairment/symptoms-causes/syc-20354578
5. F. Elizabeth Godkin, Erin Turner, "Feasibility of a continuous, multi-sensor remote health monitoring approach in persons living with neurodegenerative disease", *Journal of Neurology*, October 2021.
6. Syed Muhammad Usman, Muhammad Usman, Simon Fong "Epileptic Seizures Prediction Using Machine Learning Methods", *Computational and Mathematical Models in Machine, Hindawi Journals*, June 2017.
7. "Types of Seizures", https://www.cdc.gov/epilepsy/about/types-of-seizures.html
8. Benjamin H. Brinkmann, Philippa J. Karoly, Ewan S. Nurse, Sonya B. Dumanis, "Seizure Diaries and Forecasting With Wearables: Epilepsy Monitoring Outside the Clinic", *Frontiers in Neurology*, vol. 12, pp. 1–4, July 2021.
9. R. Wang, G. Blackburn, M. Desai, D. Phelan, L. Gillinov, P. Houghtaling, et al. Accuracy of wrist-worn heart rate monitors accuracy of wrist-worn heart rate monitors letters. *JAMA Cardiology*, vol. 2, no. 1, pp. 1–3, 2017)
10. P. F. Viana, J. Duun-Henriksen, M. Glasstëter, M. Dümpelmann, E. S. Nurse, I. P. Martins, et al. 230 days of ultra-long-term subcutaneous EEG: seizure cycle analysis and comparison to patient diary. *Annals of Clinical and Translational Neurology*, vol. 8, no. 1, pp. 288–293, 2021.
11. Yunyuan Gao, Leilei Ren, Rihui Li, Yingchun Zhang, "Electroencephalogram–Electromyography Coupling Analysis in Stroke Based on Symbolic Transfer Entropy", *Frontiers in Neurology*, vol. 8, pp. 1–10, January 2018.

12. K. Vandecasteele, T. De Cooman, Y. Gu, E. Cleeren, K. Claes, W. V. Paesschen, et al. "Automated epileptic seizure detection based on wearable ECG and PPG in a hospital environment", *Sensors*, vol. 17, pp. 1–12, 2017.
13. Paula M. Vergara, Enrique de la Cal, José R. Villar, Víctor M. González, Javier Sedano "An IoT Platform for Epilepsy Monitoring and Supervising", *Journal of Sensors, Emerging Technologies: IoT, Big Data, and CPS with Sensory Systems*, vol. 2017, 18 pages, July 2017.
14. Shivani Tiwari, Varsha Sharma, Mubarak Mujawar, Yogendra Kumar Mishra, Ajeet Kaushik, Anujit Ghosal "Biosensors for Epilepsy Management: State-of-Art and Future Aspects", *National Library of Medicine*, vol. 19, no. 1825, pp. 1–28, April 2019.
15. Itaf Ben Slimen, Larbi Boubchir, Zouhair Mbarki, Hassene Seddik, "EEG epileptic seizure detection and classification based on dual-tree complex wavelet transform and machine learning algorithms", *Journal of Biomedical Research*, vol. 34, no. 3, pp. 151–161, May 2020.
16. Xiashuang Wang, Guanghong Gong, Ni Li, Shi Qiu, " Detection Analysis of Epileptic EEG Using a Novel Random Forest Model Combined With Grid Search Optimization", *Frontiers in Human Science*, vol. 13, pp. 1–13, February 2021.
17. Z. J. Koles, M. S. Lazar, S. Z. Zhou, "Spatial patterns underlying population differences in the background EEG," *Brain Topography*, vol. 2, no. 4, pp. 275–284, 1990.
18. Z. J. Koles, J. C. Lind, P. Flor-Henry, "Spatial patterns in the background EEG underlying mental disease in man," *Electroencephalography and Clinical Neurophysiology*, vol. 91, no. 5, pp. 319–328, 1994.
19. Khaled Arbateni, Abdelhak Bennia, "Sigmoidal radial basis function ANN for QRS complex detection", *Journal of Neurocomputing*, vol. 145, pp. 438–450, May 2014.
20. Turky N. Alotaiby, Saleh A. Alshebeili, Latifah M. Aljafar, Waleed M. Alsabhan "ECG-Based Subject Identification Using Common Spatial Pattern and SVM", *Hindawi Journals*, vol. 2019, 9 pages, March 2019.
21. Isa Conradsen, Peter Wolf, Thomas Sams, Helge B. D. Sorensen, Sándor Beniczky, "Patterns of muscle activation during generalized tonic and tonic-clonic epileptic seizures", National Library of Medicine, National Centre for Biotechnology Information, November 2011.
22. Sándor Beniczky, Isa Conradsen, Mihai Moldovan, Poul Jennum, Martin Fabricius, Krisztina Benedek, Noémi Andersen, Helle Hjalgrim, Peter Wolf, "Quantitative analysis of surface electromyography during epileptic and nonepileptic convulsive seizures", National Library of Medicine, National Centre for Biotechnology Information, July 2014.
23. Sándor Beniczky, Isa Conradsen, Oliver Henning, Martin Fabricius, Peter Wolf, "Automated real-time detection of tonic-clonic seizures using a wearable EMG device", *American Academy of Neurology*, vol. 90, no. 5, pp. 428–434, January 2018.
24. Sándor Beniczky, Isa Conradsen, Peter Wolf, "Detection of convulsive seizures using surface electromyography", https://onlinelibrary.wiley.com/doi/full/10.1111/epi.14048, June 2018.
25. Jianbin Tang, Rima El Atrache, Shuang Yu, Umar Asif, "Seizure detection using wearable sensors and machine learning: Setting a benchmark", National Library of Medicine, National Centre for Biotechnology Information, July 2021.
26. Yunyuan Gao, Leilei Ren, Rihui Li, Yingchun Zhang, "Electroencephalogram–Electromyography Coupling Analysis in Stroke Based on Symbolic Transfer Entropy", National Library of Medicine, National Centre for Biotechnology Information, January 2018.
27. "Telemedicine & Epilepsy", https://practicalneurology.com/articles/2019-oct/telemedicine-epilepsy, Practical Neurology, October 2019.
28. Erika Rovini, Carlo Maremmani, Filippo Cavallo, "How Wearable Sensors Can Support Parkinson's Disease Diagnosis and Treatment: A Systematic Review", *Frontiers in Neuroscience*, vol. 11, pp. 1–41, October 2017.
29. Ritesh A. Ramdhani, Anahita Khojandi, Oleg Shylo, Brian Kope, "Optimizing Clinical Assessments in Parkinson's Disease Through the Use of Wearable Sensors and Data Driven Modelling", September 2018.
30. Haiqun Xie, Yukai Wang, Shuai Tao, "Wearable Sensor-Based Daily Life Walking Assessment of Gait for Distinguishing Individuals With Amnestic Mild Cognitive Impairment", *Frontiers in Aging Neuroscience* 22 October 2019.
31. Lu Ruirui, Xu Yan, Xiaohui Li, Yongli Fan, Weiqi Zeng, Yang Tan, Kang Ren, Wenwu Chen, Xuebing Cao, "Evaluation of Wearable Sensor Devices in Parkinson's Disease: A Review of Current Status and Future Prospects", September 2020.
32. "Essential Tremor and Parkinson's Disease: How They Differ", Abbott, November 2018.

33. F. Elizabeth Godkin, Erin Turner, "Feasibility of a continuous, multi-sensor remote health monitoring approach in persons living with neurodegenerative disease", *Journal of Neurology*, Springer, October 2021.
34. Luca Lonini, Andrew Dai, Nicholas Shawen, Tanya Simuni, Cynthia Poon, Leo Shimanovich, Margaret Daeschler, Roozbeh Ghaffari, John A. Rogers, Arun Jayaraman, "Wearable sensors for Parkinson's disease: which data are worth collecting for training symptom detection models", *NPJ Digital Medicine*, November 2018.

# 7 Artificial Intelligence-based Biosensors

*Mohamed Jebran P.*
Jain University, Bengaluru, India

*Shweta Gupta*
Woxsen University, Telangana, India

## 7.1 INTRODUCTION

Biosensors are integrated receptor-transducer devices that use a biological recognition element to provide selected quantitative or semi-quantitative analytical information. Biosensors may be broken down into a few distinct categories depending on the sort of transducer units they use, including bio-electrode sensors, semiconductor biosensors, thermal biosensors, photo biosensors, and piezoelectric crystal biosensors. Biosensors are classified according to the identifying molecules they use: enzyme, nucleic acid, microbial, cellular, tissue, and immunological sensors. Biosensors may be broken down into the subcategories of bio-affinity biosensors, metabotropic biosensors, and catalytic biosensors according to the nature of the recognition elements they use (Jin et al. 2020; Garzón et al. 2019).

For monitoring purposes, a biosensor can be used on either biological or non-biological matrices. Their applications in basic bio-research, food safety, environmental monitoring, illness diagnosis, and medication screening are broad (Qian et al. 2019; Cui et al. 2020b). Big data has vast unrealised potential that might be used in a wide variety of contexts. While it has the potential to greatly aid the research and development of new insights, harnessing its power is no easy feat. Some examples of these difficulties include an increase in background noise, false correlation, inaccurate measurements, and the need for a lot of computing power. The ability to generate data, analyse it, and derive useful insights may depend on solving any of the aforementioned issues (Cottle et al. 2013; Rein and Memmert 2016).

Biosensors have evolved due to the sophisticated processing of data collected by sensors. The integration of AI and biosensors has resulted in a novel, interdisciplinary field known as "AI biosensors". The three primary components of AI biosensors' core architecture are data collecting, signal conversion, and AI-data processing. The term "information collection" is used to describe a set of biosensors used for the real-time tracking of data of many types, including but not limited to physical, chemical, biological, environmental, and personal characteristics. Information gathered in one domain is converted into an electrical output signal with a predetermined sensitivity by the signal conversion system. An AI-data-processing stack consists of the interface, data categorisation, the data model and analysis, and the decision layer. The emphasis is on using machine learning (ML) for sensing data processing. Through the use of ML, conventional biosensors have the potential to evolve into intelligent ones, capable of autonomously predicting the species or concentration of the analyte based on a decision-making algorithm. Large amounts of sensing data, especially those involving complicated matrices or samples, may be processed efficiently with the help of ML. Moreover, it may "fix" sensor performance fluctuations brought on by biofouling and interferences in actual samples. The easy and accurate interpretation of sensing data is possible with the help of ML algorithms for uncovering latent objects and patterns (Cui et al. 2020a).

There are three main parts to a biosensor: the bioreceptor, the transducer, and the signal processor. A bioreceptor is fixed on a sensor screen to pick up the analyte of interest in bodily fluids like blood


DOI: 10.1201/9781003245346-7

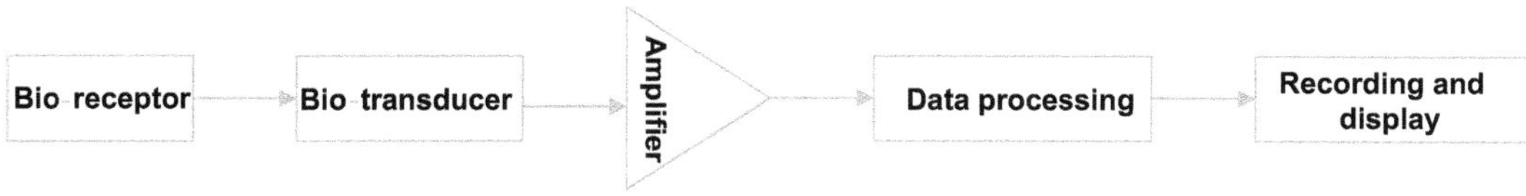


**FIGURE 7.1** The theory behind biosensors.

and plasma serum. The transducer is the physicochemical element that mediates the transformation of a biological reaction into a signal that a signal processor can record, analyse, and present. Figure 7.1 shows the theory behind biosensors. Since they find widespread use in many fields of study and industry, researchers have turned to novel, high-throughput methods, including electrochemistry, nanotechnology, bioelectronics, and hybrids thereof in an effort to improve their sensitivity, specificity, safety, and cost-effectiveness. This has led to the creation of novel biosensors that are superior to previous generations in terms of linear range, detection limit, analysis time, mobility, and cost.

## 7.2 CHARACTERISTICS OF THE IDEAL SMART BIOSENSOR

One of the requirements for a good biosensor is the assurance that it can provide a reliable response that is unique to the analyte of interest. Reaction frequency must be high, and recovery time must be minimal. These biosensors can make decisions in real time because of how they are constructed and the vast amounts of data they provide for therapies.

The focus of this chapter is on cutting-edge ML and its recent applications to biosensors, providing topical conversation and unique insights on the topic. The most recent developments in biosensing, wearable biosensing, and AI biosensing are covered in this chapter as they form the backbone of tomorrow's implantable and wearable technologies (Stefano and Fernandez 2017).

## 7.3 ML-ENABLED BIOSENSORS OF VARIOUS KINDS

### 7.3.1 Electrochemical (EC) Biosensors

It is difficult to get reliable results from EC biosensors in practical applications. The interfering substances in real samples may span a broad range of ionic strength, temperature, pH, and other conditions. The sensitive signals that are strongly linked with the analyte type and amount cannot be acquired using a one-dimensional data analysis approach. This reveals a new window of opportunity to investigate how ML might enhance the precision and dependability of EC biosensor measurements (Ni and Kokot 2008). Massah and Vakilian (2019) sought to enhance the functionality of a cyclic voltammetry-based EC biosensor using a support vector machine (SVM) regression model. Over 400 samples' worth of nitrate concentrations were predicted using a mixture of linear, polynomial, and Gaussian kernels, each with its own set of parameters (Massah and Vakilian 2019). This was accomplished without having to replace the enzyme.

Among EC biosensors, electrochemical impedance spectroscopy (EIS) is widely used. In order to reliably extract important parameters from EIS data using $\chi^2$ testing, the comparable circuit models are always utilised. In this particular instance, Rong et al. (2018) created an SVM model in order to conduct an analysis of the EIS data without making use of equivalent circuit fitting (Rong et al. 2018). The SVM that used a radial base function kernel was shown to have the best performance when it came to correctly categorising the training dataset, with an accuracy of 98%. There has not been any report of an EC biosensor that has been assisted by deep learning as of yet. The low number of datasets that are now accessible is one probable explanation for the problem. Opportunities for the implementation of deep learning will arise as a result of the development of arrays or multiplexed EC biosensors for the purpose of testing a large number of actual samples (e.g., clinical specimens). It is possible to increase the accuracy and precision of single-molecule (SM) identification by combining ML with SM electrical biosensors (Taniguchi 2020). For the purpose of determining the identity of the analyte, a maximum current, denoted by Ip, and a current duration, denoted by td, are extracted from either the tunnelling current-time waveform or the ion current-time waveform. The detection and identification of several analytes cannot be accomplished through the overlapping of current signals. This difficulty may be conquered, however, by employing ML techniques, such as SVM, random forest (RF), and convoluted neural network (CNN), to conduct an analysis of the wave shape at the present time (Albrecht et al. 2017). Analytes that are quite comparable in terms of their molecular volumes and border orbital energies exhibit Ip and td signals that are very similar to one another.

### 7.3.2 Non-invasive Biosensors

A tiny biosensor that may be worn or carried by the user is often the component that makes up a non-invasive biosensor. These sensors focus mostly on acquiring bodily fluids that may be done so in a non-invasive manner, such as perspiration, tears, saliva, and exhaled breath. Non-invasive technologies hold a great deal of potential for providing continuous health monitoring as well as quick access to information on food quality.

### 7.3.3 Wearable Biosensors

These are divisible into three categories: on-body, garment and textile-based, and in-body and accessory-based (Steinberg et al. 2016). Their ability to monitor health without interfering with daily activities is made possible by the fact that they are both non-invasive and wearable. It is commonly believed that numerous physiological signals may be monitored in real time by means of wearable electronics, such as electronic tattoos and epidermal electronic systems. Wearable electronics have several uses in fundamental biomedical research as well as clinical care. Some of these applications include human–machine interfaces, artificial skins, diagnostics, and health monitoring.

Subjective states of "tiredness" and "lack of energy" are hallmarks of mental fatigue, which can impair one's performance in a number of contexts, such as while operating a motor vehicle or conducting surgery. Thus, a non-intrusive approach for assessing mental exhaustion is urgently required. Mental tiredness levels must be monitored in a manner that is pleasant, efficient, and unobtrusive. Zeng et al. (2020) created a multimodal epidermal electronic system capable of concurrently detecting electrocardiogram (ECG), respiration rate, and galvanic skin reaction (GSR) signals as well as a fatigue-recognition procedure using ML methods. Module 1 of the epidermal electronic system (EES) has three flexible surface electrodes and a strain sensor for measuring ECG and respiration rate, while module 2 includes two flexible surface electrodes for detecting GSR on one palm. The EES instrument is used to provide reliable measurements of human physiological signals. A mental fatigue classification system based on an ML algorithm extracts features from the signals and processes them to provide precise predictions about the subject's levels of exhaustion. Supervised machine learning (SML) is an ML activity that infers a function from labelled training data and has seen extensive usage in the categorisation of tiredness levels. Figure 7.2 shows a high-level block diagram of our SML-based system for detecting tiredness. Acquiring data on tiredness, extracting relevant features from that data, and then recognising exhaustion are the three components of this method. In the fatigue data collecting phase, healthy volunteers are required to wear our epidermal electrical devices and execute a mental task. Mental exhaustion is classified into three levels: none, fatigue, and severe weariness. Cardiogram (CG), GSR, and respiration signals are used to extract six types of characteristics, including heart rate, standard deviation of the normal-to-normal (R-R) peak interval (SDNN), GSR peak number sum, GSR peak magnitude sum, GSR peak duration sum, and breathing rate. Three distinct ML algorithms – including the SVM (and the SVM linear kernel and the SVM radial basis function kernel), K-nearest neighbour (KNN), and decision tree (DT) – are

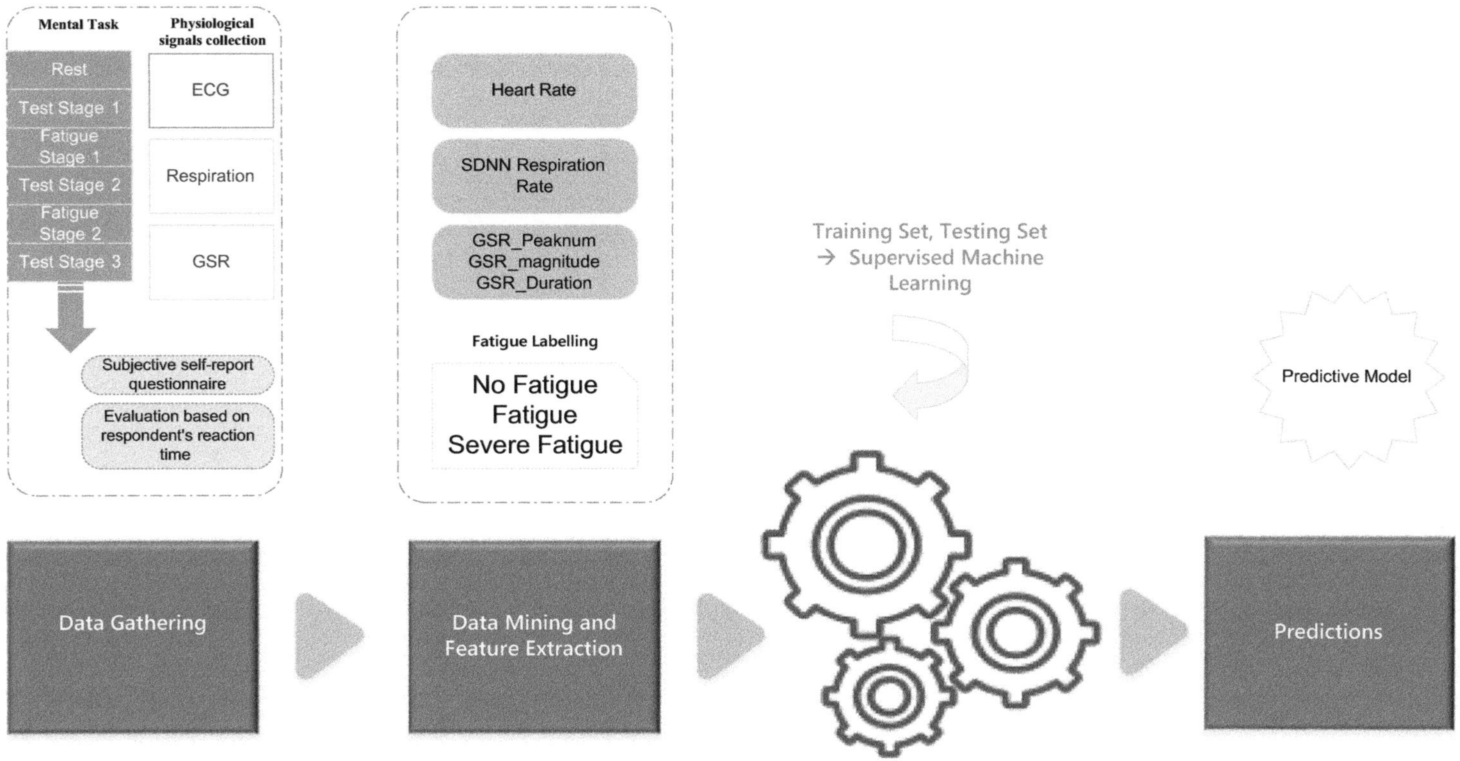


**FIGURE 7.2** Methods and outcomes of a supervised machine-learning-based system for detecting cognitive exhaustion.

utilised for model training and the construction of different predictive models that automatically detect fatigue states based on physiological features. In this research, DT algorithms had the highest level of predicted accuracy at 89%.

Electroencephalography (EEG) data may be used to obtain insight into a person's mental state, and Zeng et al. (2018) suggest that deep CNNs and deep residual learning might be used to do this. In this study, two unique classifiers called EEG-Conv and EEG-Conv-R were constructed. EEG-Conv is based on the conventional CNN, whereas EEG-Conv-R combines CNN with recent deep residual learning. Both of these classifiers were used to analyse EEG data.

The integration of wearable electronics with ML for the continuous monitoring of temperature, blood oxygenation, and respiratory biomarkers (cough frequency and intensity, and respiratory rate) of COVID-19 patients is an important example of another application of intelligent sensors for the purpose of addressing the current public health challenge. John A. Rogers's team at Northwestern University is developing a wearable sensor with a high-bandwidth accelerometer and temperature sensor to detect early indications and symptoms linked with COVID-19 patients, including temperature, coughing intensity and patterns, and heart rate (Jeong et al. 2020). These continuous and real-time biophysical assessments give significant insights into the physiological condition of COVID-19 patients. Importantly, integrating this physiological data with cutting-edge ML approaches will establish a valuable platform for detecting COVID-19 infections, predicting illness severity and life-threatening results, and providing guidelines for reopening the economy.

### 7.3.4 AI-assisted Wearable Biosensors

Figure 7.3 shows the functional parts of the AI-assisted wearable biosensing system. Biosensors perform the function of data collection units by gathering biochemical or biophysical data from body fluids and converting that data into signals that may be understood by devices that collect and analyse data. Wearable biosensors have the ability to directly collect biofluids from the surface of the body in order to analyse levels of health-related biomarkers. A bioreceptor, which may be an antibody, nucleic acid, or glucose oxidase, and a transducer, which may be an optical, electrochemical, or mechanical signal converter, are the two fundamental elements that make up a conventional biosensor. Using various biofluids as their basis, biosensors might be connected with a variety of wearable platforms, such as wristbands, contact lenses, or electronic skin. After that, personal smart readout devices or other processing terminals receive the information that was gathered by biosensors and send it through wireless connection devices. Bluetooth, near-field communication (NFC), and the fifth-generation mobile network are examples of communication technologies that might be used in wearable biosensors. The unprocessed raw sensory data is finally processed and stored in local devices or cloud servers. These are the locations where ML techniques may be employed to aid in the diagnostic process (Kim et al. 2016; Yetisen et al. 2018; Lin et al. 2022).

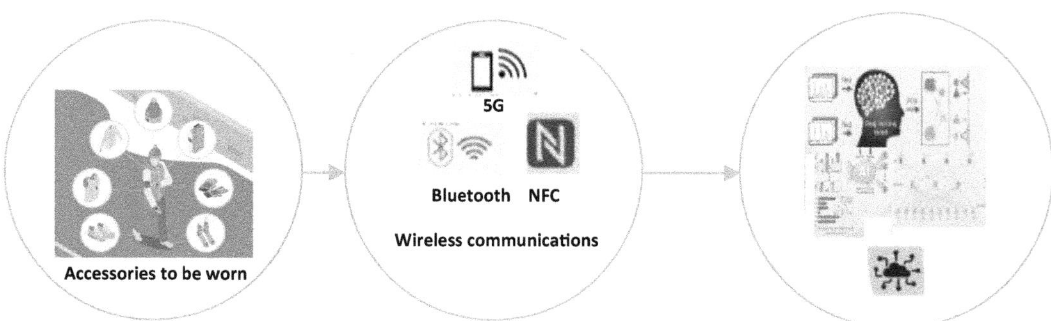


**FIGURE 7.3** Functional components of AI-assisted wearable biosensing system.

Raw sensing data can be found in a variety of forms, such as digital datasets for electrochemical biosensors and image datasets for optical sensors, depending on the type of sensor that was used to collect the information. It is possible to construct an ML model based on datasets in order to process the data more effectively. In addition, the raw sensor data frequently require various pre-processing procedures in order to improve the performance of ML models and guarantee that timely warnings are supplied following the discovery of irregularities. Preprocessing of data may have a significant impact on the accuracy of AI models as well as the amount of time they take to compute.

### 7.3.5 Surface Enhanced Raman Spectroscopy (SERS) and Spectra-based Biosensors

The SERS technique can obtain information on the inherent fingerprint of an analyte even when it is present in a complex matrix. It is extremely desirable to do single-cell and single-molecular research using SERS biosensors in conjunction with ML approaches. During inspections and quarantines, as well as during forensic investigations and wildlife protection, it is a common practice to use blood samples to identify different species. Traditional procedures include deoxidation and reduction, which include utilising reactants such as leucomalachite green, luminol, phenolphthalein, and tetramethylbenzidine (McLaughlin et al. 2014). It is becoming common knowledge that Raman spectroscopy is a method that is both practical and non-destructive, and that it can be used to qualitatively and quantitatively characterise the chemical and physical characteristics of materials (Guevara et al. 2018). Because of the intrinsic weakness of the Raman signal, background and noise can cause spectra to become distorted.

The traditional approaches often presuppose the existence of an explicit parametric model in order to account for unknown characteristics like noise and baseline. In addition, the preprocessing approaches are not dependent on the subsequent regression or classification models, therefore there is a possibility that they will not improve the models. The popularity of deep learning (Lecun et al. 2015), a method for extracting characteristics of data using numerous processing layers, has recently attracted much attention. Researchers have used CNNs for spectral analysis due to their reputation as one of the most successful deep learning models (Krizhevsky et al. 2017). CNNs have a number of advantages over other spectral analysis methods, including a low requirement for expert knowledge, the absence of a need to design explicit features, and a potent capacity to capture inner structures. To differentiate human blood from that of other animals using Raman spectra, Dong et al. (2019) created a useful CNN model they called RamanCNN. RamanCNN combines preprocessing and discrimination into a single unit that can be taught to learn its parameters adaptively from calibration data. The accuracy of the RamanCNN model was checked by its application to the classification of blood samples, and its results were compared to those of more conventional models like PLS-DA and SVM. Compared to PLS-DA and SVM, RamanCNN fared better in the experiments evaluating classification accuracy.

Damaged oligonucleotides (ONDs) on a gold gratings substrate may be detected with the help of a SERS biosensor that was built with the help of a CNN (Guselnikova et al. 2019). The SERS spectra of ONDs were gathered using a portable spectrometer by a variety of operators without prioritising the experimental conditions (such as optimal location on substrate, laser intensity, acquisition time, and manual baseline correction). Even the smallest amounts of DNA damage may be identified by SERS-CNN spectra with the help of a CNN, something that is nearly impossible with conventional methods. Findings demonstrated a confidence level of greater than 95% in OND damage categorisation, with an accuracy of up to 98%. The same team subsequently refined their SERS and CNN technique for differentiating between healthy and malignant cells in a cell culture medium (Erzina et al. 2020).

It would be ideal to use SERS biosensors in tandem with ML techniques for single-cell analysis. In order to quantify Rhodamine 800 concentrations, Thrift and Ragan (2019) introduced a CNN-based SERS. The use of ML in conjunction with a large Raman set of microbes has the potential to deliver more accurate findings. Additionally, the CNN model has the capability of converting a spectral signal into a concentration based on the deviations of the Langmuir isotherm.

### 7.3.6 Biosensors for Cardiac Health Care

Both cardiovascular diseases (also known as CVDs) and stroke are among the leading causes of mortality across the world. In order to have a good prognosis for CVD and stroke, an early and prompt diagnosis is essential. Myoglobin, B-type natriuretic peptide (BNP), cardiac troponin I (cTnI), interleukins, and interferons are some of the many biomarkers that have been found that are particular to the heart. However, although major breakthroughs in the generations of biosensors have been accomplished, these sensors still have some important limitations (Selestina et al. 2018). Recent developments in AI have opened up new domains and tools for the development of innovative modelling and forecasting approaches for clinical applications, such as the treatment of heart disorders. Chang et al. (2017) built a biosensor for the XPRIZE DeepQ Tricorder that is capable of properly diagnosing 12 different prevalent ailments.

The mining of medical data relies heavily on the use of ML techniques. ML has been able to establish its relevance in chemical and biosensing applications for clinical and pathological procedures as a result of an increase in the amount of data that has been collected as well as an expected decrease in the price of computers (Ching et al. 2018). The Long-Term ST Database, which preserves the ECG recordings of patients and may classify diseases based on those recordings, is one of the databases that is often utilised (Rani 2011).

When doing an analysis for therapeutics, preprocessing the data necessitates the elimination of noise as well as any outliers that may become problematic. Utilising a low-pass filter in conjunction with a high-pass filter that has a cutoff frequency is a viable option for noise reduction. A notch filter with a frequency of 50 Hz and an interference filter for power sources are two examples of band-rejection techniques (Dolatabadi and Khadem 2017). In addition, a notch filter and the Pan–Tompkins technique are utilised in order to get rid of the cutoff frequency of 50 Hz and find R-peaks. A dynamic temporal warping approach for segmentation is another two-way procedure that is used to examine the existence of noise in the signal (Pan and Tompkins 1985). This technique is followed by the Hampel filter, which removes the noise from the signal.

In addition, feature extraction is the method of identifying key features in datasets by means of a number of independent variables. In supervised learning, the data is labelled and the algorithm is taught to make predictions based on the labelled data. KNN, linear discriminant analysis, SVMs, RF, neural networks (NNs), and deep learning are just a few examples of the many supervised learning methods now in use. KNN is one of the most widely used classifiers for coronary artery disease (CAD) since it makes no assumptions about the data distribution. Singh et al. (2018) used KNN to produce accurate and automatic categorisation of CAD. For the purpose of recognising cardiac irregularities from ECG data, the KNN classifier functions more effectively than the SVM classifier. NN is another powerful classifier that is utilised extensively because of the simplicity with which it can be implemented. In order to make its predictions, this method takes into account 15 medical characteristics, including an individual's age, gender, blood pressure, cholesterol levels, and level of obesity. The DT is yet another non-parametric classifier that is utilised for the supervised learning approach (Mastoi et al. 2018) and for classifying data, doing regression analysis, and making predictions depending on the value of a target variable. Another type of classifier that is widely utilised for the processing of large amounts of data is called RF.

Clustering and association rule mining are the two unsupervised learning techniques that are used the most frequently. In unsupervised learning, the dataset is left unlabelled, and the algorithm learns to make a prediction about the structure or pattern based on the input data, while in the case of reinforced learning, the machine is able to autonomously learn what level of performance is optimal for a given situation. There is a rising trend toward using visual representations of patient-specific clinical data and biosensor outputs to aid clinicians in evaluating important clinical parameters (Guidi et al. 2014). In addition, when integrated with ML algorithms for categorisation and prediction, the ability of a medical practitioner to expand his or her diagnostic reach to a remote region of care becomes even more efficient and effective.

## 7.4 ML ALGORITHMS FOR BIOSENSING DATA ANALYSIS

To better assess users' health, ML systems can learn from the accumulated biosensing data. Wearable multiplexed sensors produce high-dimensional biosensing data, which may be processed and analysed using ML to reveal previously unseen patterns and relationships. Users may make better sense of the biosensing data they acquire with the aid of the system's robust pattern detection capability. In recent years, biosensors have employed both non-neural and neural algorithms to interpret biological data, allowing for the classification of users as healthy or unwell and the quantification of biomarker levels.

SVMs are supervised learning algorithms that might be used for classifying, regressing, and identifying abnormalities in the raw sensing data. The effectiveness of the SVM is solely determined by the kernel function selection, which can be linear, polynomial, sigmoid, or radial basis. As a result, SVM is capable of preserving its performance even when applied to a problem with a large dimension, which makes it appropriate for the processing of data derived from multiplexed sensing. The SVM has been utilised in a variety of biosensors, including glucose oxidase sensing (Gonzalez-Navarro et al. 2016) and nitrate sensing (Massah and Vakilian 2019).

Recent research usually assesses the performance of many ML algorithms to determine the best one to use for biosensing data, as there are currently no established guidelines for making this choice. Based on the wavelet transform-support vector machine (WT-SVM) algorithm, Wang et al. (2021) created an eye-movement controlled wheelchair system. In comparison to the standard approach, the 96.3% accuracy in recognising eye movement is rather impressive. Carbon dot-based fluorescent array sensing was utilised to recognise patterns using ML techniques. Analysing these patterns using linear discriminant analysis (LDA) allowed researchers to distinguish between eight proteins with a precision of 98%. The ECG signal, skin conductivity, and respiration rate were integrated into an AI-assisted monitoring system for mental tiredness level. AI algorithms were included in the system to extrapolate elements from raw sensor data that might be utilised to forecast user tiredness. The eight proteins may be categorised with a 100% degree of certainty using either the SVM or the KNN technique.

The architecture of human neurons serves as an inspiration for artificial neural networks (ANNs). The most significant benefit of utilising ANNs is that they are able to learn from the dataset that they are being trained on without requiring any user-defined parameters (Benardos and Vosniakos 2007). Exhaled breath was analysed using an e-nose for a feedforward neural network (FNN), which was then utilised to identify lung cancer (Goor et al. 2018). The recurrent neural network (RNN) was utilised in the process of developing a health monitoring system for diabetic patients (Alfian et al. 2018). The use of AI in the realm of medicine has the potential to dramatically cut the cost of therapy while also greatly improving diagnostic precision.

## 7.5 POINT OF CARE DIAGNOSIS USING BIOSENSORS

A procedure that is carried out in close proximity to the patient and that is characterised by its rapidity, low cost, and high level of efficiency is referred to as the point of care (POC). In situations when laboratory facilities are limited or non-existent, POC diagnostics are designed to facilitate the fast initiation of treatment or diagnosis. The integration of biosensors with wireless capabilities such as Bluetooth, Wi-Fi, and GPS has made it easier for professional medical experts to communicate with patients who are cared for in their homes. Applications that are based on POC testing can be further broken down into the categories of lab-on-a-chip, labelled, label-free, nanomaterial-based wearable, and wireless (Quesada-González and Merkoçi 2018). The wearables include electrochemical, calorimetric, and optical detection methods, respectively. It is possible to sense a limited number of micro-fluids as biosamples on the skin's epidermis using conductive ink on a screen-printed electrode on textiles or intelligent tattoos and patches (Mostafalu et al. 2017).

Real-time detection of infections aids in administering timely medical care and, more critically, allows for the management of epidemics (Sin et al. 2014). Biosensors, which are now often found in analytical instruments, use a biological molecule to translate recognition events into a usable output. Although antibodies are the original and most used affinity reagents in biosensors today, they are too time-consuming and expensive to be utilised in a pandemic. POC biosensors' ability to specifically and accurately detect target molecules is reliant on affinity reagents (Nayak et al. 2017). The need for a POC platform has spurred fast development in biosensor technology (Kaushik and Mujawar 2018).

The majority of tests performed by point-of-care test (POCT) systems rely on unmodified or minimally modified actual samples (such as blood, serum, urine, or saliva). POC diagnostic technologies are focused on making the equipment simple enough to operate that even untrained personnel can do so, as well as making the instrument portable. The whole POC system was revolutionised as a result of the widespread adoption of adaptable and wearable technology such as cellphones, drones, and Bluetooth. Because of these characteristics, POC diagnostics are ideally suited for use as a quick diagnostic instrument in the management of infectious diseases. In the event that patients are unable to obtain commercial diagnostic tests because they are unaffordable or are in short supply, POC tests are a viable alternative that can be used effectively in their place. These features make it easier for patients to monitor and diagnose their own infectious diseases in the early stages of a viral infection. Figure 7.4 shows a schematic diagram of POC instruments.

Recently, there has been a change in emphasis from intuition-based to data-based decision making (McRae et al. 2016), thanks to POC systems that incorporate ML techniques, that is, AI. The use of AI gives doctors more flexibility in tailoring patient care and keeping tabs on results. Using these AI systems, medical professionals are able to evaluate patients' risks for a variety of diseases and injuries, including heart attacks, cancer, and trauma. The AI sensors begin by carrying out the multi-step test with the help of a portable analyser, which then goes on to automatically digitise the biomarker concentrations. It is possible to make judgements on therapy based on the spectrum of illnesses that may be anticipated with the assistance of gathered data using a variety of algorithms, such as classification, cluster, pattern, and aspects of diseases. M-Health is a WHO global observatory that supports a variety of wireless devices, including mobile phones and personal digital

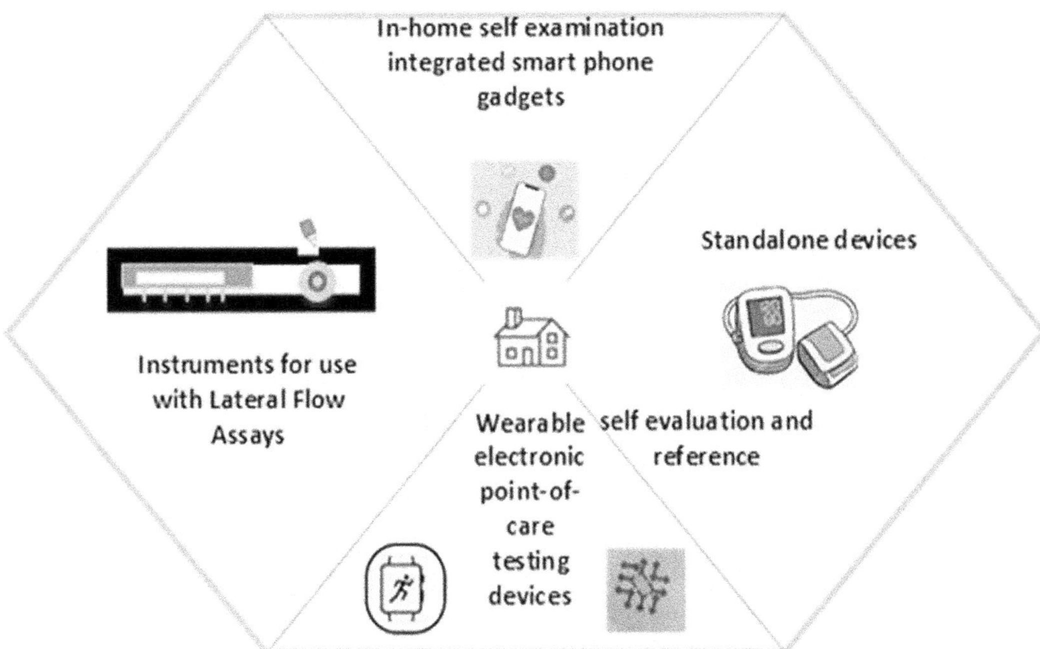


**FIGURE 7.4** POC instruments for resource-limited patient self-testing.

**Source: Shrivastava et al. 2020.**

assistants (Wang et al. 2017). M-Health is used to present findings to patients and is supported by these devices. As a result, patients receive individualised care that focuses on the active management and prevention of disease risks thanks to health analytics. Both real-time POC diagnostics and ML have had a transformative effect on the healthcare industry.

## 7.6 FUTURE OF AI-BASED BIOSENSORS

We believe that there is room for revolutionary change in the way human samples are collected. As such, implantable biosensors may play a pivotal role in hastening the development of individualised therapeutics. Saliva, exhaled condensate breath, blood, and interstitial fluid are just a few of the materials it can track with a minimally intrusive setup. This industry is becoming more self-assured, sensitive, and individualised as a result of the development of biosensors, as well as the Internet of Things, AI, and 5G wireless networks. In the future, intelligent gadgets will be able to track a wide range of health indicators all at once, and then report this information to a mobile app. Rapid expansion, including patient contentment, in the healthcare sector is anticipated as a result of this technology's development.

The mechanical understanding of biological structures at the molecular level is made possible with the use of biosensors. The applications of these types of analytic tools are virtually limitless, spanning fields as diverse as pharmaceuticals, agriculture, environmental technologies, and the study of biological processes. They are crucial in many biotech procedures, including the search for new therapeutics, the identification of pathogens, the development of vaccines, and the delivery of gene therapy.

The frequency of doctors' visits may be cut down or eliminated entirely if people could use portable biosensors to monitor their health in real time. Important steps have been taken toward the creation of bimolecular sensors for real-time monitoring of the target biomolecules. The distribution of healthcare is destined to change as a result of biosensors and care-point systems.

AI growth has spawned new domains and tools in bioscience, allowing for the development of novel modelling and predictive approaches for clinical usage, with applications ranging from cardiology to other fields.

Multiplex biosensor arrays with the capability to detect numerous biomarkers simultaneously on the same chip need to be created, along with the inclusion of microfluidics, biomarker pattern software, and AI programs in the near future. However, the most cutting-edge research must be conducted in order to further develop IoT and ML biosensing systems. Once these systems have been effectively automated, diagnostic accuracy may be improved to its highest possible level. Therefore, coupled advancements in the cutting-edge IoT technology of biosensors have the potential to revolutionise cancer care and therapy while also reducing the worldwide death rate.

The data collected by wearable biosensors is transmitted wirelessly, analysed, and stored, and an interactive user interface is also provided. Biosensors are data gathering devices that analyse body fluids for biochemical or biophysical markers. Biofluids may be collected straight from the skin's surface and used as a diagnostic tool. In order to aid in diagnosis, ML algorithms are used on the raw sensory data after it has been processed and stored in local devices or cloud servers. With the use of cutting-edge data modification techniques or completely made-up data sources, synthetic data may be used to produce different training samples that closely resemble the actual world in terms of their attributes and connections. Maintaining the representativeness of synthetic data and tying it to clinical/scientific findings are major obstacles to implementing it in medical applications. There is much room for growth in the field of AI-powered wearable biosensors, which might benefit greatly from the introduction of synthetic data-based systems.

As a branch of applied mathematics, chemometrics offers powerful mathematical tools for making sense of sensing data. Using ML approaches can enhance not only the qualitative identification of complicated overlapping signals but also the quantitative prediction of trace analytes. The use of deep learning techniques, such as CNN and RNN, is becoming increasingly common in the processing of sensing data. The development and implementation of multiplex or high-throughput biosensors can assist researchers in overcoming the data bottleneck that they are experiencing. The analysis of data obtained from the detection of a single molecule, a single particle, or a single cell presents a number of difficulties. These difficulties are mostly caused by a low signal-to-noise ratio, signal overlap, and dispersive signals.

Exploring and selecting data in the conventional way based on hypotheses may not be a good idea since it may lead unexpected signals to be overlooked. In order to enhance the accuracy of objective recognition and the precision of pattern recognition, it is necessary to develop ML approaches to filter out background noise and extract features from multi-dimensional signals.

Wearable medical biosensors that use AI will first require human intervention. An AI and human collaboration is known as an AI–human team. Mia, an AI platform for breast screening developed by Kheiron Medical Technologies, is an example of the integration of human and artificial intelligence (Kheiron Medical 2021). The AI's prognostic results must be interpretable if they are to be useful to clinicians and patients.

Wearable biosensors aided by AI are beginning to incorporate energy harvesting techniques and wireless connectivity. Through their various uses, sensors provide an opportunity to create a more individualised healthcare and telemedicine system. Ongoing health and fitness monitoring may be accomplished with the use of biosensors when integrated with smartphone-based sensing devices.

In order to function as a POCT, biosensors for infectious illnesses are hindered by the necessity for sample collection and processing. Another challenge to POC testing is the necessity to refrigerate reagents in long-shelf-life forms. As a result, scientists have begun to employ microfluidic platforms, which contain all the necessary operational steps but in an expensive and cumbersome configuration. Depending on the operating circumstances, the biosensor's performance may degrade within a few months due to the biomolecules' low stability. It is crucial to note that identified end-users do not trust POC devices due to overestimation and mistakes in results. This is mostly due to the fact that testing is conducted inside laboratories rather than in actual healthcare settings, creating a disparity between expectations and results. Quality assurance programmes must be put into place in POCT to provide reliable outcomes. These bioanalytical technologies are projected to see significant development in future years. In the long run, this will change the face of clinical diagnostics, making it possible to reduce the severity of health problems in underdeveloped nations. Integration of big data analysis is required for computer-aided diagnostic systems or the internet-of-medical-things (IoMT), where various techniques such as visualisation tools, ML, and data mining must be investigated. Market development and obstacle elimination for an AI and IoMT-supported POCT assay is substantially more difficult.

## 7.7 CONCLUSION

It is necessary to identify and diagnose a variety of human diseases at their earliest stages so that patients can be effectively treated. Therefore, it is crucial to provide accessible, highly sensitive, and economically viable diagnostic instruments like biosensors for efficient disease detection. Clinical care, preventative therapy, patient health data, and disease evaluations are just some of the ways in which biosensors have already proven useful to clinicians and their patients. To achieve the objective of providing the most effective treatment for each individual patient, advancements in AI and the use of wearable sensors are indispensable. When these two areas are combined, better wearable sensors for monitoring health, fitness, and the environment may be designed, and more accurate patient data can be collected. AI biosensors that have the right technological qualities are currently confronting new possibilities and problems. This is because the IoT, big data, and big health are all moving from the conceptual stage to the implementation stage. Patients are expected to place a higher demand on POC devices for self-diagnostics. The newly developed POC tests based on biosensors allow for a diagnosis of emergent infectious diseases in a matter of seconds, which is exactly what is required at this time. In this age of pandemics, POCT devices will make a substantial contribution to economies as a result of their accurate and affordable diagnosis.

## REFERENCES

Albrecht, Tim, Gregory Slabaugh, Eduardo Alonso, and S. M. Masudur R. Al-Arif. "Deep Learning for Single-Molecule Science." *Nanotechnology* 28, no. 42 (2017): 423001. doi:10.1088/1361-6528/aa8334.

Alfian, Ganjar, Muhammad Syafrudin, Muhammad Ijaz, M. Syaekhoni, Norma Fitriyani, and Jongtae Rhee. "A Personalized Healthcare Monitoring System for Diabetic Patients by Utilizing BLE-Based Sensors and Real-Time Data Processing." *Sensors (Basel, Switzerland)* 18, no. 7 (2018): 2183. doi:10.3390/s18072183.

Benardos, P. G., and G.-C. Vosniakos. "Optimizing Feedforward Artificial Neural Network Architecture." *Engineering Applications of Artificial Intelligence* 20, no. 3 (2007): 365–82. doi:10.1016/j.engappai.2006.06.005.

Chang, Edward Y., Meng-Hsi Wu, Kai-Fu Tang Tang, Hao-Cheng Kao, and Chun-Nan Chou. "Artificial Intelligence in XPRIZE DeepQ Tricorder." In *Proceedings of the 2nd International Workshop on Multimedia for Personal Health and Health Care*. New York, NY: ACM, 2017.

Ching, Travers, Daniel S. Himmelstein, Brett K. Beaulieu-Jones, Alexandr A. Kalinin, Brian T. Do, Gregory P. Way, Enrico Ferrero, et al. "Opportunities and Obstacles for Deep Learning in Biology and Medicine." *Journal of the Royal Society, Interface* 15, no. 141 (2018): 20170387. doi:10.1098/rsif.2017.0387.

Cottle, Mike, Waco Hoover, Shadaab Kanwal, Marty Kohn, Trevor Strome, and N. Treister. "Transforming Health Care Through Big Data Strategies for leveraging big data in the health care industry." *Institute for Health Technology Transformation*, http://ihealthtran.com/big-data-in-healthcare (2013).

Cui, Feiyun, Yun Yue, Yi Zhang, Ziming Zhang, and H. Susan Zhou. "Advancing Biosensors with Machine Learning." *ACS Sensors* 5, no. 11 (2020a): 3346–64. doi:10.1021/acssensors.0c01424.

Cui, Feiyun, Zhiru Zhou, and H. Susan Zhou. "Molecularly Imprinted Polymers and Surface Imprinted Polymers Based Electrochemical Biosensor for Infectious Diseases." *Sensors (Basel, Switzerland)* 20, no. 4 (2020b): 996. doi:10.3390/s20040996.

Dolatabadi, A. D., and S. E. Z. Khadem. "Automated Diagnosis of Coronary Artery Disease (CAD) Patients Using Optimized SVM." *Computer Methods and Programs in Biomedicine* 138 (2017): 117–26.

Dong, Jialin, Mingjian Hong, Yi Xu, and Xiangquan Zheng. "A Practical Convolutional Neural Network Model for Discriminating Raman Spectra of Human and Animal Blood." *Journal of Chemometrics* 33, no. 11 (2019). doi:10.1002/cem.3184.

Erzina, M., A. Trelin, O. Guselnikova, B. Dvorankova, K. Strnadova, A. Perminova, P. Ulbrich, et al. "Precise Cancer Detection via the Combination of Functionalized SERS Surfaces and Convolutional Neural Network with Independent Inputs." *Sensors and Actuators. B, Chemical* 308, no. 127660 (2020): 127660. doi:10.1016/j.snb.2020.127660.

Garzón, Vivian, Daniel G. Pinacho, Rosa-Helena Bustos, Gustavo Garzón, and Sandra Bustamante. "Optical Biosensors for Therapeutic Drug Monitoring." *Biosensors* 9, no. 4 (2019): 132. doi:10.3390/bios9040132.

Gonzalez-Navarro, Felix F., Margarita Stilianova-Stoytcheva, Livier Renteria-Gutierrez, Lluís A. Belanche-Muñoz, Brenda L. Flores-Rios, and Jorge E. Ibarra-Esquer. "Glucose Oxidase Biosensor Modeling and Predictors Optimization by Machine Learning Methods." *Sensors (Basel, Switzerland)* 16, no. 11 (2016). doi:10.3390/s16111483.

Goor, Rens van de, Michel van Hooren, Anne-Marie Dingemans, Bernd Kremer, and Kenneth Kross. "Training and Validating a Portable Electronic Nose for Lung Cancer Screening." *Journal of Thoracic Oncology: Official Publication of the International Association for the Study of Lung Cancer* 13, no. 5 (2018): 676–81. doi:10.1016/j.jtho.2018.01.024.

Guevara, Edgar, Juan Carlos Torres-Galván, Miguel G. Ramírez-Elías, Claudia Luevano-Contreras, and Francisco Javier González. "Use of Raman Spectroscopy to Screen Diabetes Mellitus with Machine Learning Tools." *Biomedical Optics Express* 9, no. 10 (2018): 4998–5010. doi:10.1364/BOE.9.004998.

Guidi, Gabriele, Maria Chiara Pettenati, Paolo Melillo, and Ernesto Iadanza. "A Machine Learning System to Improve Heart Failure Patient Assistance." *IEEE Journal of Biomedical and Health Informatics* 18, no. 6 (2014): 1750–56. doi:10.1109/JBHI.2014.2337752.

Guselnikova, O., A. Trelin, A. Skvortsova, P. Ulbrich, P. Postnikov, A. Pershina, D. Sykora, V. Svorcik, and O. Lyutakov. "Label-Free Surface-Enhanced Raman Spectroscopy with Artificial Neural Network Technique for Recognition Photoinduced DNA Damage." *Biosensors & Bioelectronics* 145, no. 111718 (2019): 111718. doi:10.1016/j.bios.2019.111718.

Jeong, Hyoyoung, John A. Rogers, and Xu Shuai. "Continuous On-Body Sensing for the COVID-19 Pandemic: Gaps and Opportunities." *Science Advances* 6, no. 36 (2020). doi:10.1126/sciadv.abd4794.

Jin, Xiaofeng, Conghui Liu, Tailin Xu, Lei Su, and Xueji Zhang. "Artificial Intelligence Biosensors: Challenges and Prospects." *Biosensors & Bioelectronics* 165, no. 112412 (2020): 112412. doi:10.1016/j.bios.2020.112412.

Kaushik, Ajeet, and Mubarak A. Mujawar. "Point of Care Sensing Devices: Better Care for Everyone." *Sensors (Basel, Switzerland)* 18, no. 12 (2018): 4303. doi:10.3390/s18124303.
Kheiron Medical. "Mia: Mammography Intelligent Assessment - AI Mammograms," August 10, 2021. https://www.kheironmed.com/meet-mia
Kim, Chong-Chan, Hyun-Hee Lee, Kyu Hwan Oh, and Jeong-Yun Sun. "Highly Stretchable, Transparent Ionic Touch Panel." *Science (New York, N.Y.)* 353, no. 6300 (2016): 682–87. doi:10.1126/science.aaf8810.
Krizhevsky, Alex, Ilya Sutskever, and Geoffrey E. Hinton. "ImageNet Classification with Deep Convolutional Neural Networks." *Communications of the ACM* 60, no. 6 (2017): 84–90. doi:10.1145/3065386.
Lecun, Y., Y. Bengio, and G. Hinton. "Deep Learning." *Nature* 521 (2015): 436–44.
Lin, Muyang, Hongjie Hu, Sai Zhou, and Sheng Xu. "Soft Wearable Devices for Deep-Tissue Sensing." *Nature Reviews Materials* 7, no. 11 (2022): 850–69. doi:10.1038/s41578-022-00427-y.
Massah, Jafar, and Keyvan Asefpour Vakilian. "An Intelligent Portable Biosensor for Fast and Accurate Nitrate Determination Using Cyclic Voltammetry." *Biosystems Engineering* 177 (2019): 49–58. doi:10.1016/j.biosystemseng.2018.09.007.
Mastoi, Qurat-Ul-Ain, Teh Ying Wah, Ram Gopal Raj, and Uzair Iqbal. "Automated Diagnosis of Coronary Artery Disease: A Review and Workflow." *Cardiology Research and Practice* 2018 (2018): 1–9. doi:10.1155/2018/2016282.
McLaughlin, Gregory, Kyle C. Doty, and Igor K. Lednev. "Raman Spectroscopy of Blood for Species Identification." *Analytical Chemistry* 86, no. 23 (2014): 11628–33. doi:10.1021/ac5026368.
McRae, Michael P., Glennon Simmons, Jorge Wong, and John T. McDevitt. "Programmable Bio-Nanochip Platform: A Point-of-Care Biosensor System with the Capacity to Learn." *Accounts of Chemical Research* 49, no. 7 (2016): 1359–68. doi:10.1021/acs.accounts.6b00112.
Mostafalu, Pooria, Amir Sanati Nezhad, Mehdi Nikkhah, and Mohsen Akbari. "Flexible Electronic Devices for Biomedical Applications." In *Advanced Mechatronics and MEMS Devices II*, 341–66. Cham: Springer International Publishing, 2017.
Nayak, Samiksha, Nicole R. Blumenfeld, Tassaneewan Laksanasopin, and Samuel K. Sia. "Point-of-Care Diagnostics: Recent Developments in a Connected Age." *Analytical Chemistry* 89, no. 1 (2017): 102–23. doi:10.1021/acs.analchem.6b04630.
Ni, Yongnian, and Serge Kokot. "Does Chemometrics Enhance the Performance of Electroanalysis?" *Analytica Chimica Acta* 626, no. 2 (2008): 130–46. doi:10.1016/j.aca.2008.08.009.
Pan, J., and W. J. Tompkins. "A Real-Time QRS Detection Algorithm." *IEEE Transactions on Bio-Medical Engineering* 32, no. 3 (1985): 230–36. doi:10.1109/TBME.1985.325532.
Qian, Lisheng, Qiaobin Li, Kwaku Baryeh, Wanwei Qiu, Kun Li, Jing Zhang, Qingcai Yu, et al. "Biosensors for Early Diagnosis of Pancreatic Cancer: A Review." *Translational Research: The Journal of Laboratory and Clinical Medicine* 213 (2019): 67–89. doi:10.1016/j.trsl.2019.08.002.
Quesada-González, Daniel, and Arben Merkoçi. "Nanomaterial-Based Devices for Point-of-Care Diagnostic Applications." *Chemical Society Reviews* 47, no. 13 (2018): 4697–4709. doi:10.1039/c7cs00837f.
Rani, Usha. "Analysis of Heart Diseases Dataset Using Neural Network Approach." *International Journal of Data Mining & Knowledge Management Process* 1, no. 5 (2011): 1–8. doi:10.5121/ijdkp.2011.1501.
Rein, Robert, and Daniel Memmert. "Big Data and Tactical Analysis in Elite Soccer: Future Challenges and Opportunities for Sports Science." *SpringerPlus* 5, no. 1 (2016): 1410. doi:10.1186/s40064-016-3108-2.
Rong, Y., A. V. Padron, K. J. Hagerty, N. Nelson, S. Chi, N. O. Keyhani, J. Katz, S. P. A. Datta, C. Gomes, and E. S. McLamore. "Post Hoc Support Vector Machine Learning for Impedimetric Biosensors Based on Weak Protein–Ligand Interactions." *The Analyst* 143, no. 9 (2018): 2066–75. doi:10.1039/c8an00065d.
Selestina, Lidija F., Simona Zemljić, and Vanja Strnad. "Textile-Based Biomaterials for Surgical Applications." *In Fundamental Biomaterials: Polymers*, 2018, 179–215.
Shrivastava, Sajal, Tran Quang Trung, and Nae-Eung Lee. "Recent Progress, Challenges, and Prospects of Fully Integrated Mobile and Wearable Point-of-Care Testing Systems for Self-Testing." *Chemical Society Reviews* 49, no. 6 (2020): 1812–66. doi:10.1039/c9cs00319c.
Sin, Mandy L. Y., Kathleen E. Mach, Pak Kin Wong, and Joseph C. Liao. "Advances and Challenges in Biosensor-Based Diagnosis of Infectious Diseases." *Expert Review of Molecular Diagnostics* 14, no. 2 (2014): 225–44. doi:10.1586/14737159.2014.888313.
Singh, Poornima, Sanjay Singh, and Gayatri S. Pandi-Jain. "Effective Heart Disease Prediction System Using Data Mining Techniques." *International Journal of Nanomedicine* 13 (2018): 121–24. doi:10.2147/ijn.s124998.
Stefano, George B., and Elmer A. Fernandez. "Biosensors: Enhancing the Natural Ability to Sense and Their Dependence on Bioinformatics." *Medical Science Monitor: International Medical Journal of Experimental and Clinical Research* 23 (2017): 3168–69. doi:10.12659/msm.905800.

Steinberg, Matthew D., Petar Kassal, and Ivana Murković Steinberg. "System Architectures in Wearable Electrochemical Sensors." *Electroanalysis* 28, no. 6 (2016): 1149–69. doi:10.1002/elan.201600094.

Taniguchi, Masateru. "Combination of Single-Molecule Electrical Measurements and Machine Learning for the Identification of Single Biomolecules." *ACS Omega* 5, no. 2 (2020): 959–64. doi:10.1021/acsomega.9b03660.

Thrift, William John, and Regina Ragan. "Quantification of Analyte Concentration in the Single Molecule Regime Using Convolutional Neural Networks." *Analytical Chemistry* 91, no. 21 (2019): 13337–42. doi:10.1021/acs.analchem.9b03599.

Wang, Li-Ju, Yu-Chung Chang, Rongrong Sun, and Lei Li. "A Multichannel Smartphone Optical Biosensor for High-Throughput Point-of-Care Diagnostics." *Biosensors & Bioelectronics* 87 (2017): 686–92. doi:10.1016/j.bios.2016.09.021.

Wang, Xiaoming, Yineng Xiao, Fangming Deng, Yugen Chen, and Hailiang Zhang. "Eye-Movement-Controlled Wheelchair Based on Flexible Hydrogel Biosensor and WT-SVM." *Biosensors* 11, no. 6 (2021): 198. doi:10.3390/bios11060198.

Yetisen, Ali K., Juan Leonardo Martinez-Hurtado, Barış Ünal, Ali Khademhosseini, and Haider Butt. "Wearables in Medicine." *Advanced Materials (Deerfield Beach, Fla.)* 30, no. 33 (2018): e1706910. doi:10.1002/adma.201706910.

Zeng, Hong, Chen Yang, Guojun Dai, Feiwei Qin, Jianhai Zhang, and Wanzeng Kong. "EEG Classification of Driver Mental States by Deep Learning." *Cognitive Neurodynamics* 12, no. 6 (2018): 597–606. doi:10.1007/s11571-018-9496-y.

Zeng, Zhikang, Zhao Huang, Kangmin Leng, Wuxiao Han, Hao Niu, Yan Yu, Qing Ling, Jihong Liu, Zhigang Wu, and Jianfeng Zang. "Nonintrusive Monitoring of Mental Fatigue Status Using Epidermal Electronic Systems and Machine-Learning Algorithms." *ACS Sensors* 5, no. 5 (2020): 1305–13. doi:10.1021/acssensors.9b02451.

# 8 Design of Circuits for Various Cognitive Diseases Using Various Cognitive Predictive Maintenance Tools

*N. Amuthan and M. S. Jyothi*
AMC Engineering College, Bengaluru, India

*B. Gopal Samy*
V.S.B. Engineering College, Karur, Tamil Nadu, India

## 8.1 INTRODUCTION

Over the past three decades, a huge amount of data has been produced/generated in healthcare systems and hospitals with respect to medical imaging (MI), device monitoring functions, genomic information, and others. Unfortunately, the data are unstructured and create difficulties among doctors and healthcare professionals in understanding, identifying, and even curing the therapies. However, MI and its processing tools are contributing towards the risk identification, understanding the pathogenesis, and even the challenges of therapies. Indeed, it has revolutionized the study pathways, disease prediction in quick and non-invasive pattern, management and treatment procedure. The advancements in image processing techniques have also led to low-risk and even cost-effective investigations. Analysis and treatment of cognitive or brain associated diseases has become stress free due to Magnetic Resonance Imaging (MRI), Positron Emission Tomography (PET), Computed Tomography (CT), and others.

Brain disorders refer to the non-normal functioning of the brain and include those termed bipolar disorder (BP) and schizophrenia (SZ). Some psychiatric disorders are also grounded in brain functioning, but many are diagnosed depending on the clinical interview symptom scores. Though there are no gold standards for the recognition of brain disorders, functional MRI (fMRI), PET, and Electro-Encephalography (EEG) serve as significant tools to analyze brain disorders. Nevertheless, the manual processing of any medical data and the images of brain disorders in particular are time consuming and the possibilities of interpretational errors are high. It has been found that commonplace and discrepancy errors in radiology are more than 3–5% (Brady 2017). The context has called up several advanced approaches to help medical professionals regarding efficient and effective data analysis. Regardless of available techniques and tools, the volume and complexity of data make it unfeasible to find help from regular computer-based algorithms. If we consider images from MI and lesions, it is always difficult to accurately predict the date by simple and traditional models and available equations. Even the analysis and control of disease become difficult with the available data. This is where artificial intelligence (AI) has gained importance in computational neuroscience and received immense attention in the last decade. Machine learning (ML), being a subset of AI, identifies the categories/forecasts the future/informs of unusual conditions by analyzing and processing brain diseases. Alzheimer's disease (AD), Parkinson's disease (PD), vascular dementia, and mild cognitive impairment (MCI) are some of the major brain disorders demanding predictive and maintenance tools from ML.


DOI: 10.1201/9781003245346-8

In the field of medicine, at first the usage of ML algorithms involved elementary assignment, that is, the "binary and ternary classification of patients". Binary classification assesses whether the patient is demented, whereas the other one works on the prediction of cognitive impairment, be it demented or healthy. This algorithm is still in use in the case of automated diagnosis. This chapter provides an overview of several ML approaches developed for cognitive impairment and disorders.

## 8.2 ML APPROACHES FOR COGNITIVE IMPAIRMENT AND DISORDERS

As mentioned in the preceding section, the use of ML in the medical field started with the task of basic classification. This is now done in many categories. It starts with classification based on questionnaire data and ends with classification based on MI and other relevant data.

Questionnaire data was the first and primary available data when ML algorithms were first applied to cognitive diseases. The basic types of questionnaire data available were: (1) the functional activities questionnaire (FAQ) (Pfeffer et al. 1982); (2) the mini-mental status exam (MMSE) (Folstein, Folstein, and McHugh 1975); (3) the dementia rating scale (DRS) (Schmidt et al. 2005); (4) the six-item blessed orientation, memory and concentration test (BOMC) (Fillenbaum et al. 1987). However, the selection or choice of the algorithm depends on the user and the authors. Most of the users also choose rule-based classifiers and IB1 and Naïve Bayes (NB) (Quinlan 2014, Agrell and Dehlin 1998, Duda and Hart 2006). Researchers from the University of California used customary classifiers like IB1, NB, and C4.5 (Datta, Shankle, and Pazzani 1996, Shankle et al. 1998, Shankle et al. 1997). For the classification process, they used the data collected by a research center for AD. The classification achieved nearly 80% accuracy for all the used classifiers. Though the overall accuracy was good, that for the classifier of cognitively impaired patients' data resulted in an accuracy of only 60% (Shankle et al. 1996) with a lesser discrimination of impaired patients among normal control patients. The next classification is rule based, where, depending on the generated rules, one will classify and analyze the important features and also estimate the margin values (Shankle et al. 1997, Datta, Shankle, and Pazzani 1996).

The next major evolution was MI data classification. After experimenting with algorithms of ML in various domains, MI was explored as the major data pool. This domain includes MRI scan images and PET scans. The main idea here was to extract the information from the images and differentiate the impaired functioning images from the normal functioning ones. The task was to narrow down the group and average the data, relying on the region of interest (ROI), which certainly presents the relevant or specific data for the considered medical task. With the aid of the Dynamic Bayesian Network (DBN), Burge et al. (2004) mined regular associations from fMRI (Patil and Yardi 2012). A default mode network (DMN) was extended with the time point T and the variable network's values were found. The authors developed neural-anatomical networks which could classify healthy and demented patients.

Another group used DBN for fMRI data analysis and observed some flaws when plain DBN was used to analyze the entire group of data; however, they attempted to solve the issue by applying DBN to each group distinctly (Li, Wang, and McKeown 2007). Linear programming boosting was proposed to predict AD with MRI (Hinrichs et al. 2009). Spatial constraints and L1 sparsity combined for voxels increased the accuracy in the classification. An extra study on voxels which were chosen at the training phase confirmed a concentration at the hippocampus as well as the parahippocampal gyrus. These were in association with AD. The PET voxels were divided into 67 brain portions and the metabolic activities were extracted by Kippenhan et al. (1992). Another group (Sivakumar and Kanagasabapathy 2018) evaluated the efficiency of bio and cognitive markers to predict the changes from MCI to AD.

Electroencephalography data (ECG) signals and blood sample information was used to differentiate the disease and diagnosis. The protein in blood plasma was quantified by Doecke et al. (2012). The rigorous feature selection employed protein properties (180 inputs). The method comprised two independent datasets and four varied selection features for each set. Another group used

120 proteins for the data analysis and used significant analysis of microarrays (SAM) (Ray et al. 2007). This SAM mainly deals with alterations in the proteins that are significant statistically. It performs a t-test variant on every protein and measures the relationship with respect to a response variable. The authors succeeded in identifying the 18 statistically different proteins among AD and normal control patients.

Data fusion is another type of classification that involves multi-source data integration employing a multifaceted algorithm that extracts accessible information. The data fusion pattern solving the issues is divided into early, moderate, and late integration, which rely on the point of fusion within the administered learning network. The first integration compiles all the source data and gives one single dataset table. In the intermediate/moderate fusion, the data are fused depending on the predictive models. In the last integration, the construction of predictive models is achieved for every data source. All the predictions are joined finally via model weighting.

## 8.3 CLASSIFICATION AND PREDICTION OF BRAIN DISORDERS

Cognitive diseases are a class of disorders that impair cognitive function. This chapter reviews and discusses the classification and prediction of brain disorders using modeling tools and voltage-based circuits. The cognitive diseases that have been researched so far are AD, PD, MCI, and multiple sclerosis. The research is still in its beginning stages. However, since the human brain is the most complex thing we have ever tried to study in science, and is difficult to understand even using all the data available today, it will take much more time and effort before we can understand these disorders better. "The study was published in the peer-reviewed journal *Scientific Reports*. This study can also be defined as dealing with a disease where the brain's processing of information and management of behavior is impaired. The result is that affected individuals develop impairments in cognition, behavioral disorders, mental capacity, and personality; this includes AD, SZ, and BP. Unfortunately, AD is the most common form of dementia which causes cognitive impairment. It is a progressive disorder that will eventually lead to death if not treated. Other common types of cognitive diseases are SZ, BP, traumatic brain injury, and strokes. SZ is a severe mental illness that affects thoughts, feelings, perceptions, and behavior. The causes of SZ are not known, but it is thought to be the result of either genetics or environmental factors like infection and neurological abnormalities. People with SZ have hallucinations and delusions that often interfere with their ability to live independently. It can affect anyone of any age, and it is estimated that about 1% of the population has an SZ diagnosis. Symptoms can appear at any point during a person's life, but usually start to show up in late adolescence or early adulthood. Symptoms typically include the following: hallucinations, which are seeing, hearing, smelling, or feeling things that aren't there; delusions and hallucinations can happen together and involve feelings of persecution, grandeur, or paranoia; disorganized speech, thoughts, and behavior; inability to focus on what's going on; and lack of motivation for daily activities. SZ tends to be misdiagnosed more than many other mental disorders, because there are few symptoms that are specific to the disorder. Differentiating SZ from other types of psychosis can be difficult. "We see a lot of people who are not getting treatment for schizophrenia, or they're being medicated with antipsychotics and nothing's working," says psychologist Thom Tharp. "They might just be suffering from a major depressive episode or anxiety disorder." Figure 8.1 shows the functional connectivity analysis methods and possible connectivity features used for classification/prediction.

This chapter discusses the classification and prediction of brain disorders using modeling tools and voltage-based circuits. There have been many methods developed to detect cognitive diseases, such as detecting brain waves, monitoring blood pressure, or checking blood sugar levels in diabetes. However, these methods require specialized equipment that is not readily available or may not be affordable for the general population. In this study, a model was created to predict if a person has a cognitive disease by analyzing the person's neural activity through voltage-based circuits. The model was created by using a computer program that predicted the person's mood state and then

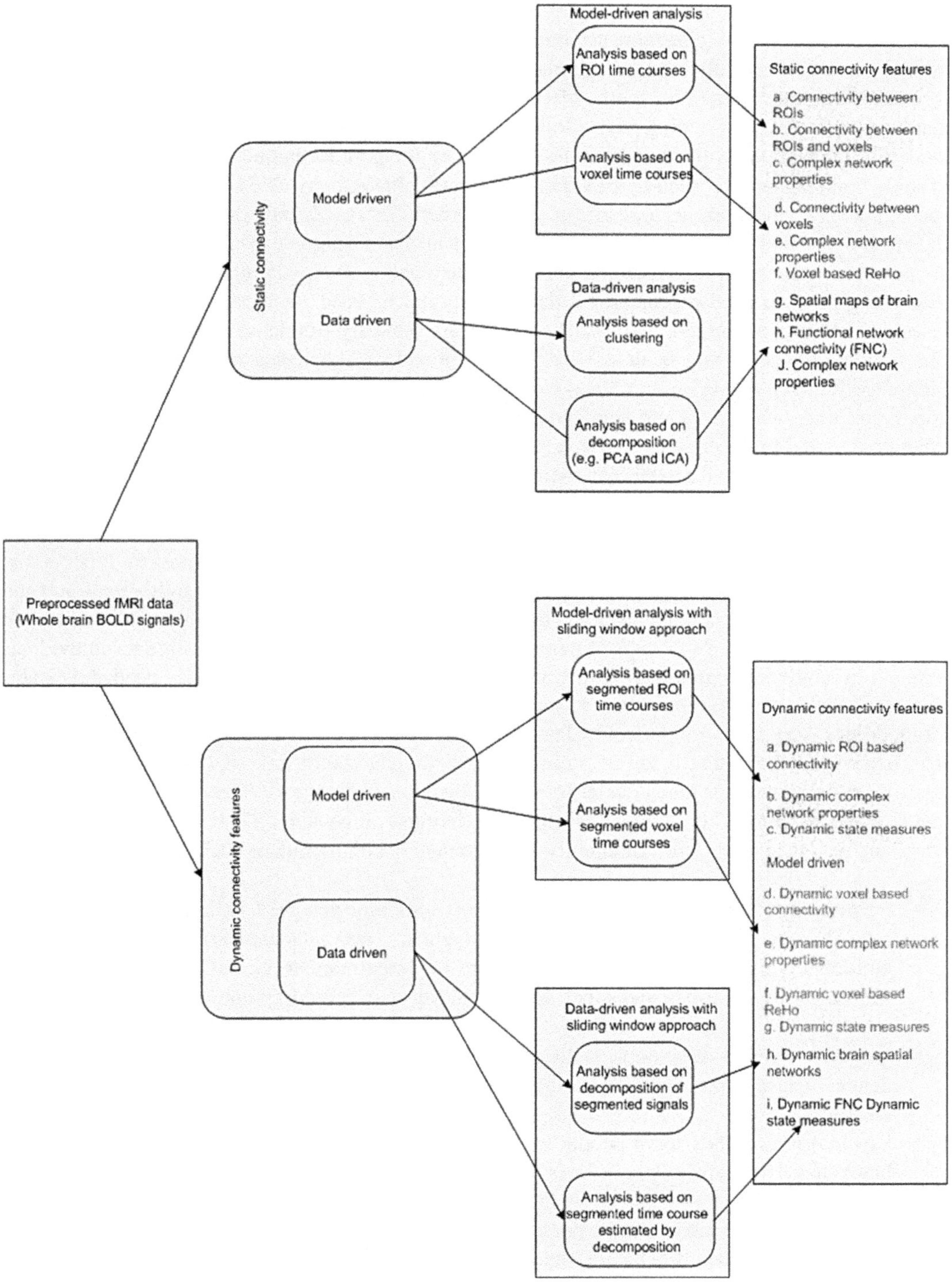


**FIGURE 8.1** Functional connectivity analysis methods and possible connectivity features used for classification/prediction.

used an algorithm to determine which specific neurons are activated, based on that state. The model was validated and found to be more accurate than conventional methods, such as using brain waves, by using a dataset of 100 subjects and classifying them into ten groups. Neuron modeling is the process of using computational methods to study neural activity in the brain. It has been applied to many different fields, including psychology, AI, neuroscience, and neuroscience research. Neuron modeling can be done with or without the use of brain imaging techniques, but it is primarily used to study brain signals recorded by EEG or magnetoencephalography (MEG). Neuron modeling has been applied to pain, learning, autism spectrum disorder (ASD), SZ, and other psychiatric disorders. In neuroscience and psychology, neuron modeling is also a technique used to produce a mathematical model of brain function. Neuron modeling is the practice of simulating models of neurons and then using them to produce functional data, which can be used for a variety of purposes, from research to testing potential therapies. The models are typically simulated in MATLAB or Python. The simulation process may be done with a variety of software packages designed for this purpose. Simulated functional data are not always used to estimate the mean and standard deviation of the population from which they are simulated. However, these quantities may be estimated from the functional model by fitting a linear regression model or an OLS or logistic regression model to it. The outputs of these fitted models can then be used to estimate the quantities of interest.

The therapeutic dilemma of either intervening or not intervening is a matter of debate. Proponents of intervention argue that treatment provides them with a greater chance for recovery and the ability to enjoy life. However, those who oppose intervention believe that it creates a significant risk of losing the personality (which might be seen as less than valuable) if they are constantly monitored and guided by others. Experts argue over whether treatment should take place on an outpatient basis or in a specialized facility. Supporters of outpatient treatment believe that it is possible for individuals to remain socially integrated with family and friends and still get the support they need. Advocates also argue that it can help the person to maintain their personal independence by not forcing them into facilities where they might feel isolated and alienated. On the other hand, opponents of outpatient treatment believe that it can be a costly and inefficient use of time and resources. They also argue that this approach is much riskier for the person than inpatient care. They argue that it's important to avoid an "abrupt" or "traumatic" change of living arrangements. There are several programs which are designed to provide community-based mental health treatment, including:

- Community mental health centers, which are specially designed buildings that provide a wide range of services for people with psychiatric and substance use disorders. These buildings typically have the capacity to care for large numbers of patients, and they are staffed by psychiatrists and other specialists who can provide treatment in a variety of settings.
- Outpatient clinics see people with psychiatric disorders, who are not in acute crisis or danger. These clinics provide treatment for individuals with milder symptoms of mental disorders.
- Psychiatric hospitals serve people with severe psychiatric disorders and acute psychotic breakouts. They typically have beds for the long-term care of patients.

Examples of diagnostic categories are personality disorder and mental disorder, in which the person has a maladaptive pattern of behavior, emotions, and thought that deviate from the culture or personal expectations or fails to live up to basic human needs.

Cognitive predictive maintenance tools are able to diagnose cognitive disorders with a high degree of accuracy by using deep learning software and models. These tools can predict when someone might develop a certain disorder before there are any symptoms present and may therefore be able to make these diseases less prevalent in the future. The ability to predict when someone might develop a disorder before there are any symptoms present is important because the earlier a condition can be identified and treated, the more likely it is that treatment will work, and patients will recover. Cognitive predictive maintenance tools use deep learning software to identify patterns in brain scans that indicate conditions such as SZ, dementia, or ADHD. Deep learning techniques are computer programs that are able to learn how to recognize patterns in a dataset without being explicitly programmed with those rules. One example of a deep learning technique is the artificial neuron or "neuron" which learns from experience and changes its behavior based on that experience. Neurons learn by adjusting their weights and thresholds. As the amount of experience the neuron has accumulated increases, so the weight of its connections to other neurons becomes more significant, and vice versa. The adjustment of weights allows for the strength or weakness of a neuron's contributions to be gradually increased or decreased in proportion to their usefulness. With enough experience, an artificial neuron will become capable of predictable outcomes that indicate whether a certain category is present within its input data. In this representation, the neuron is given a weight of 100. This means that any input with a value greater than or equal to 100 will increase the output by 1, while any input with a value less than or equal to –100 will decrease the output by 0.33333. The numbers indicate what would happen if this neuron received an arbitrary input value.

## 8.4 INTELLIGENT PREDICTIVE MAINTENANCE AND REMOTE MONITORING

A cognitive model is a representation or abstraction of the knowledge, beliefs, and desires of an agent (usually a person), which may be formally encoded in computer-readable form. They are used in AI to simulate human decision making. In general, they are used to predict the decisions and outputs of intelligent agents. Cognitive science is the study of cognitive processes such as memory, language, attention, and perception. "Cognitive dissonance" is a term in psychology used to describe the uncomfortable feeling experienced by an individual who holds two contradictory beliefs, ideas, or values at the same time. This discomfort can range from minor uneasiness to intense discomfort. A person experiencing cognitive dissonance may be motivated to reduce it by changing one of the beliefs, ideas, or values. Cognitive dissonance can also occur when a person encounters information that contradicts their worldview. This may result in cognitive dissonance because they now have to alter their worldview beliefs in order to reconcile the new information with what they already know. A person experiencing cognitive dissonance may act as if the new information is not true in order to reduce the conflict between their beliefs and the new information. In the case of a person who believes that vegetarians and vegans are unhealthy, they may try to rationalize this fact by focusing on personal health and not on social issues. Explanations for the existence of cognitive dissonance may include:

- It is caused by a conflict between beliefs;
- It is caused by a discrepancy between the actual and the ideal situation;
- A person will have cognitive dissonance if they face an obstacle that prevents them from achieving something they believe they deserve.

This is when a person is in the middle of changing their habits for the better and something prevents them from doing this. They are committed to changing their habits but have a mental block that stops them from achieving what they want. The section of intelligent predictive maintenance and remote monitoring focuses on the use of AI in modeling and engineering. The main goal is to develop a system that can predict when there will be a breakdown with the help of predictive analytic models, which are used for both preventive maintenance as well as for after-the-fact diagnostics. Figure 8.2. shows an installing predictive maintenance flow diagram.

The goal of predictive maintenance is to provide a system of monitoring, diagnosis, decision making, and prognosis that provides predictive intelligence for equipment. With the rapid advancement in technology, cognitive models and intelligent data analysis will play an important role in this field.

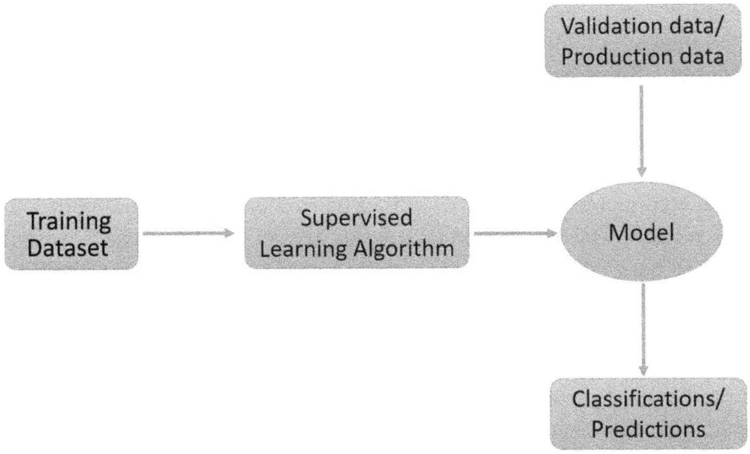


**FIGURE 8.2** Installing predictive maintenance.

Intelligent predictive maintenance tools are:

- Cognitive CoPilot: a set of tools for developing test benches with automated testing methods.
- Cognitive Flux: a system that manages information from sensors on equipment or machinery.
- Cognitive Engineering Toolkit (CoET): designed to be used by engineers to design circuits.
- Modeling tools: such as electromagnetic toolbox, which allow engineers to simulate different aspects of the electromagnetic spectrum.
- Prediction tool: is a simulation tool that helps engineers to predict the quality of systems by using cognitive models and intelligent data analysis, from which it is possible to make predictions about the health of equipment. Such predictions may include things like predicting when a machine will fail or what the expected life span for a component may be. Some companies are already adopting predictive maintenance to detect and repair small problems before they become more expensive repairs. Predictive maintenance is a process that examines a system for anomalies and predicts the likelihood of failure. It can be used to maintain optimum performance, avoid downtimes, and extend the life of a system.

Predictive equipment maintenance is designed to provide quality assurance and to reduce the need for reactive maintenance. It relies on models to predict the life of a system. This along with remote monitoring technology has made it possible for machine engineers and managers to be notified in advance when equipment is slated for failure and can therefore be repaired. The application of predictive maintenance techniques to the oil and gas industry has led to a significant saving in maintenance costs, improved product quality, and operational efficiency. Many companies have found that they can both extend the life of their equipment and reduce their overall costs by applying predictive maintenance techniques to equipment design. In an operating environment where cost reduction is the ultimate goal, predictive maintenance has been a key tool in that effort. Modern predictive maintenance primarily uses two classes of models for reliability prediction: deterministic models and probabilistic model-based predictors. Determinism allows for a high level of precision, but often only works for single failure modes or cases. Probabilistic model-based predictors can take into account the many different failure modes and case-specific failure rates and have a higher chance of accuracy. Deterministic predictive maintenance models need to be completed for all possible combinations of components and failure modes in order to be able to calculate reliability predictions accurately. These models are often large, complicated, and prohibitively expensive in terms of cost.

Predictive maintenance:

- Predictions of the life of a system are based on data collected from sensors;
- ML algorithms are used to predict how long a system will last;
- Interventions are triggered before critical failures happen;
- A condition monitoring report is generated every day or week that contains predictions about which components will fail soon;
- The machine can also be monitored remotely so that experts can detect problems before they become catastrophic failures;
- The systems are monitored with data collection and analysis tools to identify patterns in the data that pertain to the system.

## 8.5 BEHAVIORS IN CHILDREN WITH AUTISM AND COGNITIVE CONTROL

Autism is a developmental disorder of the brain and is characterized by difficulties in social interaction, verbal and nonverbal communication, and repetitive behaviors.

Children with autism often have difficulty with cognitive control which is a specific skill that regulates behavior in order to perform a task. The child needs a lot of help and guidance with things like achieving their own goals, sustaining attention, and focusing on the task at hand. They also need help developing and growing cognitive control abilities to help them stay present in the moment and inhibit certain actions, which is a skill that helps them manage their behavior better.

Cognitive control can be explained as a set of tools such as modeling tools, the design of circuits, or cognitive paths. These tools allow children to better understand how their minds work and what they should be doing to avoid risky behavior or consequences that may arise from it. In the field of education, designing tools that assist children in understanding how their minds work and what to do to avoid risky behavior is a major area of research. There are a number of techniques available for teachers to use with their students, including understanding the self-regulation theory, which helps children understand why they behave one way or another and can give them strategies on how to change their behavior. There are different strategies that a teacher can use with their students including using an occupational therapy model, which is the same model they would use to help children learn how to self-regulate and perform tasks independently or using a reward system. The use of these tools can help children better understand their own behavior when it comes to risks involved in certain tasks or activities while encouraging them to take calculated risks in other areas (see Figure 8.3).

Research has found that children with autism often have cognitive control impairments that lead to an array of behaviors, including repetitive behaviors and inattention, fidgeting, tantrums, and social withdrawal. The brain is the center of the central nervous system that controls all the actions of our body. The brain is divided into regions or lobes. Each lobe has different functions that are involved with special senses such as: sight and sound; motor control, like moving your eyes or legs; and cognitive function, such as memory or learning new things.

There are a number of symptoms and behaviors associated with ASD. These include difficulties in social interactions, repetitive behaviors, and sensory sensitivities. This can be caused by many different factors, but research has found that most cases of autism are caused by a combination of genetic and environmental factors. The diagnostic criteria for ASDs are defined on three spectrums: social communication deficits, social interaction deficits, and restricted/repetitive behavior which can be combined or can stand on their own if they occur in the majority of the three symptom areas:

- Social communication deficits: difficulties in initiating or sustaining a conversation, understanding, and using nonverbal cues, or interacting appropriately with people; difficulty with sharing interests, passions, or emotional reactions.
- Social interaction deficits: limited use of facial expressions and body language; difficulties understanding humor or sarcasm; difficulty reading social cues such as tone of voice, eye contact, or facial expression.

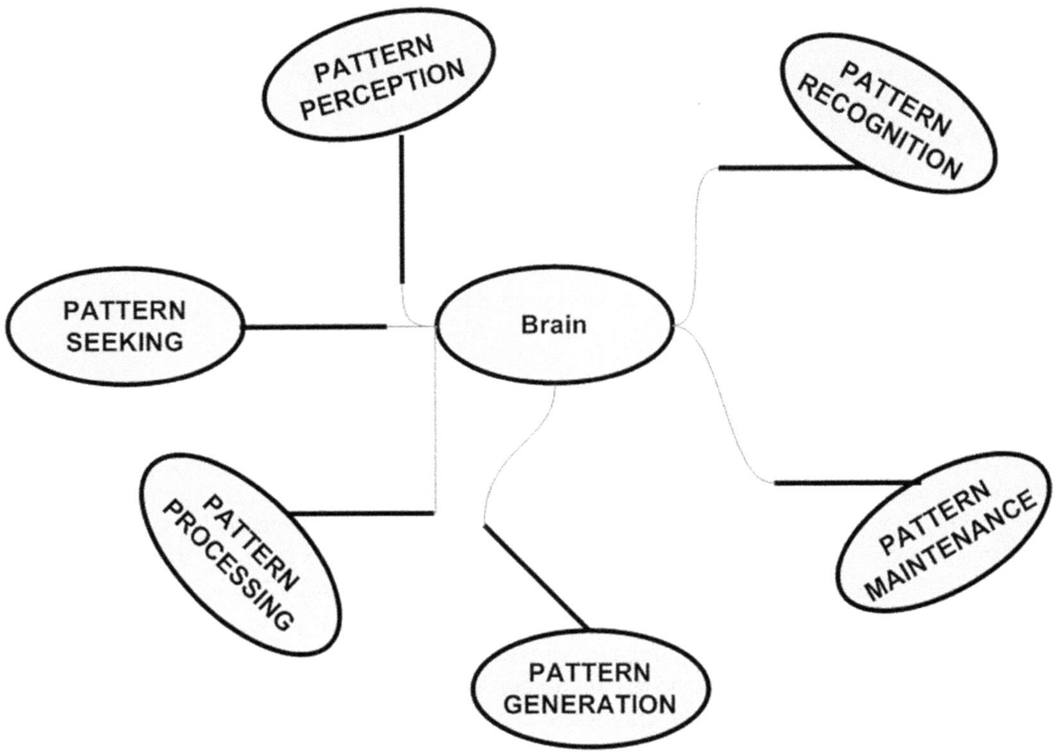


**FIGURE 8.3** Non-social dimensions of pattern in relation to relevant autism-associated phenotypes.

Autism is a spectrum disorder that affects the brain. The behaviors exhibited by children with autism and other cognitive diseases often include difficulty controlling impulses and repetitive behaviors. These behaviors can be avoided or minimized with the use of cognitive predictive maintenance tools (CPMTs), which are behavioral interventions that can help manage and prevent the behaviors found in individuals with autism. The tools include a specific set of procedures, training and coaching, computer software or hardware, and any other method that supports the individual's effort to participate. They were approved by the U.S. Food and Drug Administration (FDA) on October 1, 2016. The sponsor of the device or tool is responsible for its content and for ensuring that it complies with all applicable laws, rules, and regulations. The sponsor may be a manufacturer, distributor, or another entity approved by the FDA. A tool includes software-based tools as well as hardware-based tools, such as a device for measuring and recording drug concentrations, such as an absorbance spectrophotometer. A drug is any substance intended for use in the diagnosis, cure, mitigation, treatment, or prevention of disease or to otherwise affect the structure or function of the body. The term "therapeutically effective amount" refers to an amount of a substance that, when administered, is sufficient to lead to the desired clinical result for the treatment or prevention of a disease.

## 8.6 COGNITIVE PREDICTIVE MAINTENANCE TOOLS

CPMTs are designed to anticipate and solve these problems at an early stage in order to prevent any further possible damage. They work to model cognitive paths that involve decision making, the prediction of next steps, and risk assessment using cognitive analytics. These tools use data collected by a variety of sensors and devices to model the interactions between people and machines, including information that is not available via conventional means. For example, the tools can predict the risk of failure in buildings that have been installed with IoT sensors as well as identify cognitive paths most likely to lead to such failures. In a cognitive predictive maintenance application, the system uses data from sensors and devices to model how people interact with machines. In addition to collecting sensor data, it can also collect telemetry information, such as video or audio recordings, for further use in its prediction models. The system then uses this information to predict when and where failures are likely to happen, and to make predictive maintenance decisions. There are many different types of cognitive systems, but they all use various techniques in attempts to predict failure and improve performance. They are designed to extract insights from data, meaning that they can teach themselves new things about the world. This can be accomplished by making predictions and inferences (from data), reasoning and learning from their own experience, and simulating the behavior of a person or entity in a particular situation. These systems are often programmed as AI software, or in open-source programs using the Python programming language (see Figure 8.4).

The effects of four distinct virtual classroom layouts on the parameters of scalp EEG were measured over a short period of time (including varying window placements and room sizes). Participants in each design condition were given a battery of five cognitive tasks that needed to be completed before the end of the experiment. The Stroop Test, the Digit Span Test, the Benton Test, the Visual Memory Test, and the Arithmetic Test were some of the examinations that were administered. The results of the cognitive tests were compared to the EEG data that was collected from the different layouts of the classroom. In terms of how well people performed on cognitive tests, there were no statistically significant differences discovered between the two different room configurations. In order to get an idea of how the brain's electrical activity changed as a result of the various design choices, we carried out a number of computations on the power and connectedness of the brain's electrical frequency bands. These computations were performed in order to get an idea of how the electrical activity of the brain changed. Our objective was to determine how the electrical activity of the brain altered in response to the many design options that were shown to it. In order to investigate the reliability of the EEG characteristics, an ML classification strategy known as leave-one-out was used. The trained model's accuracy in classifying data was measured against data provided by a participant whose identity was kept secret in many evaluations (Gruz-Garza et al. 2022).

Interviews using the self-attitude technique, discussions using the transactional analysis model, free-reasoning about situations chosen according to the age and other parameters of participants,

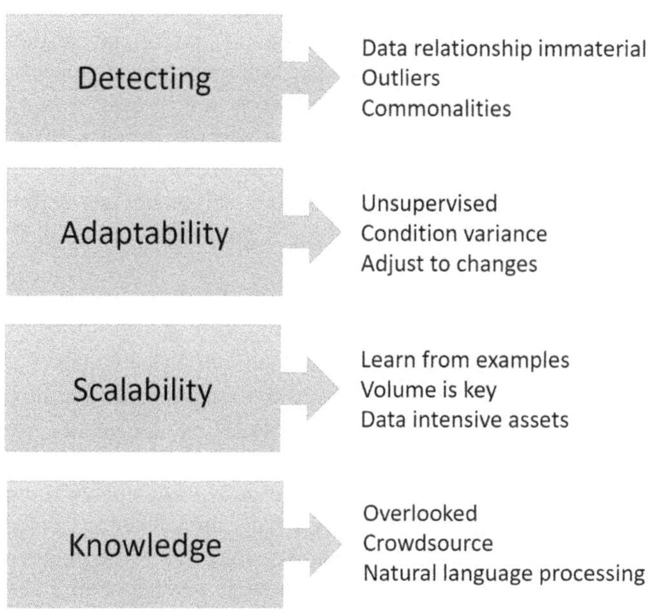


**FIGURE 8.4** Cognitive analysis capabilities.

and watching video clips with an unexpected ending were all used to provoke an outburst and remotely resolve the cognitive-emotional conflict. Other methods included: free-reasoning about situations chosen according to the age and other parameters of participants; watching video clips with an unexpected ending; and free-reasoning about situations chosen according to the age and other parameters. Other methods included using techniques from neural networks that are based on VGG16, a program developed for personal computers that can automatically categorize the emotional responses of persons seen in video footage. In addition, the P. Ekman FACS model used data that was openly available to the general public in order to pretrain the neural network in order to recognize a range of emotions. The last step in this procedure consisted of annotating video recordings with remarks that were based on the findings of the expert evaluations of the level of cognitive-emotional conflict that was occurring (Vartanov et al. 2022). A cognitive predictive maintenance model is proposed to assist in categorizing and recommending corrective methods, as well as estimating equipment failure time (Poosapati et al. 2019). Piezo electric materials are more useful for utilizing cognitive electronic circuits (Sivakumar 2019; Sivakumar and Kanagasabapath 2018).

## 8.7 CONCLUSION AND FUTURE DIRECTION

The design of circuits and the functions of these circuits can be modeled with various cognitive predictive maintenance tools. There are such tools that can assist in the design of new circuits. There are also various methods for testing a circuit without having to go under its logic board including 3D printing and testing a network of neurons. Sometimes, very complex circuit designs are required to deal with the performance of certain algorithms. In these cases, a simulator can be used in conjunction with the circuit design software to simulate how a new design would perform. Logic board testing never reveals the source of an electronic failure; however, with a simulation and lab bench test it is possible to narrow in on the problem. Logic boards are also expensive to replace and time-consuming to repair so it is important for circuits to be tested before they are released for sale.

In the future, we might be able to use this technology to prevent cognitive diseases in humans. This will involve developing non-invasive technology that can monitor electrical signals in the brain and identify any anomalies in the way they are communicated. As with any type of predictive maintenance, there are obstacles and limitations. The biggest obstacle is the understanding of what exactly causes which neural cluster to malfunction in which way. The design work that goes into a new product often includes extensive prototyping and simulations before it is taken to manufacturing levels. Prototypes are built on paper or on computer models before they are built in the real world. Prototyping is an important part of design work. A prototype is an early sample, model, or release of a product developed to test a functional concept or process or event. It is a working model intended to act as a thing to be replicated or learned from. In general, "prototype" refers to a preliminary model of something. The effects of brain development and cognition on society can include changes in behavior, mental health, or thought processes that result from changes in the structure of the brain.

The conclusion discusses how the work done could lead to better understanding of the mechanisms that cause cognitive diseases and help in designing new drugs to treat them. This may also provide insights on designing circuits for specific cognitive diseases which can be used as models for future research and drug development. To study the neural pathways in the brain related to music, Yasuaki Iwatsuki, a professor of cognitive science at Kyoto University, and his team recorded the electrical activity of neurons in the brains of mice expressing green fluorescent protein (GFP) under an "excitatory" or "inhibitory" gene. While one mouse was listening to music with a specific tempo, the other mouse was listening to silence. "When the mice listened to music, we could easily tell when neurons in their auditory cortex reacted because they lit up with pulses of light," I was said. "This showed us that the brain activity was related to what was happening externally. The waves of light reflected on a video screen demonstrated that neurons in a specific region of the brain were being repeatedly activated, a process called excitation." The study found that the light was getting in one eye and stimulating neurons in the visual cortex. They then created an algorithm to tease out which parts of the brain were seen by showing various objects on different video screens. "It was important for us to show that when people are moving their eyes, their brains are actually undergoing significant processing of the visual world," said Vann. What is neuroplasticity? Neuroplasticity is the ability of the brain to change, reorganize, and rewire itself through learning.

## REFERENCES

Agrell, Berit, and Ove Dehlin. 1998. "The clock-drawing test." *Age and Ageing* no. 27 (3):399–404.

Brady, Adrian P 2017. "Error and discrepancy in radiology: inevitable or avoidable?" *Insights into Imaging* no. 8 (1):171–182.

Burge, J., V.P. Clark, T. Lane, H. Link, and S. Qiu. 2004. "Bayesian classification of FMRI data: Evidence for altered neural networks in dementia". University of New Mexico, Tech. Rep. TR-CS-2004-28.

Datta, Piew, WR Shankle, and Michael Pazzani. 1996. Applying machine learning to an Alzheimer's database. *Paper read at Conference proceedings of the AAAI symposium.*

Doecke, James D, Simon M Laws, Noel G Faux, William Wilson, Samantha C Burnham, Chiou-Peng Lam, Alinda Mondal, Justin Bedo, Ashley I Bush, and Belinda Brown. 2012. "Blood-based protein biomarkers for diagnosis of Alzheimer disease." *Archives of Neurology* no. 69 (10):1318–1325.

Duda, Richard O, and Peter E Hart. 2006. *Pattern classification*. John Wiley & Sons.

Fillenbaum, Gerda G, Albert Heyman, William E Wilkinson, and Carol S Haynes. 1987. "Comparison of two screening tests in Alzheimer's disease: The correlation and reliability of the Mini-Mental State Examination and the Modified Blessed Test." *Archives of Neurology* no. 44 (9):924–927.

Folstein, Marshal F, Susan E Folstein, and Paul R McHugh. 1975. "'Mini-mental state': a practical method for grading the cognitive state of patients for the clinician." *Journal of Psychiatric Research* no. 12 (3):189–198.

Hinrichs, Chris, Vikas Singh, Lopamudra Mukherjee, Guofan Xu, Moo K Chung, Sterling C Johnson, and Alzheimer's Disease Neuroimaging Initiative. 2009. "Spatially augmented LPboosting for AD classification with evaluations on the ADNI dataset." *Neuroimage* no. 48 (1):138–149.

Kippenhan, Jonathan Shane, Warren W Barker, Shlomo Pascal, Joachim H Nagel, and Ranjan Duara. 1992. "Evaluation of a neural-network classifier for PET scans of normal and Alzheimer's disease subjects." *Journal of Nuclear Medicine* no. 33(8):1459–1467.

Li, Junning, Z Jane Wang, and Martin J McKeown. 2007. A framework for group analysis of fMRI data using dynamic Bayesian networks. *Paper read at 2007 29th Annual International Conference of the IEEE Engineering in Medicine and Biology Society.*

Patil, MM, and AR Yardi. 2012. "MLP classifier for Dementia levels." *International Journal of Modeling and Optimization* no. 2 (5):567.

Pfeffer, Robert I, Tom T Kurosaki, CH Harrah Jr, Jeffrey M Chance, and S Filos. 1982. "Measurement of functional activities in older adults in the community." *Journal of Gerontology* no. 37 (3):323–329.

Quinlan, J Ross. 2014. *C4. 5: programs for machine learning*. Elsevier.

Ray, Sandip, Markus Britschgi, Charles Herbert, Yoshiko Takeda-Uchimura, Adam Boxer, Kaj Blennow, Leah F Friedman, Douglas R Galasko, Marek Jutel, and Anna Karydas. 2007. "Classification and prediction of clinical Alzheimer's diagnosis based on plasma signaling proteins." *Nature Medicine* no. 13 (11):1359–1362.

Schmidt, Kara S, Paul J Mattis, Jane Adams, and Paul Nestor. 2005. "Alternate-form reliability of the Dementia Rating Scale-2." *Archives of Clinical Neuropsychology* no. 20 (4):435–441.

Shankle, William Rodman, Piew Datta, Michael Dillencourt, and Michael Pazzani. 1996. "Improving dementia screening tests with machine learning methods." *Alzheimer's Research* no. 2 (3).

Shankle, William Rodman, Subramani Mani, Michael J Pazzani, and Padhraic Smyth. 1997. Detecting very early stages of dementia from normal aging with machine learning methods. *Paper read at Conference on artificial intelligence in medicine in Europe.*

Shankle, William Rodman, Subramani Mania, Malcolm B Dick, and Michael J Pazzani. 1998. "Simple models for estimating dementia severity using machine learning." In *MEDINFO'98*, 472–476. IOS Press.

Sivakumar, N., and H. Kanagasabapathy. 2018. "Optimization of parameters of cantilever beam using novel bio-inspired algorithms: A comparative approach." *Journal of Computational and Theoretical Nanoscience* no. 15(1): 66–77. https://doi.org/10.1166/jctn.2018.7057

# 9 Advances in the Treatment of Cognitive Diseases Using IOT-based Wearable Devices

*Sangeeta Avinash Tripathi and M. S. Rohokale*
SKN Sinhgad Institutes of Technology and Science, Pune, India

*Sanjay Kumar*
Amity University, Rajasthan, India

## 9.1 INTRODUCTION

Many sectors of the healthcare industry are teaming up with the technology sector, and this will strengthen the connection between the two in the years to come. Recently, we have witnessed the explosive growth and deployment of the Internet of Things (IoT) approach, as well as the introduction of miniature wearable biosensors and the development of big data techniques for the efficient manipulation of large datasets that are multiscale, multilayer perceptron, dispersed, and diverse. The treatment of cardiovascular disease, high blood pressure, and muscle disorders, as well as neurobehavioral disorders such as Parkinson's disease and Alzheimer's disease (AD), are just some of the conditions that can be helped by the widespread use of wearable medical technology, which is based on biofluidics, tattoos, and textiles. Wearable technologies that combine antennas and sensors and are based on textiles are also included in this category. The effectiveness of wearables as drug delivery systems has increased, leading to a rise in the field of personalized medicine. There are several problems that are inherent to these wearables that need to be handled before they can be commercialized as a completely individualized healthcare system. This chapter introduces the various IoT-based healthcare personalized devices used to make human life more productive and safer to track. Numerous healthcare devices are being designed and studied for tracking purposes, and an emphasis is placed on the efficacy of these devices for the monitoring of a variety of diseases, as well as their applications in the diagnosis and treatment of various conditions. Future prospects for these wearable technologies in healthcare, as well as the challenges they currently face, are discussed.

## 9.2 DRIVING FORCE BEHIND THE WORK

The IoT is the next logical transition in the accelerated growth of the internet. It involves the linking of devices that can communicate data to a larger network, where it can be used to increase profitability. All gadgets must have unique IDs and use embedded technology to sense and gather data about themselves and their environment. Data must be connected and examined to make smarter decisions. The IoT provides great potential to harness previously undiscovered information and insight to alter industrial processes and business models. This is more than a link. Several companies have defined the IoT, and it is important to compare their definitions.

The medical industry is currently undergoing a significant transition, due to the aging of the population, toward the study, development, and design of biosensors for the real-time monitoring of


DOI: 10.1201/9781003245346-9

human health, the prevention of illness, and the individualized treatment of both chronic and acute disorders. The management of patients who suffer from chronic illnesses such as cardiovascular disease, diabetes, or neurological disorders requires monitoring that is both continual and instantaneous. This is a vital component of the care that these patients receive. Point-of-care technology (POCT) provides quick and patient-centered diagnostics, especially for those with limited access to health services.

According to the research that was conducted by Pantelopoulos and Bourbakis (2010) and published in the *Bulletin of the World Health Organization* (WHO), chronic diseases are to blame for 75% of all fatalities that occur around the world and they impose tremendous financial costs. Wearable technology is any electronic device that may be worn on or in clothing. They have a receptor as well as a transducer. A receptor is responsible for recognizing the target analytic. The industry is attempting to extract clinically relevant information by applying physical signals to explore such factors as heart rate, blood pressure, skin temperature, respiratory rate, and body motion (Pantelopoulos and Bourbakis 2010; Chan et al. 2012; Patel et al. 2012; Kim et al. 2019).

The ever-increasing incidence of dementia poses a significant problem for the state of global health on a variety of fronts. According to the findings of Hurd et al. (2013) and Wimo et al. (2013), on the level of the economy, dementia and, more specifically, AD are among the diseases that are most costly for the West, with an estimated price tag of $160 billion per year. This is a significant amount of money. AD is a type of degenerative brain illness that generally and gradually advances through three primary stages, which are referred to as early, middle, and moderate or late, as shown in the study by Patel et al. (2012). Because this disease affects people in a variety of different ways, it is possible that each person who contracts it will have a unique set of symptoms and will progress through the stages in a different way, as shown by Gupta et al. (2016).

Over the course of the last decade, wearable biosensors have received a significant amount of attention, most of which has been focused on the healthcare industry. Wearable sensors are predicted to expand at a compound annual growth rate (CAGR) of roughly 38% globally from 2017 to 2025, with the development of smart watches growing at a particularly fast rate. The global market for these sensors is predicted to reach $1.7 billion over the same period. This growth will be driven in large part by the trend toward personalized medicine in healthcare systems, as shown by Massaroni et al. (2018). Bio-diagnostic components and tools are heavyweight, expensive, and require specialist employees to operate in the area of the IoT. Wearable technologies could transform bio-diagnostics into a patient-centered approach instead of a hospital-centered one, though present techniques and the generation of smart technology have a few drawbacks, some of which include a restricted amount of relevant biometric information, poor aesthetics and comfort, and a bulky structure. Because the human body is a soft and curvilinear system, disruptive soft wearable technologies are highly desirable in this context, whereas the majority of today's electronics are rigid and planar (Ling et al. 2019).

Current stiff wearable gadgets, despite being continuously downsized, cannot conform to and contact the delicate skin of humans for collecting correct information; they also fail mechanically or electrically to accommodate human dynamics. Feiner and Dvir (2017) and Someya et al. (2016) have shown that, over the past decade, soft bioelectronics research has grown. The development of microelectronic epidermal or electronic skin (e-skin) sensors for the monitoring of biometric signals has brought us one step closer to personalized medical management. Figure 9.1 shows the IoT-based wireless body area network system with closed-loop feedbacks. The feedback system is utilized to capture the real-time data for the monitoring system. Electroencephalography (EEG), electrocardiography (ECG), and electromyography (EMG) are employed to communicate important body signals, regarding the signs of urgent attention, to the sensors, as shown. Wearable sensors are then utilized to send these signals to the healthcare server through internet connectivity. Once the signals are received by the server decisions can be taken whenever needed. During Stage I, conformal wearable sensors are employed to capture critical indications such as physiological, electrophysiological, and biochemical signals. The obtained biometric information is communicated to the internet via

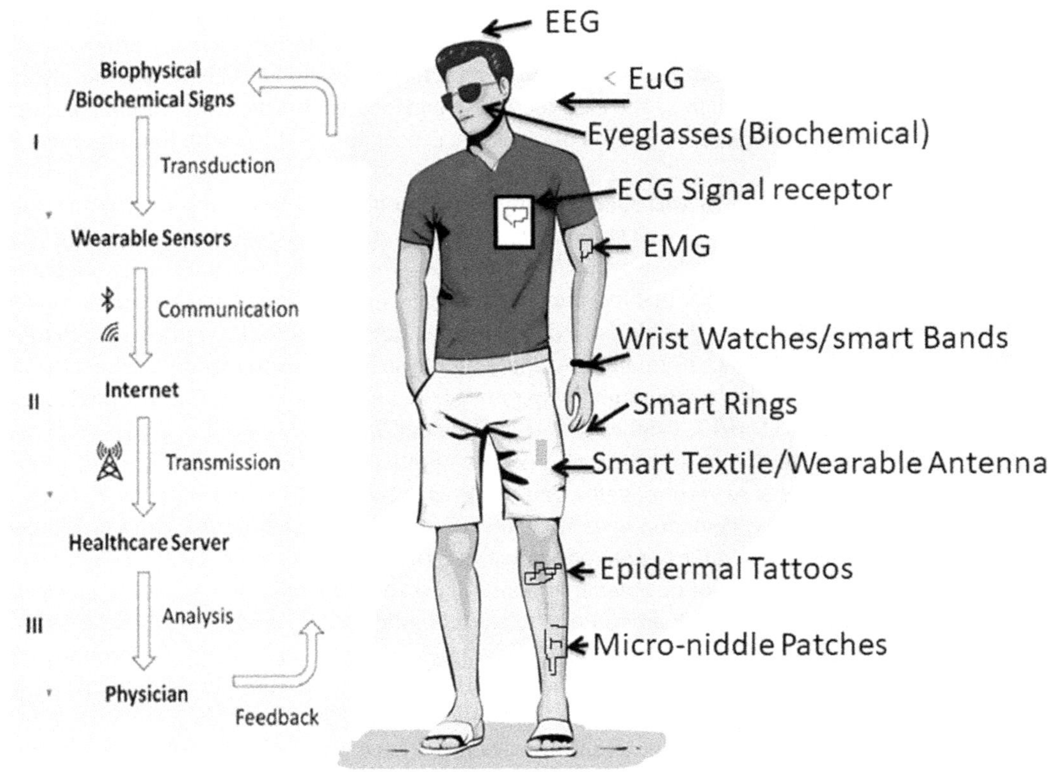


**FIGURE 9.1** Simple geometric illustration of how the IoT depends on wireless body area network (WBAN) devices can be used to manage individualized medical treatment. (Based on Pantelopoulos and Bourbakis, 2010).

wireless communication units in the middle stage so that it can be analyzed remotely for medical purposes.

Depending on the health information obtained, related medicine interventions or therapies are carried out at the Stage III level by closed-loop wearable devices or by medical personnel, as explored by Pantelopoulos and Bourbakis (2010), Elhayatmy et al. (2017), and Lin et al. (2021).

## 9.3 CLASSIFICATION OF HEALTHCARE WEARABLE DEVICES (HWDs)

Monitoring that is both continuous and performed in real time is absolutely necessary for the efficient management of patients who suffer from chronic conditions such as cardiovascular diseases, neurological disorders, and diabetes. According to the WHO, chronic diseases account for 75% of all mortality globally and impose significant economic burdens as a result. As a matter of fact, a wide range of approaches is needed for the monitoring and diagnosis of these diseases; one approach that is helpful in this respect is the utilization of HWDs, as discussed by Someya et al. (2016).

Wearable technology refers to any electronic device that can be attached to or worn on an individual's body or clothing. These devices include a target receptor as well as a transducer. A target analytic can be recognized by a receptor, which then triggers an appropriate response. The response from the receptor is transformed into a signal that can be utilized by the transducer (Xie et al. 2020; Bhalla et al. 2016).

These HWDs contribute to providing better knowledge of the variations that take place inside the human body, which in turn can assist in the prevention and treatment of diseases. This was the case prior to their introduction into the wearable sensor market. In 1956, Leland C. Clark, now commonly known as the "father of biosensors", was the first person to employ electrodes for the purpose of assessing the amount of oxygen present in blood. His experiment was successful. During cardiovascular surgery, this device's primary function was to provide continuous as well as real-time measurements of oxygen levels in the operating room. In 1969, G.G. Guilbault and J.G. Montalvo Jr. developed a potentiometric biosensor for the detection of urea. This was made possible by the introduction of electrodes for use in the healthcare industry. The year 1975 was when consumers could purchase their very first glucose analyzer, which was modeled after Clark's electrochemical biosensor. The introduction of electrodes into the medical field was the catalyst for the development discussed in Bhalla et al. (2016).

## 9.4 CATEGORIES OF VARIOUS HWDs

Skin, which covers most of the body, is ideal for non-invasive HWDs. These devices on the skin can monitor physiological and psychological factors to treat diseases like cardiovascular and neuromuscular ones. Sweat can be analyzed qualitatively and quantitatively to diagnose diseases. Textile or epidermal materials may be utilized in the construction of skin-based wearable devices. This distinction is made according to the nature of the skin contact. Wearables that are based on textiles incorporate sensors in clothing, whereas those that are based on the epidermis are applied in a manner comparable to that of a tattoo and are referred to as electronic skin (e-skin). Various popular categories of HWDs are shown in Figure 9.2. They are broadly categorized in two parts as fully flexible and partially flexible. Fully flexible may be completely printable or wearable on the body, as in the form of a tattoo, and are also popular in drug delivery systems.

In the following sections, we will explore how HWDs based on tattoos and textiles can be used to monitor and diagnose diseases. Fabrics can be found almost anywhere and have been around for many years and centuries. Textiles and clothing have historically been thought of as a means of maintaining human body temperature and as an aesthetic necessity. Because of the simplicity

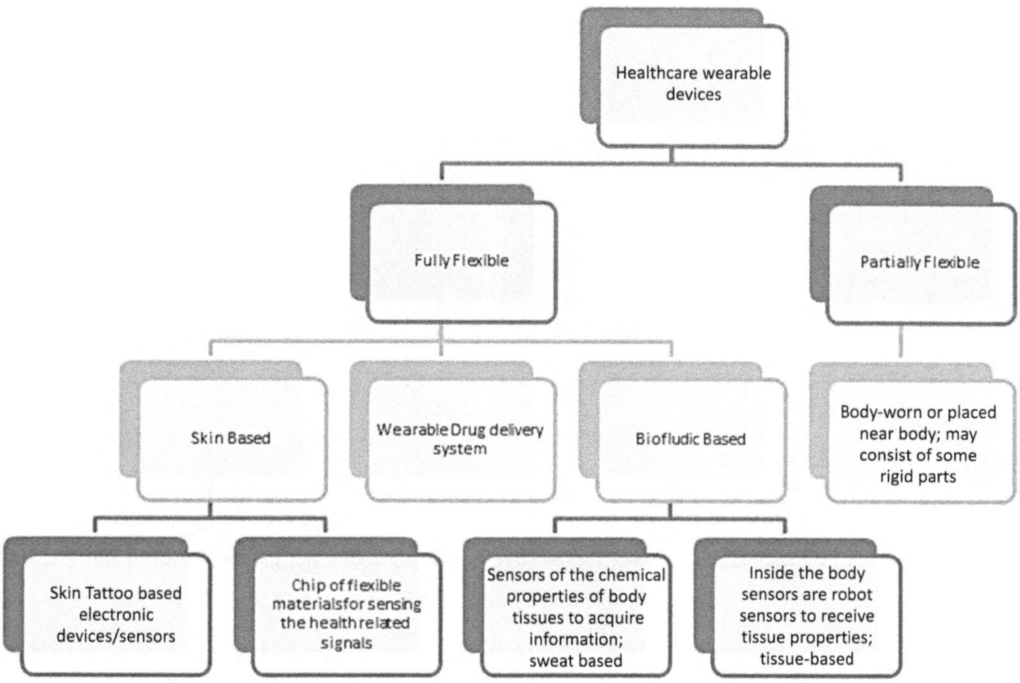


**FIGURE 9.2** Classification of various popular flexible HWDs along with their applications.

with which they may be installed and the amount of comfort that they provide, they can be used for detecting essential parameters like the temperature of the human body, the rate of the heart, and the respiratory system rate (Massaroni et al. 2018; Alizadeh Meghrazi et al. 2020). This allows them to be utilized for the purpose of sensing the body. Electronic textiles or just plain e-textiles are the terms that are most used to refer to this category of HWDs. E-textiles are articles of clothing that are woven with electronic components and sensors. These components allow the garment to perform a variety of functions. Textiles are a great medium for HWDs because of their ability to stretch and their close contact with the skin on a large scale (Choudhry et al. 2020).

Since the discovery of graphene, carbon nanotubes, and nanowires, numerous attempts have been made to integrate sensors into clothing for the purpose of performing continuous monitoring. One such endeavor was undertaken by Yapici and Alkhidir, who developed an intelligent textile-based HWD for the monitoring of ECGs. ECGs are traditionally monitored with gel-based Ag/AgCl electrode cables, which can be uncomfortable for the person who is wearing them. Graphene-functionalized fabric that is embedded with ECG sensors has been developed for use in textile-based ECG monitoring. Since graphene possesses remarkable material qualities and has a strong correlation with conventional gel-based ECG monitoring, it was decided that it would be the best material to be used for this application (Gong et al. 2019; Jayathilaka et al. 2019; Modali et al. 2016; Yapici and Alkhidir 2017; Hajizadegan et al. 2017).

A wearable shirt is depicted in Figure 9.3 and is made up of six electrodes in a dry condition that are sewn into a shirt in order to calculate and measure electrical muscle activity (EMG). After that, the signal processing of these EMG readings is done by a monitoring system that receives them via Bluetooth. If the system detects muscle fatigue, which it does by utilizing the Dimitrov fatigue index (FI), it will notify the user. The results of HWDs made from textiles are distorted because of the lack of tight contact that exists between the skin and the device. To get clean signals, it is necessary to apply further signal processing techniques to the raw data. Only then is it possible to acquire

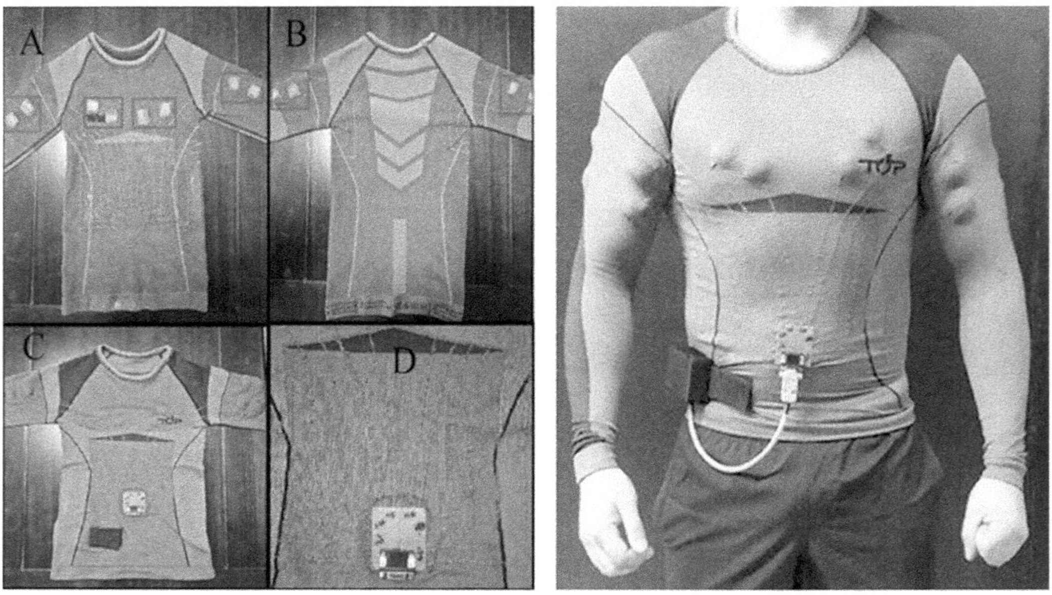


(a) (b)

**FIGURE 9.3** Shirt with hardware connector and textile sensors. (a) A front, B back, C front, D hardware connector and conductive thread. (b) Front view of an EMG shirt with textile electrodes and an acquisition box.

**Source: Dimitrov et al. (2006).**

them. Fabric-based HWDs also provide continuous monitoring in real time and are comfortable to wear. However, due to the incorporation of bio-recognizable molecules, the stability of textile-based HWDs decreases with repeated washing. This is the situation, although these HWDs give continuous and real-time monitoring of the person who is wearing them. Tattoo-based HWDs have the potential to resolve, at least in part, the instability that is associated with textile-based HWDs (Dimitrov et al. 2006).

Due to the adaptability and versatility of the medium, tattoos have long been considered a form of body art. These characteristics are amenable to analysis, which can then provide monitoring and diagnostic data. E-skins are currently being employed to a large extent for the detection of a wide variety of physical and electrical characteristics, including ECG, EEG, and EMG. The easiest of them to recognize is the ECG, which has an amplitude of the order of 1 mV despite its very low voltage. As a result of this, it is now feasible to perform the detection of heart signals via the skin and that is both accurate and non-invasive. In the case of cardiovascular arrhythmias such tachycardia and bradycardia, the ECG is the reference for the diagnosis and management of the condition. To acquire a signal, conventional ECG monitors, as was noted previously, require the connection of a gel-based electrode with cables in addition to other external electronic instrumentation. This can be uncomfortable for the person who is wearing the monitor. It is not possible for the wearer to carry the ECG monitor around with them at all times because they are intended to be used exclusively in clean environments such as medical centers and laboratories. Many patients who are afflicted with heart disease could reap the benefits of continuous monitoring of their heart rhythm; however, a daily visit to a hospital presents both a financial and a logistical challenge. Despite these obstacles, continuous monitoring of heart rhythm could be beneficial to patients. In addition, due to the miniaturization and stretchability of tattoo-based ECG monitoring systems, they are able to resolve the issues of instability and sensitivity that are present in textile-based systems. Additionally, they provide the wearer with increased flexibility and comfort. Figure 9.4 shows a tattoo-based HWD; an ECG monitor provides a notable illustration of this type of monitor (Someya and Amagai 2019; Kabiri Ameri et al. 2017). Also shown are graphene-based electronic tattoo sensors, a gel-based ECG sensor, and the transmission of EMG signals from the forearm using a GET system.

Sweat, saliva, tears, and urine are all examples of secretions that come from the body and contain significant indicators that are necessary for monitoring and diagnostic purposes. These secretions are necessary for purposes such as monitoring and identifying a condition. Direct use of HWDs is possible, as is usage of the devices via their interaction with other platforms. For instance, microfluidic platforms have the potential to be combined to derive relevant information from a wide variety of biofluids (Padash et al., 2020). HWDs have the potential to make use of microfluidic platforms fabricated from a wide variety of materials. Some examples of these platforms include microfluidic devices that are based on polymers, on paper, and on micro-needles (Padash et al. 2020; Li et al. 2020), which are needles that have been shrunk down to a micronized size.

The rest of this section provides an overview of recent efforts on HWDs that are based on biofluids and are organized according to the type of biofluid. Sweat, which is an epidermal biofluid, is a vital indicator of changes taking place inside the human body and can, as a result, serve as an important parameter for chemical and biological sensing. Biomarkers found in sweat include metabolites (such as glucose, lactate, and urea), proteins, nucleotides, and electrolytes (such as chlorine and sodium), all of which have major diagnostic repercussions (Li et al. 2020). Sweat is composed of several biomarkers and is produced by more than 100 glands per square centimeter of skin, making it readily available for chemical analysis. It is dispersed across the entirety of the body. It can therefore be utilized for the extraction of various chemical and biological factors that engage HWDs to provide monitoring and diagnostics in point-of-care settings. This can be accomplished by employing sweat as a solvent (Rhomas et al. 2020).

Tears are another vital biofluid that can be used for the diagnosis and monitoring of a variety of diseases. Diabetes is an example. Moreover, a variety of HWDs have been created specifically for the goal of diagnosing this condition.

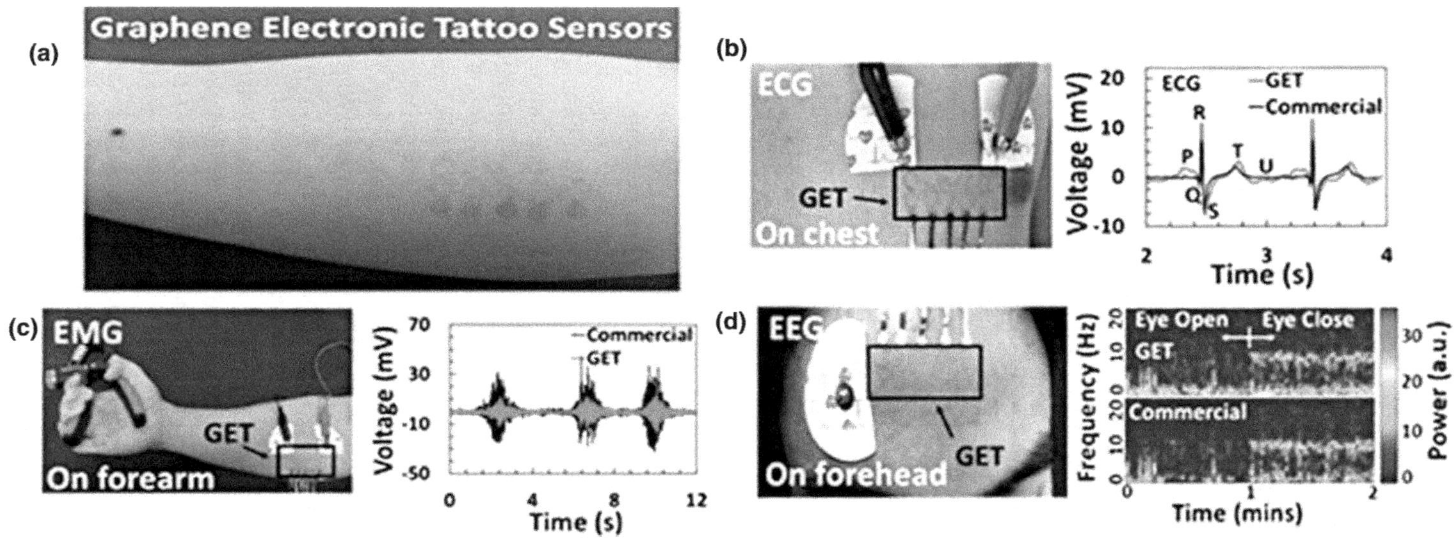


**FIGURE 9.4** (a) Forearm inscribed with a graphene electronic tattoo (GET). (b) The GET ECG is compared to a commercial chest-mounted ECG monitor. (c) Transmission of EMG signals from the forearm using a GET system. (d) The frequency response of EEG under open and closed eye conditions, as measured by GET from the forehead, demonstrates the presence of alpha waves solely when the eyes are closed. This is the case regardless of whether the eyes are open or closed.

**Source: Someya and Amagai (2019) and Kabiri Ameri et al. (2017).**

Diabetes is a metabolic disease that is characterized by excessive levels of glucose or blood sugar and is a chronic condition. If it is not managed, it can lead to serious damage to multiple organs, including the heart, eye, kidneys, nerves, and blood vessels. It is anticipated that the number of diabetic patients will rise, particularly in countries with middle-income and low-income levels, if the appropriate measures are not put in place. From 108 million in 2000 to 463 million in 2020, the number of diabetic patients across the globe has more than quadrupled.

As recommended by the WHO, preventing the complications of diabetes requires maintaining a healthy lifestyle in addition to closely monitoring blood glucose levels. In order to determine the amount of glucose present in the blood, the traditional portable glucometer was developed. However, it requires the patient to endure painful finger sticks, which can expose them to blood-borne pathogens and increase their risk of infection. Urine is another method that can be used to monitor blood glucose; however, it is harder to work with and can impose constraints such as only being useable in the home. The testing done with urine is not nearly as accurate as when blood samples are used. Tears, not blood or urine, can be used as a source for glucose measurement in HWDs, which makes them a more convenient and comfortable alternative to traditional monitoring methods. Because of this, HWDs are an appealing alternative to the more conventional techniques. Researchers led by Sen and Sarin carried out a study in which they measured the amount of glucose present in samples of tear fluid and then connected those findings to the amount of glucose found in blood samples. This proved that tears are an effective method for glucose measurement (Sen and Sarin 1980).

## 9.5 COGNITIVE DISEASE TREATMENT WITH THE ADVANCEMENT OF THE IOT

The twenty-first century is witnessing a rapid digital revolution (Uppal et al. 2021) in which the IoT has become the buzz term in recent years. The notion that real-world physical devices or entities can be managed remotely through the use of the internet is a relatively recent one. The IoT serves humans in many aspects of life; applications include the remote controlling of smart homes, alerts for natural disasters, the health monitoring of patients, and location tracking.

The phrase "Internet of Things" (IoT) is commonly used to refer to anything that can communicate and exchange data with other devices along the course of a network. "Things" or "objects" can refer to any embedded systems or sensors that interact with other systems to collect data, such as the heart rate of a patient, location information, picture recognition, or movement patterns. In this sense, "things" or "objects" can also refer to the same item.

Wearable technology is one of the most essential technologies that is driving the IoT (Izmailova et al. 2018). In a similar vein, wearable computing has implemented and introduced new techniques, more productive processes, and creative goods in a wide variety of fields, such as the entertainment industry, industrial logistics, and sports (Gupta et al. 2012). No other industry anticipates and absorbs wearable technology as fully as healthcare (Amit et al. 2018). A wearable IoT device combined with a smartphone app could be a practical option for healthcare services, operating as a patient's intelligent personal assistant. Well-being, illness prevention, chronic patient care, and other medical disciplines are examples. Wearable assistive technology describes systems or technologies that help people with physical, cognitive, or communicative limitations to improve their quality of life. In recent years, wearable technology has encouraged and empowered healthcare providers to go beyond the clinic or office to help in identifying and recognizing health concerns and tracking illness progression.

## 9.6 PORTABLE/WEARABLE TECHNOLOGIES SPECIFICALLY USED BY AD PATIENTS

Wearable technologies are sensors that can be put to use in order to collect data related to health remotely. These electronics have the potential to play a significant role in the future of healthcare research and development as they are made to monitor round-the-clock and transmit data in real time or on an as-needed basis. An accelerometer built into a bracelet is one type of sensor used to passively collect data on a person's physical activity (Izmailova et al. 2018).

AD is characterized by a slow decline in cognitive abilities over time, including a person's inability to remember recent events or understand spatial relationships between objects. A person who has this disease struggles not only with their memory but also with their ability to process visual information and even with their awareness and the ability to recognize their loved ones. Recent advances in information and communications technology have made it feasible to link everything that is around us on Earth to the internet. The IoT is what has made this feasible, and it could record and store a tremendous quantity of data that is deemed to be both very significant and very helpful. This knowledge, in turn, has the potential to be useful when training various cutting-edge machine learning and deep learning algorithms. When it comes to the ongoing health screening of a patient, helpful mobile health applications and wearable gadgets based on the IoT are giving assistance and support.

In addition to relieving stress on healthcare systems and cutting costs, these technological solutions have the potential to vastly improve the quality of life for those with AD. In the early stages of the disease, wearable gadgets and the IoT strategy aim to keep patients intellectually active in all aspects of life without the assistance of carers or family members. For patients diagnosed with AD, for example, care can be provided in the form of therapy or guidance (Gupta et al. 2016).

Many people are now using wearable devices, but we still need to incorporate the IoT with more advanced AI-based techniques (Obulesu et al. 2012) to improve the quality of life for people who have AD (Salehi et al. 2022). AD and other forms of neurodegeneration are characterized by the gradual decline in cognitive abilities and, ultimately, death as a result of the brain's inability to maintain neural connections. Two significant physiological changes that are associated with neurodegeneration are a rapid loss of brain tissue, known as atrophy, and an expansion of the lateral ventricles. AD patients had a whole-brain atrophy rate of 1.9% (+/– 0.9%) annually, according to a single study, while the rate in healthy elderly people was only 0.44% annually (Sluimer et al. 2008 and Spulber et al. 2010).

According to a report that was compiled for the project by the Centre for Neuroscience and Cell Biology of the University of Coimbra (Chan et al. 2012) AD begins to show its symptoms in a variety of behavioral shifts in the disease's early stages. As seen in Table 9.1, observable changes are presented in descending order according to their frequency.

**TABLE 9.1**
**Observable changes in AD**

| | Shifts in Perception | Ratio of Occurrences (%) | Observed Changes | Percentage |
|---|---|---|---|---|
| 1. | Amnesic deficit | 100 | Psychomotor agitation | 80 |
| 2. | Psychological alterations | 50 | Psychological alterations | 70 |
| 3. | Language alterations | 40 | Psychological symptomatology | 60 |
| 4. | Depressive symptomatology | 30 | Sleep Disturbances | 40 |
| 5. | Anxious symptomatology | 20 | Depressive symptomatology | 20 |
| 6. | Disorientation | 20 | Repetition of the same questions or conversations | 20 |
| 7. | Lack of criticism | 20 | Apraxic changes | 10 |
| 8. | Lack of capacity to organize one's daily schedule | 10 | Executive function skills deficit | 10 |
| 9. | Attention deficit | 10 | Difficulty in identifying one's own family members | 10 |
| 10. | An acute state of confusion | 10 | | |
| 11. | Giving up on leisure pursuits and activities | 10 | | |

These changes in behavior have different repercussions for both the patient's quality of life and the level of assistance required by their caregivers. This analysis ranks the many observable manifestations of the disease according to the impact that is associated with each one.

When it comes to making a diagnosis of the disease, doctors rely on the patient's responses to periodic questionnaires that they give them. These are subject to the patient's subjectivity, the relative importance he or she attributes to events to recall them, and the fact that the patient will leave out some details.

In the case of decline in health in the early stages of disease while the individual is at home or going out, as the patient's condition worsens over time, they will eventually require assistance from their caregivers on occasion. The unpredictability of these times makes it necessary for caregivers to maintain a constant presence and be alert to the possibility that a crisis may develop at any moment.

The development of automatic ways to detect some of the symptoms and/or critical times would have a number of benefits: it could help the doctor make a better diagnosis because he or she would have access to the records of all the detected events, their frequency, severity, etc.; the patient would feel safer because alarms would be sent to caregivers or family members; and caregivers wouldn't have to watch the patient all the time.

The procedure of early diagnosis might become more accurate with the implementation of such a system. Because of this, early treatment, which is the kind of medication known to slow down the progression of the disease, would be possible. On the other hand, if patients are given the idea that they are safe, it is possible for them to progress toward developing typical day-to-day activities. This would reduce the stress that they are experiencing, which is known to influence the advancement of the disease. Because of this, the patient may develop a fear of being committed to a mental institution.

Utilizing Table 9.1 will allow us to try to select symptoms that can be detected by sensors. It is now abundantly clear that "psychomotor agitation" can be measured with accelerometers, whereas all the other variables appear to be difficult to measure with the usual quantities. This is because accelerometers measure acceleration, and psychomotor agitation refers to the amount of that acceleration. Despite this, there are some authors, such as Wendy Mendes (Patel et al. 2012), who state that there is a connection between psychological states and fluctuations in heart rate. They call the connection between the two things electrodermal activity (EDA). This may be a substantial advantage since it may make it possible to design monitoring systems that can assist with the diagnosis of the condition. If this is the case, it would be a significant benefit with the potential to be an asset.

We can recognize two symptoms of AD', namely "psychological alterations" and "psychomotor agitation", which are ranked second and fifth, respectively, in terms of the relative frequency with which they are observed. Both symptoms are ranked in the top five in terms of the severity with which they are observed. The right-hand side of Table 9.1 shows that, among observable symptoms, psychomotor agitation has the greatest effect on both the patient's as well as the caregiver's quality of life. As a result of its potential for detection, it could be used to alert medical staff of the need to assist patients.

## 9.7 DILEMMAS AND POSSIBILITIES IN THE PRACTICAL DESIGN OF WEARABLE MICROWAVE SENSORS/ANTENNA FOR VARIOUS BIOMEDICAL APPLICATIONS

Diagnostic equipment like MRI and CT scans are currently available, but they can be cumbersome, expensive, and challenging for patients to use. Against this, there is a need for new wearable and portable gadgets that can help patients to monitor neurodegeneration without compromising their comfort. In addition, having a portable and wearable device can help doctors assess a patient's neurodegenerative symptoms whenever it is most convenient for them, be it at home or in a clinic. Recent studies have placed microwave radar technology at the forefront of exploration for use in head imaging systems. When compared to other, more conventional ways of diagnosis, microwave radar technology offers several benefits, including low cost, portability, and absence of radiation exposure. Microwave imaging can distinguish between normal and pathological human tissues by measuring their distinct electrical properties.

The major challenge starts here, for the instrument which has to be worn by the patient should be efficient, compact, lightweight, and comfortable for the patient.

In Figure 9.5 the wearable sensor cap is used to capture the signals of the brain (Saeedi et al. 2019). These sensors could be utilized in the area of defense application, rescues in urgent situations, as well as communicating the present situation for real-time tracking.

Radio frequency antennas play a crucial role in microwave head imaging systems. Figure 9.6 depicts the experimental setup. It consists of a vendor neutral archive (VNA), a wearable device with six hybrid silicone-textile sensors and two flexible switching circuits, a host PC, and a skull model with bio-phantoms that mimic the characteristics of the brain when it is damaged by neurodegenerative illnesses (i.e., with different levels of brain atrophy and lateral ventricle enlargement).

In this research, the case of moderate neurodegeneration is linked with a patient who has been afflicted with neurodegeneration for four to five years, whereas the case of severe neurodegeneration is associated with a patient who has been afflicted for nine to ten years. Figure 9.7 shows the

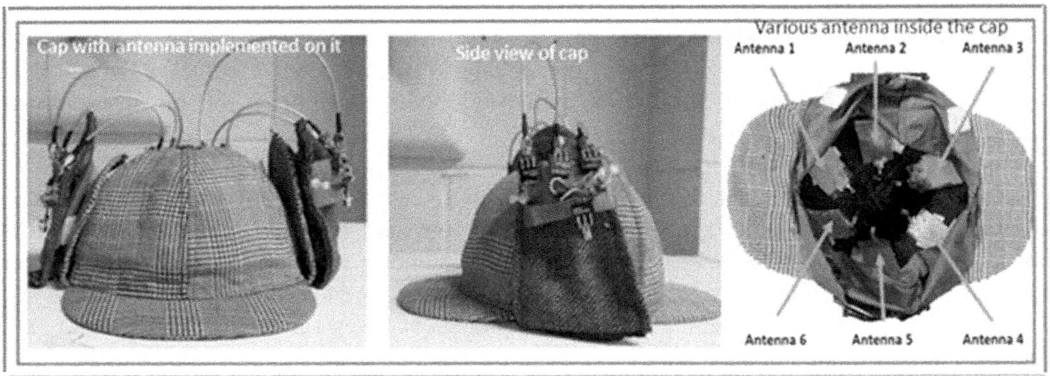


(a) (b) (c)

**FIGURE 9.5** Pictures of a wearable device for monitoring neurodegeneration, showing (a) its front and back, (b) its sides, and (c) its interior.

**Source: Saeedi et al. 2019.**

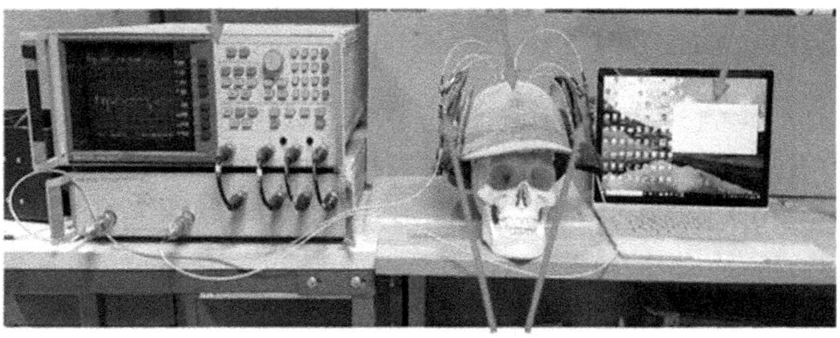


**FIGURE 9.6** The experimental setup.

**Source: Choudhry et al. (2020).**

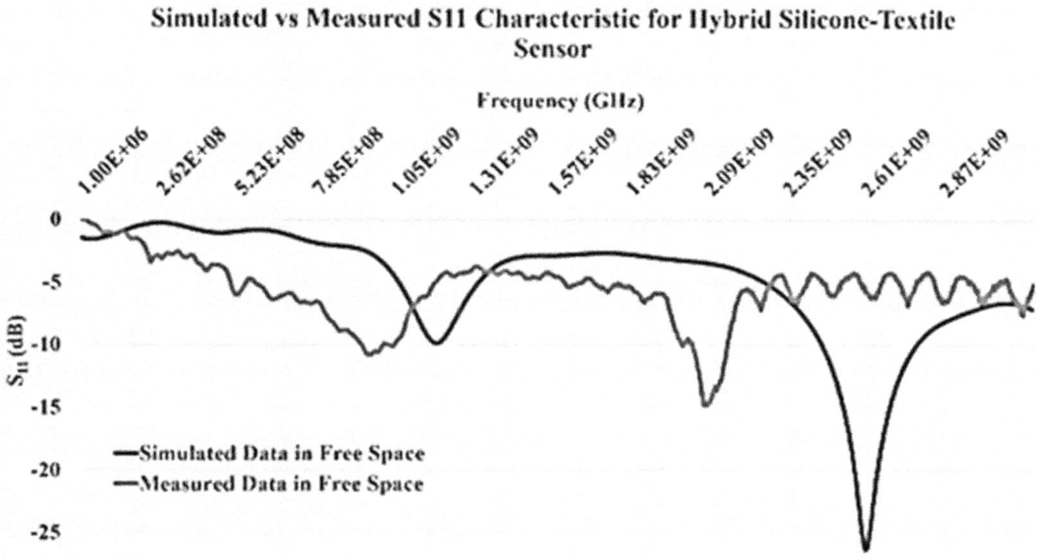


**FIGURE 9.7** Simulated and measured reflection coefficients of the sensor in free space.

**Source: Data taken from Gupta et al., 2016.**

reflection coefficient of the comparison of the measurements and simulation results. This comparison shows a good approximation of the practical device.

The presence of brain shrinkage, also known as a decrease in total brain volume, and lateral ventricle enlargement are two major changes that must be detected so as to identify whether neurodegeneration is happening in an individual's brain. Researchers built many bio-phantoms of varied sizes and volumes and placed them within the skull model to replicate the consequences of brain atrophy. For the sake of emulation, this was carried out. In addition to the thinning of the brain that was seen, the studies also replicated the characteristic of enlarged lateral ventricles. This was accomplished by generating samples of varied sizes using solidified coconut oil to imitate the cerebrospinal fluid (CSF) that collects in the lateral ventricles as they grow larger.

These samples were used to study the effects of the expansion of the lateral ventricles on the brain. This was done in order to simulate the condition of lateral ventricle enlargement. Between 500 and 800 MHz, the relative permittivity of CSF was measured to fall somewhere in the range of 70.0 to 68.9 (Choudhry et al. 2020). On the other hand, the relative permittivity of the solidified coconut oil was at its highest possible level of 364. In order to ensure that the samples of solidified coconut oil and CSF had comparable dielectric characteristics, salt was added to the coconut oil before it was solidified. Approximately 36 milliliters of salt and 56 milliliters of coconut oil were mixed to create the CSF phantom that would be used in the experiment. This was done to simulate the effects of moderate neurodegeneration.

In a similar manner, in the case of severe neurodegeneration, 96 milliliters of salt and 150 milliliters of coconut oil were combined to produce the CSF phantom that was used in the experiment. This phantom was used to simulate the CSF that would be found in a patient with severe neurodegeneration. This technique was used because it was derived from research conducted by Gupta et al. (2016).

In that study, the authors generated CSF objects of varying sizes to simulate the characteristics of enlarged lateral ventricles. This method was used since it was based on that research. Even though the fabricated CSF objects do not accurately represent the fluidic nature of CSF, the samples provide a convenient way to perform the experiments for lateral ventricle enlargement to evaluate the performance of the sensors and switching circuit. These experiments are necessary to determine whether the lateral ventricle enlargement was successful. Experiments like these are required to assess whether the expansion of the lateral ventricle was successful. The CSF distribution will therefore also fit this complex geometry in real life, and therefore the S-parameters that are measured will be different. The true geometry of the lateral ventricles in the brain is far more complex than the sphere object that is used in the experiment, which is an important point to keep in mind. The experiment uses a sphere. In particular, since the S-parameters are influenced by shifts in the dielectric constants, there is a possibility that the S11 measurements taken at different frequencies will differ.

These discrepancies in S11 measurements occur since some of the ventricles in the brain are in closer proximity to the sensor than the cases that were utilized in the studies. These cases were employed in the research. Despite this, it is vital to keep in mind that CSF exhibits a stronger dielectric constant when compared to both gray and white matter. This is the case because CSF is composed of a higher concentration of proteins. When there is a big increase in the amount of CSF in the brain, particularly in the lateral ventricles, there is going to be a major shift in the values of the S-parameters.

Regardless of the geometry of the CSF distribution, microwave imaging techniques provide an alternative to the conventional imaging modalities including computed tomography, magnetic resonant imaging systems, and ultrasound for the diagnosis of a wide range of disorders that can occur inside the human body. Radar-based systems that make use of ultra-wideband (UWB) antennas to produce a usable image of diseases inside the human body are one of the areas of medical microwave imaging that are the subject of extensive research.

There have been several documented attempts at employing microwave systems based on radar for the early diagnosis of breast cancer (Candefjord et al. 2017; Porter et al. 2016; Bond et al. 2003). The findings of a clinical trial that was performed on actual patients for the purpose of diagnosing breast cancer suggest that it may be possible to use microwave technology to supplement the already existing medical imaging systems in the not-too-distant future. The trial was carried out to learn more about breast cancer (Preece et al. 2016).

Recently, microwave technology has also been used for scanning the skull and diagnosing conditions such as stroke and traumatic brain damage (Mobashsher et al. 2014; Candefjord et al. 2017; Persson et al. 2014).

This application of the technology is relatively new. In comparison to the breast, the human head has a more complicated biological structure due to the fact that it is made up of several layers of tissue in addition to the skull (Ireland and Bialkowski 2011). An investigation into the practicability of using UWB microwave technology for head imaging approaches has been carried out with the aid of simulation tools (Zhang et al. 2012). The findings of this inquiry are presented here. It has been hypothesized that the scattered signals produced by a healthy head can be distinguished from those produced by a head that contains cancer cells since there is a discernible difference between the two sets of signals. This is because a healthy head does not contain any tumor cells. The depth of penetration of the electromagnetic wave within the head model is limited because of the employment of a high operating frequency range emitted by the suggested Vivaldian antenna. As a result, it was only possible to identify tumors near the head's periphery.

In addition, there was no switching system employed because the antenna had to be physically positioned around the head for it to work. Mohammed et al. (2014) offer a stroke detection system that makes use of microwave head imaging with UWB Vivaldian antennas. The artificial head phantom was surrounded by an array of 16 Vivaldi antennas, and the distance between the antennas and the head phantom was always kept at half a centimeter. To simulate the effects of a hemorrhagic stroke, an ellipsoidal-shaped target of two centimeters long, one centimeter wide, and half a centimeter thick was placed inside the head phantom.

Figure 9.8 shows that the proposed method was successful in revealing the location of the target stroke. It also shows the connection in a micro-programed controlled system. RF coaxial cable was utilized to receive and send the signal from and to the devices for real-time transmission.

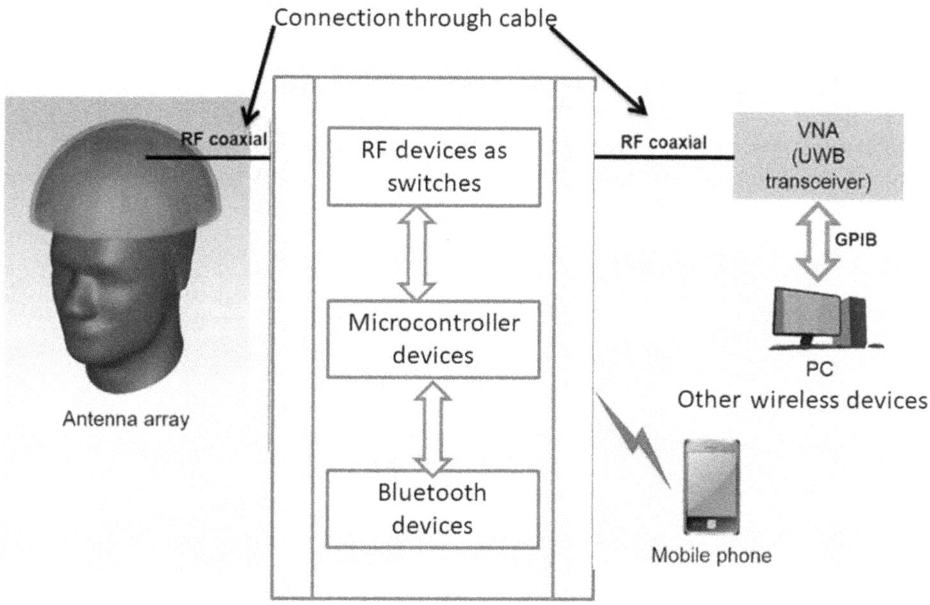


**FIGURE 9.8** Schematic representation of the proposed radio frequency switching system.

**Adopted from: Mohammed et al., 2014.**

In order to develop a wearable head imaging system, it is necessary to design an RF switching circuit for an antenna array (sensors) that is compact and lightweight, and which must make use of components that are readily available for purchase in the marketplace for chronic opioid therapy (COTS). We decided to go with Analog Device's 1P8T switch, HMC321LP4E and 1P4T switch, and HMC241ALP3E evaluation boards designed by Alizadeh Meghrazi et al. (2020) and Choudhry et al. (2020) for our monolithic microwave integrated circuit (MMIC) 1P8T switch and 1P4T switch, respectively. The switches provide a broad operating frequency range that extends from DC to 1 GHz. This frequency range is adequate to handle the operating frequency that is often utilized for head imaging applications. Many of the studies that can be found in the scientific literature use a frequency band that ranges from 1 to 4 GHz (Wimo et al. 2013; Someya et al. 2016; Gong et al. 2019). To achieve sufficient penetration and resolution within the human cranium, the above therapy is performed.

An Arduino Nano board was selected for the purpose of operating the switches based on a number of criteria, among which the most significant are the circuit board's miniature size and the low amount of power consumption. The board and the switches both function at 5 V, and it would be very simple to supply them with a 9 V battery if necessary. The Atmel ATMega328 microcontroller that is built in the Arduino Nano has a very low power consumption of only 0.2 mA while it is in its operational state. To further prove the wearable concept for the head imaging system, which would eventually be integrated with an ultra-wide band UWB transceiver, a microcontroller was integrated with the switches so that it could be used as part of the system on a chip in the future. In contrast, the primary purpose of the microcontroller in this investigation was to exercise control over the switches while the system is being operated and tested.

The selection of each specific port is controlled by the five pins that come from the Arduino board and which are attached to both switches. A wireless link is also established on the system so that a smartphone running Android may be used to control the proposed switching circuit through the utilization of a Bluetooth module. The decision to use a Bluetooth module, rather than a Wi-Fi module, was made due to the former's significantly lower power consumption when compared to the latter. This helped bring the whole system's power consumption down to an even lower level. An Android application was developed and then installed on a mobile phone in order to provide a graphical user interface.

To investigate the capabilities of the RF switches, the insertion losses in the frequency spectrum up to 3 GHz were measured by a vector network analyzer. This is shown in Figure 9.9 as illustration of this measurement. After that, the performance of their impedance matching was evaluated

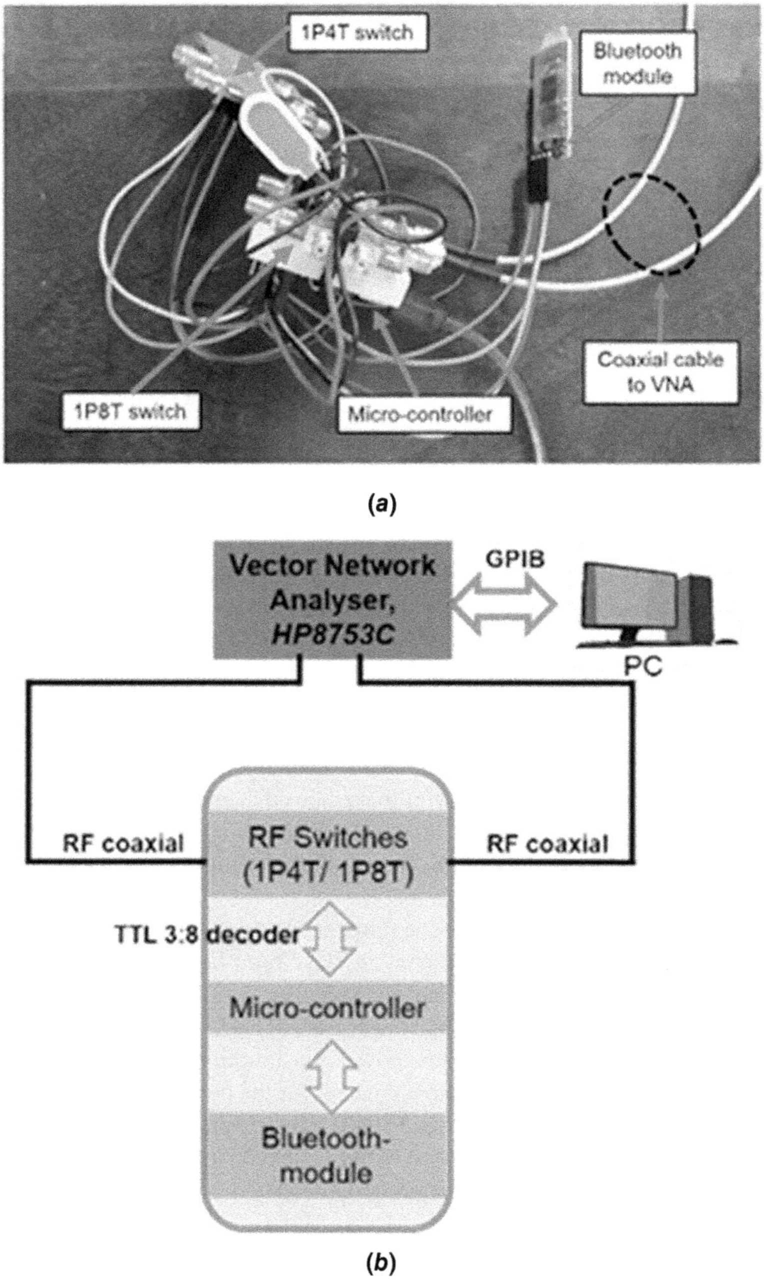


**FIGURE 9.9** The suggested measurement test configuration for the RF switching system. (a) Photograph of the measurement test setup of RF switches; (b) Diagram of the RF switches. (Based on the measurement setup designed in Mohammed et al., 2014).

using the reflection coefficient as the metric. In conclusion, a connection was made between the suggested switching system and a collection of 12 UWB monopole antennas. For performing additional research, measurements of the reflection and transmission coefficients were carried out while an artificial head phantom was present. Figure 9.10 illustrates the positioning of the antennas that were attached to the head phantom. For the sake of clarity, the lossy dielectric absorber has been omitted from the figure.

The absorber was attached to the antennas during the measurements in order to dampen the back lobe effect. The aim was to prevent the system from picking up on any unwanted background noise. Figure 9.11 shows that the values of the reflection coefficients of the three antennas (Antenna1,

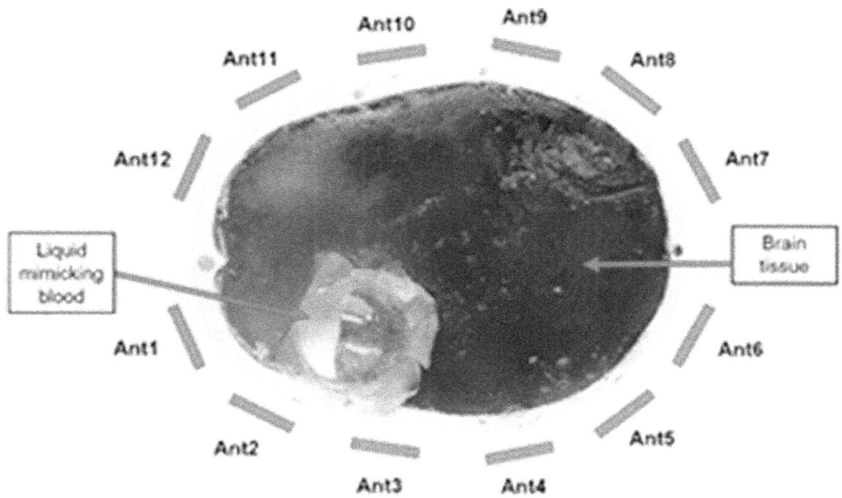


(a)

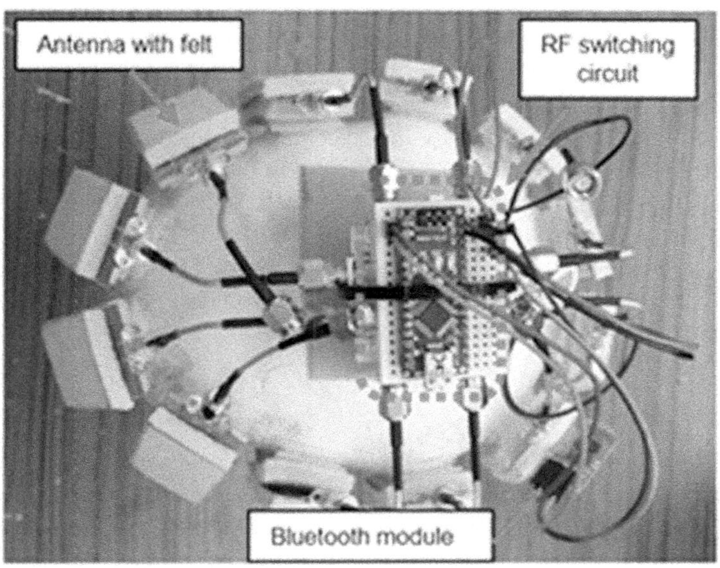


(b)

**FIGURE 9.10** (a) Position of the blood clot phantom within the cranium of the patient; (b) The positioning of the antennas as well as the switching system (top view).

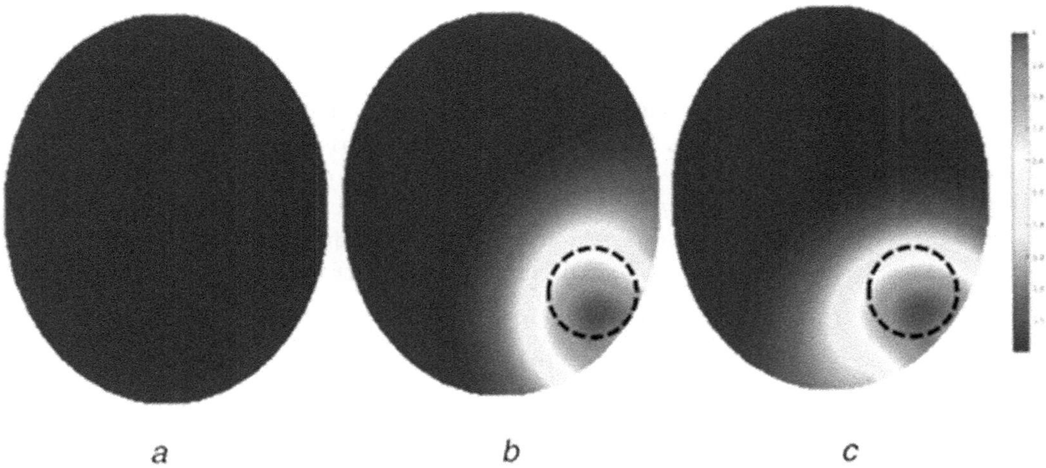


**FIGURE 9.11** (a) The head of the healthy human being; (b) the diseased head without switching the circuit head; and (c) the head with the switching circuit – the dashed black circles pinpoint the exact positions of the blood spots on the map reported in Mobashsher and Abbosh (2016).

Antenna2, and Antenna3) closest to the spherical target differ significantly between the healthy and unhealthy head, corroborating the finding reported in Mobashsher and Abbosh (2016).

Depicted in Figure 9.11 are the heads of individuals who are healthy as well as those who are unwell. Another picture of the head with the stroke, which was made without using the switching circuit, is also shown here. This one was also produced. This picture is intended to serve as a point of comparison with a system that does not contain the RF switching circuit. Both images demonstrate that the stroke has been identified and positioned precisely in the brain. This suggests that the performance of the RF switching circuit that has been presented is comparable to that of the system which does not have the switching circuit. It is possible to improve the imaging system's resolution and accuracy by increasing the number of antennas that are used; however, doing so will necessitate the utilization of a more substantial wearable device in order to accommodate the additional antennas, in addition to an increase in the amount of time that is required for the data acquisition process.

The most promising feature (polymers which are used for flexible antennas) is also being incorporated in the field of flexible electronics for the detection of biomedical purposes (Sangeeta et al. 2022; Yempally et al. 2022; Yempally et al. 2021). The most important discovery made by Sangeeta et al. (2022), which linked to the selection of flexible materials, particularly polymers, for the flexible antenna, was that polymers were the best option. The application is for the identification of biological signals, namely for the purpose of patient monitoring. There is a wealth of opportunities to discover the flexible sensors and antenna designing as a component of the IoT system for early stage detection and to make a patient's life significantly better.

## 9.8 CONCLUSION

The era of centralized IT systems for storing, processing, producing, and managing health-related data is giving way to a new model period of distributed data sharing between patients and caregivers or doctors, and wearables are assisting in this transition. Second, data from wearables and the IoT might be used to educate AI to make more accurate automated diagnoses and more effective medicines. Wearable computing enables the incorporation of dispersed data into a personalized healthcare system. Health data updates and preventative measures are encouraged. Wearable technologies and digital health care have enormous promise to improve health while also advancing technology. This chapter has presented an overview of the wearable devices that have been created to help people with AD. Various applications of flexible electronic sensors and antennas have been described in depth. The extensive study's main takeaway is the design of a comfortable and lightweight system to detect certain signals. The biomedical applications of such flexible sensing systems and antennas have been primarily investigated using performance metrics such as efficiency, comfort, light weight, return loss, and radiation characteristics. Wearable computing is undergoing a significant paradigm shift in the field of digital health. The goal here was to investigate cutting-edge technology solutions and IoT-based wearable gadgets that can help AD caregivers and patients. Future healthcare advancements will be heavily reliant on current research, particularly in the areas of the IoT and wearable applications. Future research should address the study's weaknesses, and consumer perceptions about IoT-based wearables should be examined. Similarly, when searching for a helpful, desirable, and user-friendly instrument, consider its form, size, and functionality.

## REFERENCES


Alizadeh Meghrazi, M. et al. 2020. Multichannel ECG recording from waist using textile sensors. *Biomedical Engineering* 19: 1–18.

Amft, O. 2018. How wearable computing is shaping digital health. *IEEE Pervasive Computing* 17: 92–98.

Bhalla, N., Jolly, P., Formisano, N., Estrela, P. 2016. Introduction to biosensors. *Essays Biochemistry* 60: 1–8.

Bond, E. J., Li, X., Hagness, S. C. et al. 2003. Microwave imaging via space-time beamforming for early detection of breast cancer. *IEEE Transactions on Antennas and Propagation* 51: 1690–1705.

Candefjord, S., Winges, J., Malik, A. A. et al. 2017. Microwave technology for detecting traumatic intracranial bleedings: tests on phantom of subdural hematoma and numerical simulations. *Medical & Biological Engineering & Computing* 55: 1177–1188.

Chan, M., et al. 2012. Smart wearable systems: Current status and future challenges. *Artificial Intelligence Medical* 56: 137–156.

Choudhry, N. A., Rasheed, A., Ahmad, S., Arnold, L., Wang, L. 2020. Design, development and characterization of textile stitch-based piezoresistive sensors for wearable monitoring. *IEEE Sensor Journal* 20: 10485–10494.

Dimitrov, G. V. et al. 2006. Muscle fatigue during dynamic contractions assessed by new spectral indices. *Medicine & Science in Sports & Exercise* 38: 1971–1979.

Elhayatmy, G., Dey, N., Ashour, A. S. 2017. *Internet of Things and Big Data Analytics toward Next-Generation Intelligence*. Springer.

Fear, E. C., Stuchly, M. A. 2000. Microwave detection of breast cancer. IEEE Trans. Microw. *Theories of Technology* 48: 1854–1863.

Feiner, R., Dvir, T. 2017. Tissue–electronics interfaces: from implantable devices to engineered tissues. *Nature Reviews Materials* 3: 165–176. https://doi.org/10.1038/natrevmats.2017.76

Gong, Z. et al. 2019. Wearable fiber optic technology based on smart textile: a review. *Materials* 12: 3311.

Gupta, G. et al. 2016. Mobile health applications and android toolkit for Alzheimer patients. *Caregivers and Doctors* 11(1): 199–205.

Gupta, M. et al. 2012. An intelligent session key-based hybrid lightweight image encryption algorithm using logistic-tent map and crossover operator for internet of multimedia things. *Wireless Personal Communications* 121: 1857–1878.

Hajizadegan, M. et al. 2017. Graphene sensing modulator: toward low-noise, self-powered wireless micro sensors. *IEEE Sensor Journal* 17: 7239–7247.

Hurd, M. D. et al. 2013. Monetary costs of dementia in the United States. *New England Journal of Medicine* 368(14): 1326–1334.

Iqbal, S. M. A., Butt, N. Z. 2019. Design and analysis of microfluidic cell counter using spice simulation. *Applied Physics* 1: 1–10.

Ireland, D., Bialkowski, M. E. 2011. Microwave head imaging for stroke detection. *Prog. Electromagn. Res. Magn.* 21: 163–175.

Izmailova, E. S., Wagner, J. A., Perakslis, E. D. 2018. Wearable devices in clinical trials: hype and hypothesis. *Clinical Pharmacology & Therapeutics* 104: 42–52.

Jayathilaka, W. A. D. M. et al. 2019. Significance of nanomaterial in wearables: a review on wearable actuators and sensors. *Advance Material* 31: 1–21.

Kabiri Ameri, S. et al. 2017. Graphene electronic tattoo sensors. *ACS Nano* 11: 7634–7641.

Kim, J., Campbell, A. S., de Ávila, B. E. F., Wang, J. 2019. Wearable biosensors for healthcare monitoring. *National Biotechnology* 37: 389–406.
Kozitsina, A. N. et al. 2018. Sensors based on bio and biomimetic receptors in medical diagnostic, environment, and food analysis. *Bio-sensors* 34: 1–34.
Li, S., Ma, Z., Cao, Z., Pan, L., Shi, Y. 2020. Advanced wearable microfluidic sensors for healthcare monitoring. *Small* 16: 1903822.
Lin, Y., Bariya, M., Javey, A. 2021. Wearable biosensors for body computing. *Advanced Functional Materials* John Wiley & Sons Ltd.
Ling, Y. et al. 2019. Disruptive, soft, wearable sensors. *Advance Materials* 32(18).
Massaroni, C. et al. 2018. Smart textile for respiratory monitoring and thoracoabdominal motion pattern evaluation. *Journal of Biophotonics* 11: 1–12.
Mobashsher, A. T., Abbosh, A. M. 2016. Compact 3-D slot-loaded folded dipole antenna with unidirectional radiation and low impulse distortion for head imaging applications. *IEEE Transaction Antennas Propagation* 64: 3245–3250.
Mobashsher, A. T., Abbosh, A. M., Wang, Y. 2014. Microwave system to detect traumatic brain injuries using compact unidirectional antenna and wide band transceiver with verification on realistic head phantom. *IEEE Transactions on Microwave Theory and Techniques* 62: 1826–1836.
Modali, A., Vanjari, S. R. K., Dendukuri, D. 2016. Wearable woven electrochemical biosensor patch for non-invasive diagnostics. *Electro Analysis* 28: 1276–1282.
Mohammed, B. J., Abbosh, A. M., Mustafa, S. et al. 2014. Microwave system for head imaging. *IEEE Transactions on Instrumentation and Measurement* 63: 117–123.
Obulesu, O., Kallam, S., Dhiman, G. et al. 2012. Adaptive diagnosis of lung cancer by deep learning classification using Wilcoxon gain and generator. *Journal of Healthcare Engineering* doi: 10.1155/2023/9765029
Padash, M., Enz, C., Carrara, S. 2020. Microfluidics by additive manufacturing for wearable biosensors: a review. *Sensors* 20: 1–28.
Pantelopoulos, A., and Bourbakis, N. G. 2010. A survey on wearable sensor-based systems for health monitoring and prognosis. *IEEE Transactions on Systems Man and Cybernetics Part C* 40: 1–12.
Patel, S., et al. 2012. A review of wearable sensors and systems with application in rehabilitation. *Journal of NeuroEngineering and Rehabilitation* 9: 1–17.
Persson, M., Fhager, A., Dobsicek Trefna, H. et al. 2014. Microwave-based stroke diagnosis making global pre-hospital thrombolytic treatment possible. *IEEE Transactions on Biomedical Engineering* 61:2806–2817.
Porter, E., Bahrami, H., Santorelli, A. et al. 2016. A wearable microwave antenna array for time-domain breast tumor screening. *IEEE Transactions on Medical Imaging* 35: 1501–1509.
Preece, A. W., Craddock, I., Shere, M. et al. 2016. MARIA m4: clinical evaluation of a prototype ultra wide-band radar scanner for breast cancer detection. *Journal of Medical Imaging* 3: 33502.
Saeedi, P. et al. 2019. Global and regional diabetes prevalence estimates for 2019 and projections for 2030 and 2045: Results from the International Diabetes Federation Diabetes Atlas, 9th edition. *Diabetes Research and Clinical Practice* 157: 107843.
Saied, M., Chandran, S., Arslan, T. 2019. Integrated flexible hybrid silicone-textile dual-resonant sensors and switching circuit for Wearable Neurodegeneration Monitoring Systems. *IEEE Transactions on Biomedical Circuits and Systems* 13: 1304–1312.
Salehi, W., Baglat, P. 2020. Alzheimer's disease diagnosis using deep learning techniques. *International Journal of Engineering and Advanced Technology* 3: 874–880.
Salehi, W. et al. 2022. IoT-based wearable devices for patients suffering from Alzheimer disease. *Contrast Media & Molecular Imaging* 1–15: 3224939.
Sen, D. K., Sarin, G. S. 1980. Tear glucose levels in normal people and in diabetic patients. *British Journal of Ophthalmology* 64: 693–695.
Shekhawat, S., Singh, S., Singh, S. K. 2022. A review on bending analysis of polymer-based flexible patch antenna for IoT and wireless applications. *Materials Today Proceeding* 66: 3511–3516.
Sluimer, J. D. et al. 2008. Whole-brain atrophy rate in Alzheimer disease: identifying fast progressors. *Neurology* 70: 1836–1841.
Someya, T., Amagai, M. 2017. Toward a new generation of smart skins. *Nature Biotechnology* 37: 382–388.
Someya, T., Amagai, M. 2019. Toward a new generation of smart skins. *Nature Biotechnology* 37: 382–388.
Someya, T., Bao, Z., Malliaras, G. G. 2016. The rise of plastic bioelectronics *Nature* 540: 379–385.
Spulber, G., Niskanen, E., MacDonald, S. et al. 2010. Whole brain atrophy rate predicts progression from MCI to Alzheimer's disease. *Neurobiology of Aging* 31: 1601–1605.
Thomas, S. 2020. Research highlights. *Nature Electronics*. https://doi.org/10.1039/c1lc90074a

Uppal, M. et al. 2021. Cloud-based fault prediction using IoT in office automation for improvisation of health of employees. *Journal of Healthcare Engineering* 24: 100–113.
Wearable Sensors Market Worth $2.86 Billion by 2025|CAGR: 38.8%. Available online: http://www.webcitation.org/73HUXmOKl (Accessed on 19 October 2018).
WHO. Diabetes. https://www.who.int/es/news-room/fact-sheets/detail/diabetes (2018).]
Wimo, A., et al. 2013. The worldwide economic impact of dementia 2010. *Alzheimer's and Dementia* 9(1): 1–11.
Xie, J., Chen, Q., Shen, H., Li, G. 2020. Review-wearable graphene devices for sensing. *Journal of the Electrochemical Society* 167: 1–11.
Yapici, M. K., Alkhidir, T. E. 2017. Intelligent medical garments with graphene functionalized smart-cloth ECG sensors. *Sensors* 17: 1–12.
Yempally, S., Singh, S. K., Velliangiri, S. 2021. Review of an IoT-based remote patient health monitoring system. Smart technologies, communication and robotics (STCR). *Sathyamangalam* 10: 1–5.
Yempally, S., Singh, S. K., Velliangiri, S. 2022. Analytical review on deep learning and IoT for smart healthcare monitoring system. *International Journal of Intelligent Unmanned Systems.*
Zhang, H., Flynn, B., Erdogan, A. T. et al. 2012. Microwave imaging for brain tumor detection using an UWB Vivaldi antenna array *Loughborough Antennas & Propagation Conference (LAPC)*, Loughborough.

# 10 Prediction and Maintenance of Alzheimer's Disease using Ultrasound and Infrared Spectroscopy Sensors/Augmented Reality Techniques

*Sasi Smitha and B. V. Srividya*
Dayanand Sagar College of Engineering, Bengaluru, India

## 10.1 INTRODUCTION

Minimal progress has been made in therapy despite research deepening our understanding of the cellular pathology of Alzheimer's disease (AD) because the signs and symptoms appear gradually, masking the continuous decline until a diagnosis can be made. Clinical dementia tests use neurological, cognitive, and imaging data to make diagnoses of probable AD or senile dementia of the Alzheimer type. The only method to definitively diagnose AD in such cases is a post-mortem neuropathological analysis of the brain tissue (Gupta et al. 2018).

Positron emission tomography (PET) and magnetic resonance imaging (MRI) have dramatically changed how AD is studied and how medical diagnoses are made (Gupta et al. 2018). High quality pictures that accurately reflect the neuropathological features of AD can be created, such as neurofibrillary tangles and amyloid plaques in the case of PET and cortical atrophy indicative of the progressive neurodegeneration of AD in the case of MRI. Measurements of endogenous CEST MRI cannot substitute for pHe measurements with acido-CEST MRI. Whereas endogenous CEST MRI may still have good utility for evaluating some specific pathologies, exogenous acido-CEST MRI is more appropriate when evaluating pathologies based on pHe values. Evaluation of dynamic AD processes including regional haemoglobin oxygenation and glucose uptake can be done using FDG-PET and BOLD-MRI, respectively (Sendra et al. 2018).

## 10.2 DETECTION OF AD USING INFRARED ANALYSIS SENSORS

### 10.2.1 Infrared Spectrography Sensors

The investigation of a molecule's interactions with infrared light is known as infrared spectroscopy. This can be looked at using measurements of absorption, emission, and reflection in three different ways (Xu et al. 2001).

Quick identification and evaluation of the results of early interventions may be made possible by a non-invasive technology that looks for changes in the structure and makeup of brain tissue. This might significantly speed up the creation of cures and preventative measures. Near-infrared spectroscopy, in particular, can be beneficial in probing deeper layers of tissue. Optical spectroscopy


DOI: 10.1201/9781003245346-10

can non-invasively capture chemical and structural information (Varatharajan et al. 2018). Since these wavelengths are only weakly absorbed and heavily forward dispersed, near-infrared light must travel several centimetres through tissue to reach the brain from the surface of the scalp. The clinical spectrometer system we are building was used to gather diffuse scattering spectra between 650 and 1050 nm (Chong et al. 2017). Fibre guide manufacturing has optical fibre components, which are two fibre optic probes with an internal design and manufacture.

A specially made spacing template and an elastic headband were used to position the fibre optics at the subject's temple region. A continuous-wave tungsten halogen source was used as the source probe (single fibre, low-OH, 600 mm core, NA = 0.22) to deliver near-infrared light. The detector probe was used to collect diffusely scattered light at different source-detector separations (10–30 mm in 5 mm increments) and send it to an imaging spectrograph connected to a charged-coupled device (CCD) detector cooled to −50 °C (Chong et al. 2017).

Over the past 20 years, the optical imaging method known as functional near-infrared spectroscopy (fNIRS) has been used more and more in the field of neuroimaging. It measures the variations in the concentrations of oxygenated haemoglobin (HbO) and deoxygenated haemoglobin (HbR) linked to the metabolic activity of neurons in the outer layers of the cortex using near infrared lasers at two different wavelengths (between 600 and 1000 nm). Previous research has demonstrated a strong association between the blood oxygen level dependent (BOLD) response produced by fMRI and the haemodynamic response assessed by fNIRS, making the two modalities roughly equivalent (Agüera-Ortiz et al. 2017).

However, fNIRS has many advantages over fMRI and PET, including being non-invasive, having a higher temporal resolution, being highly portable, being less expensive, being less susceptible to movement artefacts, being free of ionising radiation, and putting less strain on subjects during the measurement (Ishii et al. 2016). By monitoring cerebral haemodynamic responses, fNIRS also offers functional imaging. Due to these advantages, fNIRS may be used in place of fMRI and PET for the quick, non-invasive diagnosis or treatment monitoring of AD patients in clinic settings (Ruiz-Rizzo et al. 2017).

### 10.2.2 Digit Verbal Span Task

To minimize environmental disturbance, all studies were conducted in a small space. Subjects were advised to relax for three minutes while keeping their eyes closed before starting the experimental task. During this time, a baseline fNIRS measurement was taken. After that, subjects underwent a digital verbal span task (DVST) comprised of 30 distinct blocks as shown in Figure 10.1(a). Each block began with an encoding assignment that required the subjects to memorize a series of numbers that were displayed on a computer screen 1.5 metres in front of them, as shown Figure 10.1(b).

Number sequences, which ranged in length from four to six digits and had digits ranging from 1 to 9, were displayed for ten seconds before fading. After encoding, there was a ten-second resting time during which the patient was instructed to maintain their composure. After that, participants were told to recall the number verbally, and their responses were recorded for performance evaluation (Atkinson et al. 2015). All 30 sequences were distinct and randomly shown to the subjects during the experiment in order to reduce the subject-expectancy effect. The job was well explained to participants before the experiment's start, and enough time was given for practice so that everyone was comfortable with the methods.

### 10.2.3 fNIRS Configuration

A multi-channel NIRScout system (NIRx Medizintechnik GmbH, Germany) comprising 15 emitters and 16 detectors at a sampling rate of 3.91 Hz was used in this study to measure the fNIRS signals. At 760 and 850 nm, respectively, oxy- and deoxy-haemoglobin were identified. Inter-optode distances were established at 3 cm in accordance with the global 10-20 electroencephalography

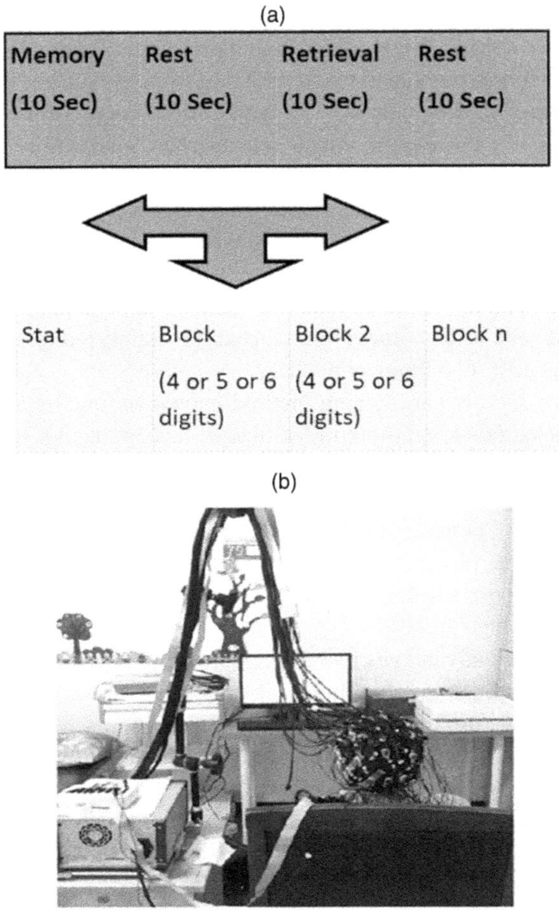


**FIGURE 10.1** Block encoding assignment of FNIRS. (a) The subjects memorize a series of numbers that were (b) displayed on a computer screen 1.5 metres in front of them.

(EEG) placement scheme, and a total of 46 measurement channels were evenly distributed over the frontal and bilateral parietal regions as shown in Figure 10.2(a). Using plastic grommets and holders, all emitters and detectors were fastened to an elastic cap to ensure the optodes made sufficient contact with the subject's cranium. As seen in Figure 10.2, an emitter–detector pair was used to describe an fNIRS channel as shown in Figure 10.2(b).

### 10.2.4 Data Pre-processing

MATLAB was used to analyse and examine the fNIRS data for each subject separately. Each fNIRS channel was visually examined, and those with significant spikes were designated as "noisy" and disregarded for further study. In order to reduce artefacts like respiration (0.2–0.3 Hz) and cardiac interference from the fNIRS data, a fourth-order Butterworth band-pass filter with cut-off frequencies of 0.01–0.20 Hz was used in the processing (0.8 Hz). When the differences in haemoglobin concentration were computed using the Modified Beer–Lambert Law, the differential path length factors for the higher (850 nm) and lower (760 nm) wavelengths were 6.38 and 7.15, respectively (HbO and HbR).

This is due to the fact that the HbO signal has a greater connection with the fMRI BOLD response and is thought to be a more reliable and sensitive fNIRS parameter compared to HbR to

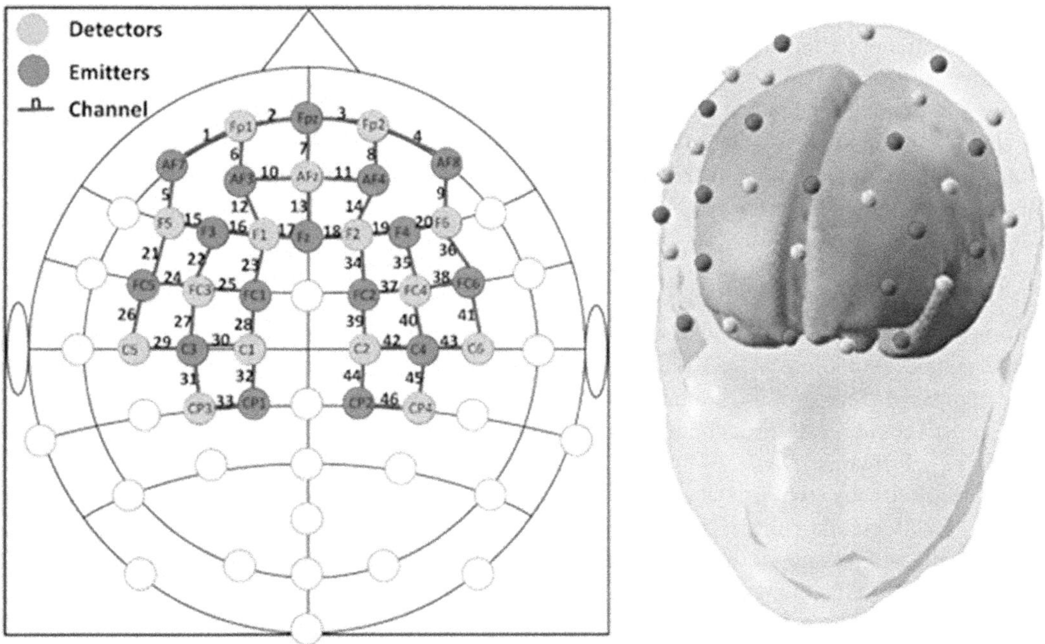


(a) (b)

**FIGURE 10.2** (a) The layout of the channels and fNIRS optodes. Purple lines and numbers define fNIRS channels, while red circles define the emitters and green circles describe the detectors. The worldwide 10-20 EEG placement locations are identified by labels inside of the circles. Channels 1–20 in the frontal area, 21–33 in the left parietal, and 34–46 in the right parietal. (b) An example of the common 3-D head model with nirsLAB-produced emitters (red dots) and detectors (yellow dots) (NIRx Medizintechnik GmbH, Germany).

task-associated changes. Additionally, in pertinent ageing investigations, HbO has been described as a more preferable marker for defining the ageing effect.

Each block's HbO signal was divided into 30 trials with a 20-second interval beginning at the start of the encoding task for each cleaned fNIRS channel. A grand-averaged HbO signal was then obtained for each channel and each subject by averaging all segmented HbO signals. These averaged HbO signals were used for further research.

### 10.2.5 Data Analysis

The frontal, left parietal, and right parietal regions of the brain have been of interest in this investigation because of prior work that yielded significant results in the mild cognitive impairment (MCI)/AD group. Researchers thus manually assigned a predetermined number of fNIRS channels to the pertinent locations, as illustrated in Figure 10.2. These active channel selection strategies, including a t-values-based approach and an amplitude-based approach, that were applied in other studies were ineffective for this one due to the anomalous haemodynamic responses from four different groups that were at variance with canonical haemodynamic responses.

In order to obtain a single, representative HbO signal for each area of interest (ROI) for each person, this study averaged the HbO signals from all cleaned fNIRS channels in the same brain region.

Two parameters – the mean change in HbO concentration (MHbO) and the slope of the HbO change (SPHbO) – were calculated for each of the four groups based on the pre-processing techniques previously mentioned. Previous research has shown that variations in HbO concentration frequently correspond to changes in the metabolic activity of nearby neurons, which is related to their functional activity and may take up to 10 seconds to reach a substantial level of activation.

A 3–12 second frame was employed to calculate the MHbO out of each area of the brain. The SPHbO, on the other hand, was described as the linear rate at which the HbO signal varies so that it reaches its peak or nadir within 10 seconds beginning at the task's onset. It demonstrated how a certain part of the brain reacted to the task. Before performing a simple linear regression to calculate the slope between the task's start and the observed peak, researchers first determined the time point at which the absolute value of the HbO signal peaked. The coefficient of the linear regression model was then determined to be the SPHbO in each ROI.

### 10.2.6 Statistical Analysis

By considering two-sample t-tests with a Bonferroni–Holm multi-comparison adjustment, mini-mental state examination (MMSE) scores and task performance differences between the four groups were compared (four groups, a total of six comparisons). The number of accurate sequences that each subject could recall throughout the retrieval test – up to a maximum of 30 – was used to assess their task performance.

In a nutshell, any two groups were compared using the two-sample t-test, which produced six p-values for all comparisons. The multi-comparison Bonferroni–Holm correction was then carried out. The adjusted p-value of the *i*th comparison (p′i p′i) was determined by first sorting all p-values from the lowest to the highest (pi, I = 1, 2, … 6).

$$\text{p}'\text{i} = \text{ptargetn} - \text{i} + 1\text{p}'\text{i} = \text{ptargetn} - \text{i} + 1$$

where ptarget is the target significant level in the test, which was set to 0.05 in this research, and n denotes the total number of comparisons in this study. Researchers considered the difference of the *i*th comparison was significant if pi is less than p′ip′i.

$$\frac{d^2R}{dt^2} = \frac{3P_0}{\rho R} + \frac{3\sigma}{4\Pi\rho R^2} \tag{10.1}$$

Because of small variations of radius, equation (10.1) can be written as

$$\frac{d^2R}{dt^2} = \frac{3P_0}{\rho}\left(\frac{1}{R_0} - \frac{(R-R_0)}{R_0^2}\right) + \frac{3\sigma}{4\Pi\rho}\left(\frac{1}{R^2} - \frac{2(R-R_0)}{R_0^2}\right) \tag{10.2}$$

or

$$\frac{d^2R}{dt^2} = -\left(\frac{3P_0}{\rho R_0^2} + \frac{3\sigma}{2\Pi R_0^3}\right)R + \left(\frac{6P_0}{\rho R_0} + \frac{9\sigma}{4\Pi\rho R_0^2}\right) \tag{10.3}$$

So the natural frequency of the oscillation of the holes is

$$f_0 = \frac{1}{2\Pi R_0}\sqrt{\frac{3P_0}{\rho} + \frac{3\sigma}{4\Pi\rho R_0}} \tag{10.4}$$

The MHbO and SPHbO for each brain region were among the fNIRS-derived indexes that were similarly evaluated using two-sample t-tests with a Bonferroni–Holm multi-comparison adjustment (four groups, six comparisons in total). Finally, Pearson's correlation coefficients between the

MMSE scores and the fNIRS-derived indexes were calculated with a significance threshold of 0.05 in order to assess the relationship between haemodynamic signals and clinical rating scores.

A predictive maintenance programme needs sensor data to work effectively. IoT sensors collect data on a variety of machine characteristics, such as temperature, pressure, and sound. When comparing the temperature differences between devices in a single image or across numerous views over time, infrared sensors are specifically used. Sensors use infrared radiation (IR) to detect current or impending problems with many kinds of assets, parts, and materials. The sensor determines an element's temperature by measuring the variable intensities of light from a radiation's wavelength, which is invisible to human sight. In one or more views, IR can compare temperature differences between components.

An IR sensor is a piece of technology that produces light to identify items that are close. An IR sensor may detect movement in addition to tracking an object's temperature. Typically, all objects emit some form of infrared thermal radiation. Despite being undetectable to the human eye, these radiations can be detected by infrared sensors (Szczésniak and Rymaszewska, 2016).

The emitter is only an IR LED, and the detector is only an IR photodiode (light emitting diode). The most significant difference between an LED and a photodiode is in the way they function. An LED converts electrical energy into light, while a photodiode converts light energy into electrical energy. A photodiode can pick up infrared light at the same wavelength as an IR LED emits. When IR light strikes the photodiode, the resistances and output voltages change in direct proportion to the amount of IR light received. The five essential elements of a typical infrared detection system are an infrared source, a transmission channel, an optical component, infrared detectors or receivers, and signal processing. Infrared lasers and LEDs with a specific wavelength are examples of infrared sources. The three most common types of infrared transmission medium are a vacuum, an atmosphere, and fibre optics (Teipel et al. 2015).

## 10.3 AD EARLY DIAGNOSIS METHODS USING AR/VIRTUAL REALITY FOR COGNITIVE ASSESSMENT

The deterioration of numerous cognitive functions is a hallmark of the dementia syndrome. Its implications include a high fatality rate as well as considerable expenses for patient care, tests, and therapies. While there is currently no known cure for dementia, receiving a fast diagnosis can help patients get the necessary care, medication, and, to the greatest extent feasible, continue to participate in intellectual, social, and physical activities. Early AD detection is believed to significantly improve the quality of life for patients and their relatives. Virtual reality (VR) is an emerging method, specifically for testing cognitive capacity while navigating a virtual world (Parsons 2015).

In addition to the invasive/non-invasive division, cognitive and non-cognitive tests can also be used to identify AD (Cruz-Oliver et al. 2014). The techniques used to evaluate a patient's intellect are referred to as cognitive tests, and they are non-invasive and simple to use. Contrarily, non-cognitive tests comprise all additional techniques for identifying and diagnosing dementia (Cordell et al. 2013).

Numerous non-invasive non-cognitive techniques are utilized to detect AD in its early stages (Muessig et al. 2013).

### 10.3.1 Neuroimaging Techniques

Neuroimaging techniques like computed tomography (CT) or magnetic resonance imaging (MRI) are used to detect disease-related alterations in patients' brains. Using machine learning techniques, the patient's head MRI data is compared to data from patients with AD (Unay and Ekin 2011).

There are white and grey matter alterations in AD patients. They were discovered via research that there is a connection between bilateral corpus callosum and internal capsule damage and thinking impairment (DT). Additionally, researchers assert a link between right-sided brain injury and

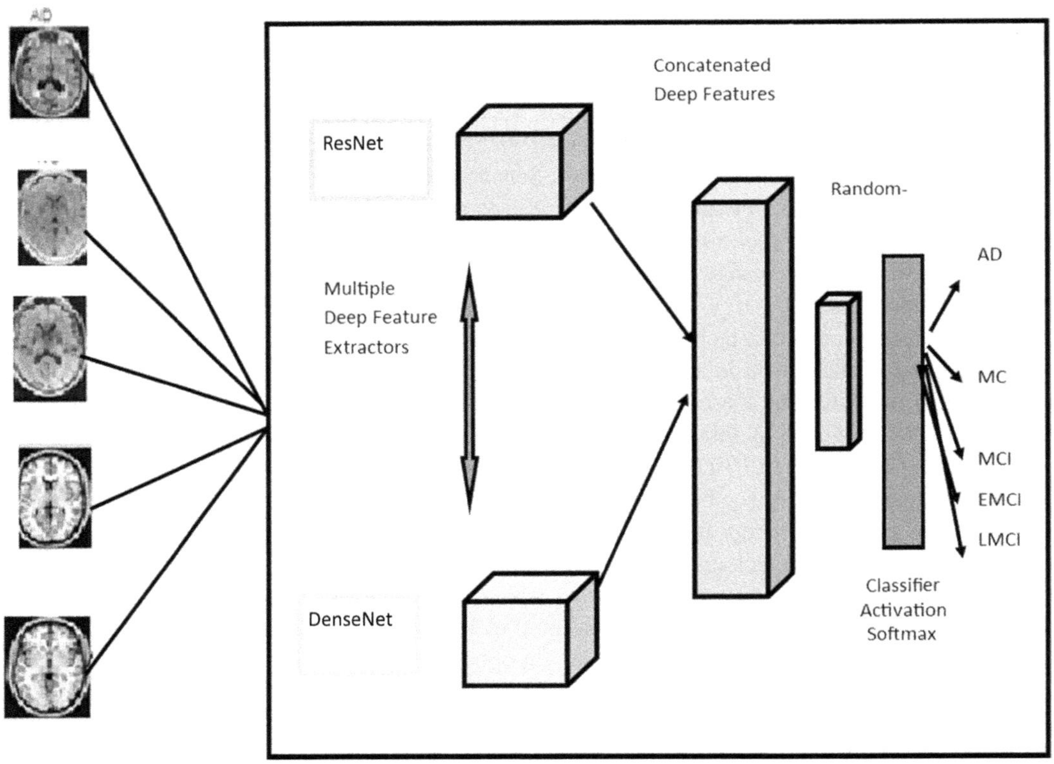


**FIGURE 10.3** Weight-randomized concatenated deep features from ResNet18 and DenseNet121 networks deliver an early diagnosis of AD.

apathy, linking the latter to the right hemisphere's role in initiating behaviour and observing the surroundings (Campbell et al. 2009).

However, due to the cost, time, and uncomfortable nature of the process, these approaches are not suitable for testing large populations. Additionally, obtaining these images frequently necessitates the use of medical equipment that is not always available (it is claustrophobic and noisy). For their own safety and discomfort, patients with mental problems are recommended not to use them (Zeng et al. 2009).

The proposed method weight-randomizes concatenated deep features from ResNet18 and DenseNet121 networks to deliver an early diagnosis of Alzheimer's disease, as shown in Figure 10.3 (Campbell et al. 2009).

### 10.3.2 Behaviour Analysis

Approaches to behaviour analysis look for unusual responses to typical situations or issues with ordinary activity. The methods used to evaluate cognitive deficits in daily activities typically call for the use of outside equipment for a period of time in order to observe patient behaviour (Crutcher et al. 2009). A sensor is attached to the patient's foot to measure gait (step height and length), which is a good indicator of the patient's level of dementia (Liu and Wang 2006). The gait measuring approach still has significant limitations, such as the patient's requirement to wear a gadget for extended periods of time. Moreover, despite being encouraging, the results are still useless because they haven't been tested on Alzheimer's sufferers (Liu and Arcone 2005).

Another form of detection employs sensors installed in patients' houses to detect specific events. The patient's assent is all that is needed to place the sensors in this non-invasive method.

The fundamental problem with these approaches is that the values are not reliable enough (detection rates are below 75%), making it difficult to develop a strategy for early stage dementia diagnosis (Clement et al. 2005). There are two problems with these systems (Duchek and Balota 2005): the requirement for patients' consent to install the sensors and security difficulties that could lead to a compromise of personal information.

Sensor-based automatic AD diagnosis systems can analyse participants' behaviour by watching them go about their daily routines at home. They keep track of sleep duration, the frequency of extensive coverage, and the length of intense activity. They conclude that the automated screening diagnosis approach is interesting but that the reliability of the sensors needs to be improved and that some customized aspects need to be taken into consideration because, occasionally, problems other than AD can impair the patients' mobility (Pernot et al. 2003).

The method for identifying AD when employing wearable technology. To analyse the participant's stride, specialized motion-detecting sensors are used that are worn on the feet. The number of steps taken, walking velocity, stride frequency, and cadence are just a few of the gait-related data that these devices collect about users.

The researchers were able to detect abrupt changes in foot movement patterns by using the intermediate-level cross-identification function (Marshall et al. 2003). The authors propose utilizing dynamic temporal warping (DTW) to align the signal in time and distinguish between participants with AD and healthy participants because the individuals' walking speeds vary throughout time. They contrast the results' sensitivity and specificity with those of other classifiers such as support vector machine (SVM), k-nearest neighbours (kNN), and inertial navigation algorithm (INA). Their results support the diagnostic efficacy of using DTW for gait categorization in AD.

### 10.3.3 Emotion Analysis

Emotion analysis is one of the additional ways relating to behaviour. Other methods, conversely, examine how patients respond to particular stimuli. Due to the significance of emotion recognition in various fields, including neuroscience and psychology, many methods have been developed for identifying human emotions. There have been several suggestions that attempt to analyse these responses or emotions using various data, including EEG, eye-tracking, audio, or facial gestures. Facial expression analysis would not be possible in cases of dementia that cause loss of facial expression, such as Lewy Body dementia (Atkinson et al. 2002).

### 10.3.4 Evaluation Techniques and Metrics for AD Diagnosis

The various AD diagnosis evaluation methods and metrics are discussed in this section. The approaches based on score and threshold as well as methods based on machine learning classification were found to be the two main strategies used to evaluate the participant's impairments (Lindeboom et al. 2002).

### 10.3.5 Machine Learning Techniques for AD Diagnosis

The goal of machine learning, a branch of artificial intelligence, is to provide methods that let machines learn. In order to predict reactions to new input variables, machine learning seeks to identify relationships between input variables and related responses (Ter Haar 2001).

Machine learning techniques could be used on data from patient tests and tasks or medical data and their related classifications, such as healthy or non-healthy subjects, to uncover relationships between data and labels (Xu et al. 2001).

Various approaches use classification techniques that can be grouped into three: one-class, binary, and multi-class, depending on the number of labels to be identified. Most approaches to AD detection that classify enormous amounts of data use these techniques. Two of them are MRI and behaviour/sensor techniques (Fountoulakis et al. 2000).

#### 10.3.5.1 Binary/Multi-class Classification

The two classification categories that are most frequently employed are binary and multi-class. Binary classification problems, or dividing data into two categories, are the easiest to solve. Among binary classifiers, SVM is one of the most often used (Rösler et al. 2000).

Separating the provided data into more than two categories is necessary for multi-class problems. Either a multi-class classifier or several binary classifiers can be used to overcome this issue. With an accuracy of 92%, an SVM classifier can distinguish between AD patients and healthy individuals using information from an MRI. Gait data from AD and healthy participants were classified using DTW, SVM, and kNN binary classifiers. While reading text paragraphs, a naive Bayes classifier is used to differentiate between healthy and MCI patients by utilizing variables including gaze length, saccade amplitude, and the overall number of fixations. In order to identify correlations between MRI scans and potential explanatory variables for AD, the general linear model is introduced (Loomis et al. 1999).

#### 10.3.5.2 One-class Classification

One-class classification (OCC) aims to isolate one category of items and distinguish it from others when the data are extremely imbalanced (with training data mainly from one class). The data from this class are used as positive samples. There may also be data from other classes, but acquiring access to it can be difficult for ethical and financial reasons (Wang et al. 1999).

Density estimation techniques make up the first family. These require a lot of training data and aren't resistant to outliers contained in the training data. Clustering-based techniques are the focus of the second category. These are robust to outliers and take into account the data's structure, but they need training data to adequately represent the entire class. The methods in the third family, which is the last one, define a boundary between the desired class and the other classes.

The latter gathers all OCC classifiers that exclusively use positive data for training, whereas the former adds data from certain outliers to the model. When the data from the classes overlap, it is often more practical to use conforming methods (Sun and Hynynen 1998).

Because it can be difficult to compare OCC and multi-class classifiers for the identification of acoustic input for the early detection of AD, due to the limited number of cases in some circumstances, one of the best uses for OCC is automatic illness diagnosis (Kohonen 1984).

Aphasia (deficits in speaking and comprehension) and issues with emotional response are two speech-related symptoms of Alzheimer's. A database called AZTIAHO was produced and consists of video recorded data from 50 healthy and 20 AD participants. Both the multi-class classifier and the OCC employ a multi-layer perceptron (MLP). While the multi-class classifier models two classes – healthy and AD – OCC produces a model that represents the healthy group. The results of their tests show that when there are few AD data, OCC performs better than the multi-class (Fry and Barger 1978).

The primary objective of using OCC is to assist people with dementia by detecting errors in daily tasks. In order to assist both patients and carers with daily tasks, they advise using OCC classifiers along with information gathered from sensors placed inside the patient's house. Because it is difficult to specify all of the possible issues that could occur during those activities, the researchers use the data from participants who successfully completed the activities without making any errors to train an OCC and the data from participants who made errors to test the OCC. The OCC is trained using a variety of features, including the quantity of sensors, event pauses, and event time probabilities.

The classifier employed is the one class support vector machine (OCSVM), a boundary approach that identifies a hyperplane that divides the positive class from the other classes. In addition, two more classifiers – one OCC and one MCC – are suggested for error classification after the outliers from the healthy model are discovered. As a result of the classifier's frequent false positive detection, the OCSVM performs poorly in the evaluation. The authors explain this as a result of incorrect error annotation. They contrast the application of OCSVM-OCSVM and OCSVM-MCC to identify mistakes and categorize them; the classification outcomes are comparable.

## 10.4 ALZHEIMER'S TREATMENT BY APPLYING ULTRASOUND WAVES

Investigation into a few Alzheimer's disorders has shown that brain shrinkage is their primary cause. The brain's holes are smaller than they would be in their normal state (Prince et al. 2015). It is established that an ultrasound wave produced at 2–18 MHz can oscillate at the width of the holes and, as a result, can restore the health of the brain for both healthy and Alzheimer's brains. Due to the method's novelty, it has been tested on sheep with healthy brains, and it has been found to be effective.

The primary and second fields of acoustic wave applications in biomedical research, respectively, are diagnostic imaging and therapy. The applied acoustic wave's power, intensity, and interval time vary between these domains. The underlying physics that controls the transmission of acoustic waves is the same in both scenarios (Van den Stock et al. 2015). This paper presents theoretical and experimental discoveries from the skulless brain. It is difficult for acoustic waves to go through the skull and into the brain. In a new technique, an acoustic "window" was made by cutting a little portion of the skull's bone. Based on the prevalence of brain lesions, recent research proposes a potential Alzheimer's treatment approach (Mitchell 2017).

### 10.4.1 Dependence of Alzheimer's Physical Symptoms on Brain Shrinking

Figure 10.4(a) illustrates brain shrinkage, which is one of the key symptoms of AD and a source of a number of issues. Brain shrinkage has unfavourable effects (as shown in Figure 10.4(b). Researchers mention two phenomena to improve our understanding of them. The first phenomenon has to do with measuring dimensions. Analysing an object's proportions is an application of brain structure. For instance, Figure 10.5 shows a few sensors (1, 2, 3, and 4) at the tips of two fingers that transmit information about an item to the brain and receive signals from the brain in relation to the duration of movement. Two fingers can move an object, and the brain receives the information the fingers have recorded (Yang et al. 2016).

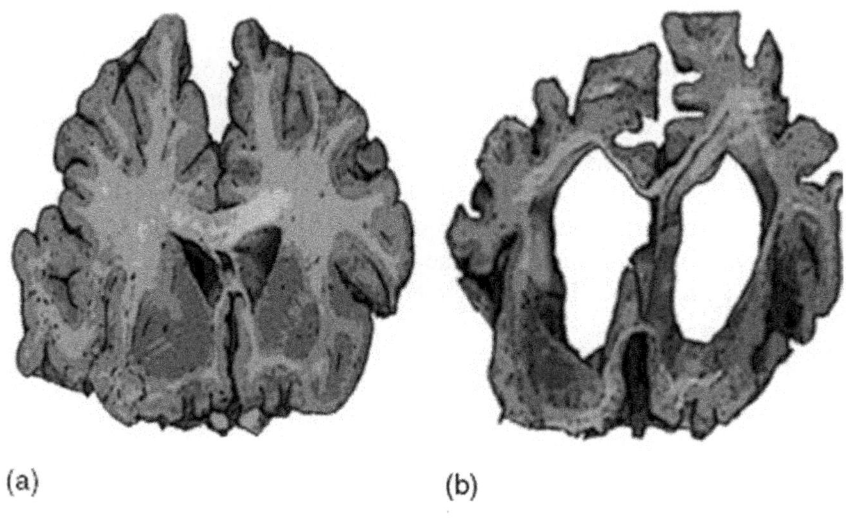


**FIGURE 10.4** (a) Cross-section of a normal brain; (b) with Alzheimer's disease.

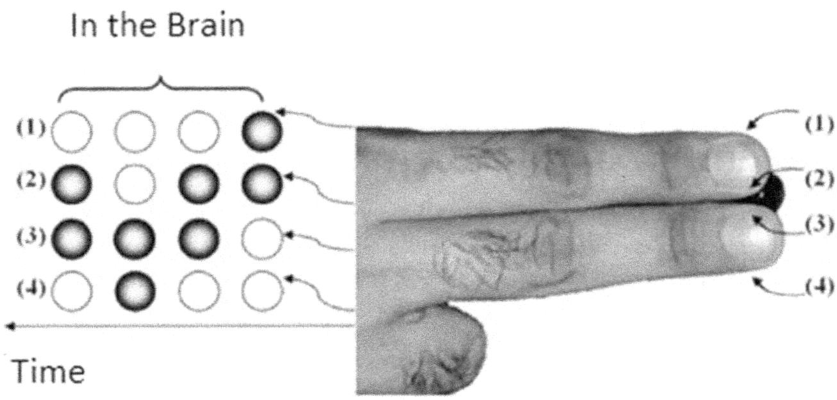


**FIGURE 10.5** Brain and finger sensors that detect objects based on movement duration are related. The white circles (off) represent no signals received, while the black circles (on) represent signals received.

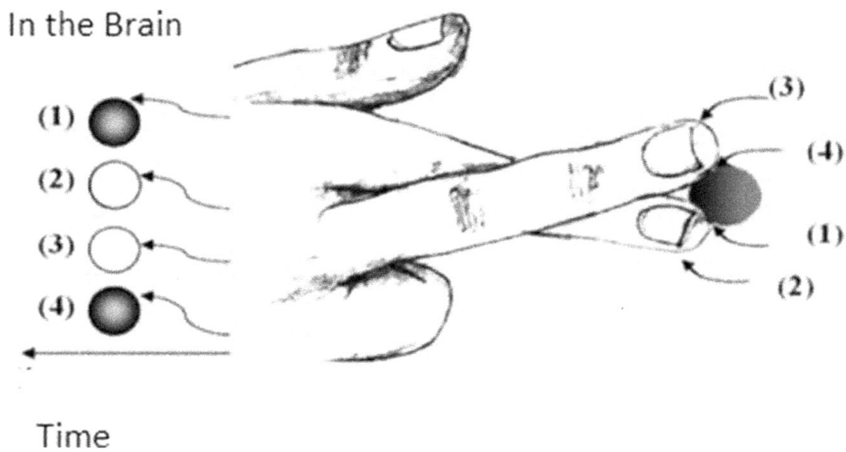


**FIGURE 10.6** Crossed fingers and the signals received by the brain.

When an object is moved, the circles 1 and 2 turn on first, then as time goes on, circle 1 turns off, and the circles 2 and 3 turn on, and so on, as shown in Figure 10.5. As a result, the brain discerns the object's dimensions and velocity. However, as illustrated in Figure 10.3, the brain is unable to accurately identify an item when two fingers are crossed. When the white circles 1 and 4 turn on while 2 and 3 are off, the brain interprets this as the presence of two objects.

This amazing experiment demonstrates that the brain will recognize an object's dimensions if the circles that are next to each other turn on. As a result, as illustrated in Figure 10.6, as the brain gets smaller, circles get smaller and more turn on due to signal interference from the object. Receiving information from a brain that was healthy and a brain that had advanced Alzheimer's is shown in Figure 10.7.

The brain interprets the thing as being larger in this scenario (Ishii et al. 2016). Alzheimer patients develop errors in distance perception as their brains shrink. Memory disturbance is the second phenomenon. There are 1011 neuron cells in the human brain, and they communicate with one another electrically. One or two axons that serve as the output and numerous dendrites that serve as the input of electrical signals make up each neuron (Ruiz-Rizzo et al. 2017). To be activated, neurons require a specific level of signal input that accumulates from all of the dendrites. Once activated, the neuron sparks and transmits a signal to neighbouring neurons via its axon (Allen 2017).

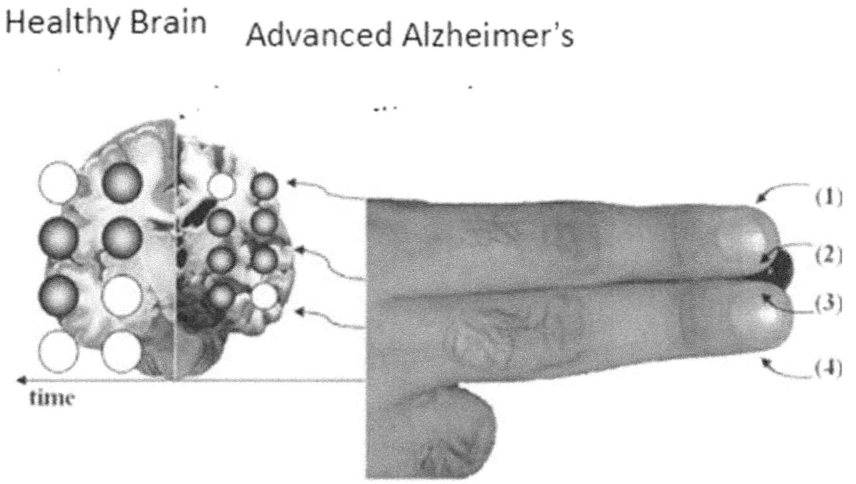


**FIGURE 10.7** Receiving information from a brain that was healthy and a brain that had advanced Alzheimer's.

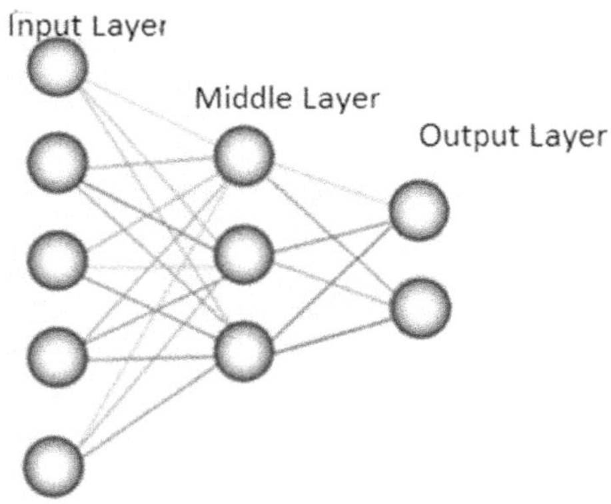


**FIGURE 10.8** Neuron organization in layers. (Left: neural networks, right: neurons in the brain).

The weight of the link and the values of the neurons in the layer above will determine the value of each neuron in that layer (Mitchell 2017), as shown in Figure 10.8. Therefore, as the brain shrinks, the weight of the connections changes and they affect one another, disrupting memory. Given these illustrations, it is evident that brain shrinkage is the primary cause of the aforementioned symptoms of AD.

### 10.4.2 Influence of Ultrasound Waves on Brain Holes

There are several holes in the brain, according to scientific finding (Yang et al. 2016). A healthy brain's majority of holes have micrometer-sized dimensions, whereas those in an Alzheimer's brain are smaller, as depicted in Figure 10.9. These holes feature particular vibration modes and are dense with tau. When one of these patterns of ultrasonic waves is applied to the brain, the vibration of the holes is resonant, and their diameters will grow (Van den Stock et al. 2015).

This procedure improves brain health. The brain's holes have a fluid-like bubble-like behaviour, as shown in Figure 10.10. The density of the brain causes ultrasound waves to move through it isothermally. Given the size of the holes, their oscillation is adiabatic and raises the brain's temperature. Therefore, the length of the process should not be too long at any time. The differential equation for the size of a hole in the brain, R, with a steady state radius, R0, and surface tension, and oscillations

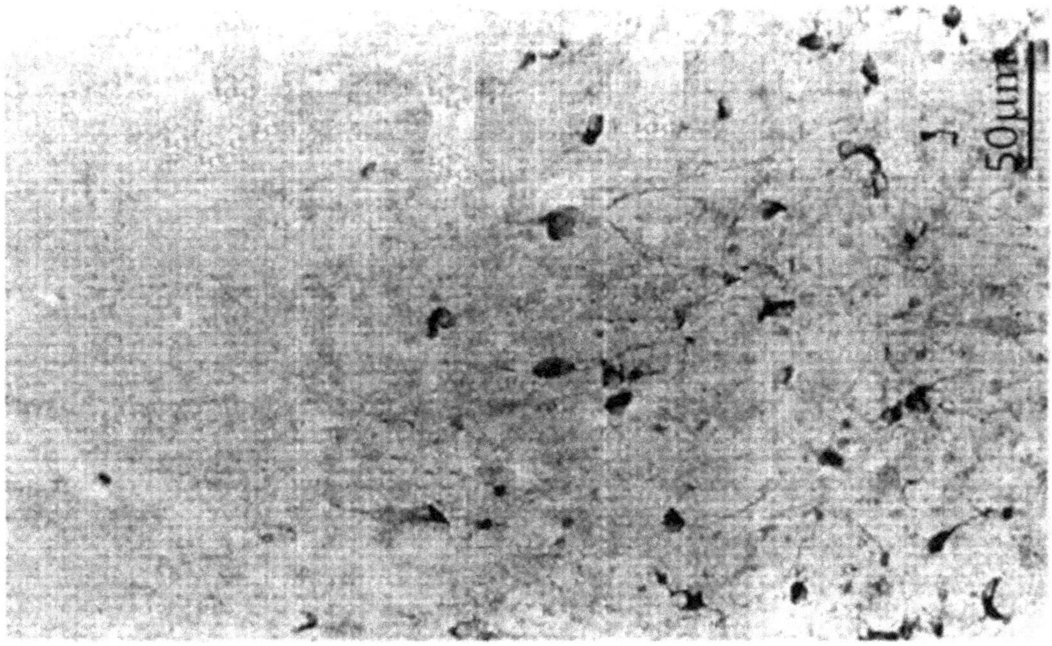


FIGURE 10.9 Alzheimer's brain and its holes.

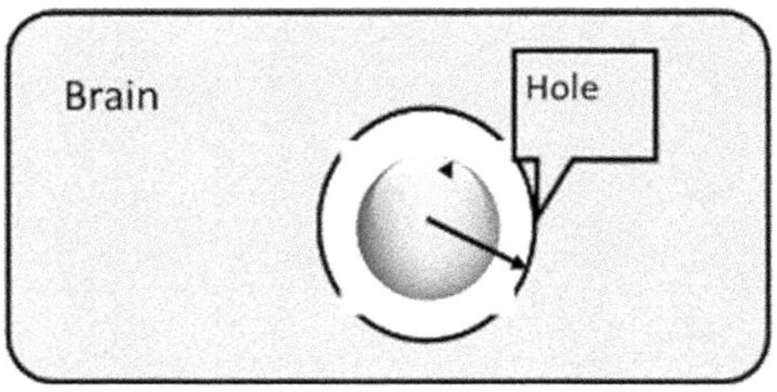


FIGURE 10.10 The oscillation of holes in the brain.

of modest amplitude in the brain's volume is caused by density and atmospheric pressure (Sapey-Triomphe et al. 2015):

$$\frac{\partial R}{\partial R0} = V\tau$$

## 10.5 CONCLUSION

With a focus on cognitive, VE/VR-based, and ultrasonic and infrared analytical sensor approaches for AD early detection, this chapter has offered a thorough assessment of the most recent and significant research in the field. Various AD diagnosis criteria were established and metrics offered, and there has been discussion surrounding them, along with a summary of the various datasets. Additionally, summaries of related VR technologies and frameworks were offered, giving practitioners a method to include modern solutions in virtual settings and get beyond limitations imposed by the old cognitive approaches to AD diagnosis, such as the ceiling effect. There has also been provided an overview of non-cognitive techniques, including a look at MRI and biomarker techniques. However, we have focused on the cognitive because many non-cognitive treatments are obtrusive and disagreeable.

## REFERENCES


Agüera-Ortiz, Luis, Juan A. Hernandez-Tamames, Pablo Martinez-Martin, Isabel Cruz-Orduña, Gonzalo Pajares, Jorge López-Alvarez, Ricardo S. Osorio, Marta Sanz, and Javier Olazarán. (2017). "Structural Correlates of Apathy in Alzheimer's Disease: A Multimodal MRI Study." *International Journal of Geriatric Psychiatry* 32, no. 8: 922–30. https://doi.org/10.1002/gps.4548

Allen, C. (2017). On (not) defining cognition. *In Synthese*. Berlin, Heidelberg, Germany: Springer, 1–17.

Atkinson, J., J. Marshall, A. Thacker, and B. Woll. (2002). "When Sign Language Breaks down: Deaf People's Access to Language Therapy in the UK." *Deaf Worlds* 18: 9–21.

Atkinson, Joanna, Tanya Denmark, Jane Marshall, Cath Mummery, and Bencie Woll. (2015). "Detecting Cognitive Impairment and Dementia in Deaf People: The British Sign Language Cognitive Screening Test." *Archives of Clinical Neuropsychology* 30, no. 7: 694–711. https://doi.org/10.1093/arclin/acv042

Campbell, Z., K. K. Zakzanis, D. Jovanovski, S. Joordens, R. Mraz, and S. J. Graham. (2009). "Utilizing Virtual Reality to Improve the Ecological Validity of Clinical Neuropsychology: An fMRI Case Study Elucidating the Neural Basis of Planning by Comparing the Tower of London with a Three-Dimensional Navigation Task." *Applied Neuropsychology* 16, no. 4: 295–306. https://doi.org/10.1080/09084280903297891

Chong, Z. H. K., Y. X. Tee, L. J. Toh, S. J. Phang, J. Y. Liew, B. Queck, and S. Gottipati. Aug. 10–11 (2017). "Predicting Potential Alzheimer Medical Condition in Elderly Using IOT Sensors-Case Study." In *Proceedings of the IRC Conference on Science, Engineering, and Technology*, Singapore.

Clement, Gregory T., P. Jason White, Randy L. King, Nathan McDannold, and Kullervo Hynynen. (2005). "An MRI-Compatible Large Scale Array for Trans-skull Ultrasound Surgery and Therapy." *Journal of Ultrasound in Medicine* 24, no. 8: 1117–25. https://doi.org/10.7863/jum.2005.24.8.1117

Cordell, Cyndy B., Soo Borson, Malaz Boustani, Joshua Chodosh, David Reuben, Joe Verghese, William Thies, Leslie B. Fried, and Medicare Detection of Cognitive Impairment Workgroup. (2013). "Alzheimer's Association Recommendations for Operationalizing the Detection of Cognitive Impairment During the Medicare Annual Wellness Visit in a Primary Care Setting." *Alzheimer's & Dementia* 9, no. 2: 141–50. https://doi.org/10.1016/j.jalz.2012.09.011

Crutcher, Michael D., Rose Calhoun-Haney, Cecelia M. Manzanares, James J. Lah, Allan I. Levey, and Stuart M. Zola. (2009). "Eye Tracking During a Visual Paired Comparison Task as a Predictor of Early Dementia." *American Journal of Alzheimer's Disease & Other Dementias* 24, no. 3: 258–66. https://doi.org/10.1177/1533317509332093

Cruz-Oliver, Dulce M., Theodore K. Malmstrom, Michael Roegner, Nina Tumosa, and George T. Grossberg. (2014). "Cognitive Deficit Reversal as Shown by Changes in the Veterans Affairs Saint Louis University Mental Status (SLUMS) Examination Scores 7.5 Years Later." *Journal of the American Medical Directors Association* 15, no. 9: 687.e5–10. https://doi.org/10.1016/j.jamda.2014.05.004

Duchek, Janet M., and David A. Balota. (2005). "Failure to Control Prepotent Pathways in Early Stage Dementia of the Alzheimer's Type: Evidence from Dichotic Listening." *Neuropsychology* 19, no. 5: 687–95. https://doi.org/10.1037/0894-4105.19.5.687

Fountoulakis, K. N., M. Tsolaki, H. Chantzi, and A. Kazis. (2000). "Mini Mental State Examination (MMSE): A Validation Study in Greece." *American Journal of Alzheimer's Disease & Other Dementias* 15, no. 6: 342–5. https://doi.org/10.1177/153331750001500604

Fry, F. J., and J. E. Barger. (1978). "Acoustical Properties of the Human Skull." *Journal of the Acoustical Society of America* 63, no. 5: 1576–90. https://doi.org/10.1121/1.381852

Gupta, D., S. Sundaram, A. Khanna, A. E. Ella Hassanien, and V. H. C. de Albuquerque. (2018). "Improved Diagnosis of Parkinson's Disease Using Optimized Crow Search Algorithm." *Computers & Electrical Engineering* 68: 412–24. https://doi.org/10.1016/j.compeleceng.2018.04.014

Ishii, H., K. Kimino, M. Aljehani, N. Ohe, and M. Inoue. (2016). "An Early Detection System for Dementia Using the M2 M/IoT Platform." *Procedia Computer Science* 96: 1332–40. https://doi.org/10.1016/j.procs.2016.08.178

Kohonen, T. (1984). *Self-Organization and Associative Memory*. New York: Springer-Verlag.

Lindeboom, J., B. Schmand, L. Tulner, G. Walstra, and C. Jonker. (2002). "Visual Association Test to Detect Early Dementia of the Alzheimer Type." *Journal of Neurology, Neurosurgery, & Psychiatry* 73, no. 2: 126–33. https://doi.org/10.1136/jnnp.73.2.126

Liu, L., and S. A. Arcone. (2005). "Propagation of Radar Pulses from a Horizontal Dipole in Variable Dielectric Ground: A Numerical Approach." *Subsurface Sensing Technologies & Applications* 6, no. 1: 5–24. https://doi.org/10.1007/s11220-005-4223-2

Liu, L., and L. V. Wang. (2006). "High Fidelity Simulation of Ultrasonic Wave Propagation in a 2-Dimensional Brain Model for Microwave-Induced Thermoacoustic Tomography." In *Proceedings of the 9th Western Pacific Acoustics Conference; 2006*; Seoul, South Korea.

Loomis, J. M., J. J. Blascovich, and A. C. Beall. (1999). "Immersive Virtual Environment Technology as a Basic Research Tool in Psychology." *Behavior Research Methods, Instruments, & Computers* 31, no. 4: 557–64. https://doi.org/10.3758/bf03200735

Lynch, G., and X. Bi. "Model for Alzheimer's Disease and Other Neurodegenerative Disease". US Patent 6, 803, 233 vol. B2

Marshall, Jane, J. Atkinson, Alice Thacker, and Bencie Woll. (2003). "Is Speech and Language Therapy Meeting the Needs of Language Minorities? The Case of Deaf People with Neurological Impairments." *International Journal of Language & Communication Disorders* 38, no. 1: 85–94. https://doi.org/10.1080/1368282030481 2

Mitchell, A. (2017). "The Mini-Mental State Examination (MMSE): Update on Its Diagnostic Accuracy and Clinical Utility for Cognitive Disorders." In *Cognitive Screening Instruments*, 37–48. Berlin, Heidelberg, Germany: Springer.

Muessig, Kathryn E., Emily C. Pike, Sara Legrand, and Lisa B. Hightow-Weidman. (2013). "Mobile Phone Applications for the Care and Prevention of HIV and Other Sexually Transmitted Diseases: A Review." *Journal of Medical Internet Research* 15, no. 1: e1. https://doi.org/10.2196/jmir.2301

Parsons, T. D. (2015). "Ecological Validity in Virtual Reality-Based Neuropsychological Assessment." In *Encyclopedia of Information Science and Technology*. 3rd ed., 1006–15. Hershey, PA: IGI Global. https://doi.org/10.4018/978-1-4666-5888-2.ch095

Pernot, M., J. Porquet, C. Saint Olive et al. (2003). 3D Finite Difference Simulation of Coupled Acoustic Wave and Bio-heat Equation. *Skull Heating Prediction for Non-invasive Brain HIFU Therapy: 2003: Proceeding of WCU* vols. 7–10. Paris, France.

Prince, M., A. Wimo, M. Guerchet, G. Ali, Y. T. Wu, and M. Prina. (2015). *World Alzheimer Report 2015: The Global Impact of Dementia. An Analysis of Prevalence, Incidence, Cost and Trends*. London, UK: Alzheimer's Disease International.

Rösler, A., M. E. Mapstone, A. K. Hays, M. M. Mesulam, A. Rademaker, D. R. Gitelman, and S. Weintraub. (2000). "Alterations of Visual Search Strategy in Alzheimer's Disease and Aging." *Neuropsychology* 14, no. 3: 398–408. https://doi.org/10.1037//0894-4105.14.3.398

Ruiz-Rizzo, Adriana L., Peter Bublak, Petra Redel, Timo Grimmer, Hermann J. Müller, Christian Sorg, and Kathrin Finke. (2017). "Simultaneous Object Perception Deficits Are Related to Reduced Visual Processing Speed in Amnestic Mild Cognitive Impairment." *Neurobiology of Aging* 55: 132–42. https://doi.org/10.1016/j.neurobiolaging.2017.03.029

Sapey-Triomphe, Laurie-Anne, Rolf A. Heckemann, Nawele Boublay, Jean-Michel Dorey, Marie-Anne Hénaff, Isabelle Rouch, Catherine Padovan, Alexander Hammers, Pierre Krolak-Salmon, and Alzheimer's Disease Neuroimaging Initiative. (2015). "Neuroanatomical Correlates of Recognizing Face Expressions in Mild Stages of Alzheimer's Disease." *PLOS ONE* 10, no. 12: e0143586. https://doi.org/10.1371/journal.pone.0143586

Sendra, S., L. Parra, J. Lloret, and J. Tomás. (2018). "Smart System for Children's Chronic Illness Monitoring." *Information Fusion* 40: 76–86. https://doi.org/10.1016/j.inffus.2017.06.002

Sun, J., and K. Hynynen. (1998). "Focusing of Therapeutic Ultrasound Through a Human Skull: A Numerical Study." *Journal of the Acoustical Society of America* 104, no. 3 Pt 1: 1705–15. https://doi.org/10.1121/1.424383

Szczésniak, Dorota, and Joanna Rymaszewska. (2016). "The Usefulness of the SLUMS Test for Diagnosis of Mild Cognitive Impairment and Dementia." *Psychiatria Polska* 50, no. 2: 457–72. https://doi.org/10.12740/PP/OnlineFirst/43141

Teipel, Stefan, Alexander Drzezga, Michel J. Grothe, Henryk Barthel, Gaël Chételat, Norbert Schuff, Pawel Skudlarski, Enrica Cavedo, Giovanni B. Frisoni, Wolfgang Hoffmann, Jochen René Thyrian, Chris Fox, Satoshi Minoshima, Osama Sabri, and Andreas Fellgiebel. (2015). "Multimodal Imaging in Alzheimer's Disease: Validity and Usefulness for Early Detection." *Lancet Neurology* 14, no. 10: 1037–53. https://doi.org/10.1016/S1474-4422(15)00093-9

Ter Haar, G. 2001. "Acoustic Surgery." *Physics Today* 54, no. 12: 29–34. https://doi.org/10.1063/1.1445545

Unay, D., and A. Ekin. Apr. 2 (2011). "Dementia Diagnosis Using Similar and Dissimilar Retrieval Items." In *Proceedings of the (2011) IEEE International Symposium on Biomedical Imaging: From Nano to Macro*, Chicago, IL, March 30: 1889–92. https://doi.org/10.1109/ISBI.2011.5872777

Van den Stock, Jan, François-Laurent De Winter, Beatrice de Gelder, Janaki Raman Rangarajan, Gert Cypers, Frederik Maes, Stefan Sunaert, Karolien Goffin, Rik Vandenberghe, and Mathieu Vandenbulcke. (2015). "Impaired Recognition of Body Expressions in the Behavioral Variant of Frontotemporal Dementia." *Neuropsychologia* 75: 496–504. https://doi.org/10.1016/j.neuropsychologia.2015.06.035

Varatharajan, R., G. Manogaran, M. K. Priyan, and R. Sundarasekar. (2018). "Wearable Sensor Devices for Early Detection of Alzheimer Disease Using Dynamic Time Warping Algorithm." *Cluster Computing* 21, no. 1: 681–90. https://doi.org/10.1007/s10586-017-0977-2

Wang, L. V., X. Zhao, H. Sun, and G. Ku. (1999). "Microwave-Induced Acoustic Imaging of Biological Tissues." *Review of Scientific Instruments* 70, no. 9: 3744–48. https://doi.org/10.1063/1.1149986

Xu, M., G. Ku, and L. V. Wang. (2001). "Microwave-Induced Thermoacoustic Tomography Using Multi-sector Scanning." *Medical Physics* 28, no. 9: 1958–63. https://doi.org/10.1118/1.1395037

Yang, L., Jing Yan, Xiaoqing Jin, Y. Jin, Wei Yu, Shanhu Xu, and Haibin Wu. (2016). "Screening for Dementia in Older Adults: Comparison of Mini-Mental State Examination, Mini-Cog, Clock Drawing Test and AD 8." *PLOS ONE* 11, no. 12: e0168949. https://doi.org/10.1371/journal.pone.0168949

Zeng, Zhihong, Maja Pantic, Glenn I. Roisman, and Thomas S. Huang. (2009). "A Survey of Affect Recognition Methods: Audio, Visual, and Spontaneous Expressions." *IEEE Transactions on Pattern Analysis & Machine Intelligence* 31, no. 1: 39–58. https://doi.org/10.1109/TPAMI.2008.52

# 11 Deep Learning in Mental Illnesses

## *Understanding Networks*

*Priya Dev and Abhishek Pathak*
Banaras Hindu University, Varanasi, India

## 11.1 INTRODUCTION

The World Health Organization has defined mental illness as a broader array of mental health disorders and conditions affecting an individual's thinking, behaviour, emotions, and mood, and which also impacts a person's physical health (Sagar et al. 2020). Mental illnesses have been linked to distress and present challenges of function within work and social contexts, and family activities. Notable mental illnesses include depression, anxiety disorders, addictive behaviours, attention-deficit hyperactivity disorder (ADHD), eating disorders, and schizophrenia. Presently, mental illnesses are increasingly prevalent and it is approximated that, globally, 450 million individuals suffer from the problem (Su et al. 2020). Moreover, children and adolescents below 18 years of age and adults also face a high risk of mental illnesses risks (Singh et al. 2021). Mental illnesses are among the most severe and increasingly prevalent public health problems. For instance, depression is currently among the foremost causes of disability and may result in heightened risk of suicide attempts and suicidal ideations (Trofimova and Sulis 2018).

Though individuals might have mental health concerns regularly, such concerns only become illnesses when the enduring symptoms and signs result in frequent stress and negatively impact on the aptitude to function normally (Al-Rousan et al. 2017). Globally, mental illnesses are the second major cause of disease burden with regards to the number of years lived with disability, as well as the sixth foremost cause of disability-adjusted life-years. Thus, mental illnesses pose severe challenges to healthcare systems, especially in middle-income and low-income nations. As a result, mental health has been acknowledged as a key priority area with regard to health policies across the globe, in addition to being included in the United Nations' Sustainable Development Goals (Insel 2018).

## 11.2 OVERVIEW OF THE DIFFERENT CATEGORIES OF MENTAL ILLNESSES

The categorization of mental illnesses conventionally began from pragmatic efforts to discover the differences and similarities in patient groups. At present, mental illness categorization is used for reimbursement and administrative purposes. Additionally, the classifications are used by researchers in the identification of the homogenous groups within patient populations to enable the exploration of their attributes and probable determinants of mental illnesses that include the causes, treatment responses, and results/outcomes (Martland et al. 2020). Further, the use of classification has, in recent times, gained significance as a clinical practice and teaching guide. The initial behavioural medicine and psychiatry practices were mostly based on criminal judgement and speculative theories regarding etiology; the introduction of operational diagnostics has demystified the varied aspects of practice, and the clinical features identified have to be defined, perceived, and if possible evaluated in a manner that is assessor-independent. Among the notable achievements of mental

 DOI: 10.1201/9781003245346-11

illness categorization is the ability to explain mental illness as a brain dysfunction. For example, schizophrenia, which was initially perceived as a societal label and a myth, has been defined as the integration of different mental functions that originate within the brain, including thought processing errors capable of leading to mental disorders (Graham et al. 2019).

The classification of mental illnesses is representative of the major aspects of psychiatry along with other mental health careers, and is considered a vital issue for individuals who might get diagnosed. At present, there are two broadly established and commonly used systems for the categorization of mental illnesses, namely Chapter 5 of the *Tenth International Classification of Disease* (ICD-10), and the American Psychiatric Association (APA)'s *Diagnostic and Statistical Manual of Mental Disorders* (DSM-5) (Bernardini et al. 2017). The two systems list mental disorder categories believed to be distinct kinds in addition to deliberately converging their distinctive codes to ensure comparability of the manuals, despite the existence of considerable differences. Some of the notable categories of mental illness are discussed below.

### 11.2.1 Neurocognitive Disorders

These cognitive disorders are a class of mental illnesses primarily affecting the cognitive aptitudes that include memory, learning, problem solving, and perception. Disorders like delirium, as well as major and mild neurocognitive disorders, were initially referred to as dementia. Cognitive disorders are mainly defined by cognitive ability deficits acquired rather than developmental, and characteristically represent decline in addition to having an underlying brain pathology (Ekhtiari et al. 2021). According to DSM-5, the cognitive function's six main domains include memory and learning, executive functioning, social cognition, language, perceptual motor function, and complex attention. Despite Alzheimer's disease accounting for a larger proportion of the cognitive disorder cases, different medical conditions affecting mental functions like reasoning, thinking, and memory exist, and include prion disease, Lewy body disease, Parkinson's disease, Huntington's disease, frontotemporal degeneration, traumatic brain injury, and dementia. Cognitive disorders are often diagnosed as major or mild, based on the severity of the symptoms. The primary causal symptom of cognitive disorders is the loss of cognitive function even though the cause tends to vary among the disorders, though most are linked to damages to the brain's memory portions (Yochim and Mast 2021). Treatment is mainly dependent on the cause and resultant damage.

### 11.2.2 Substance-abuse-related Disorders

Substance-abuse-related disorders are mainly addictive problems. Thus, certain individuals are increasingly predisposed to develop such disorders compared to others. Aspects such as dysfunctional family settings, genetics, and sexually and emotionally abusive milieus in the course of childhood are among the notable triggers and causes of these mental disorders (Bzdok and Meyer-Lindenberg 2018). Substance abuse often induces symptomatology resembling mental illness. This often occurs during intoxication and withdrawal. In certain instances, substance-abuse-related mental disorders may persist for some time, following detoxification, as observed in prolonged depression and psychosis that occur after cocaine and amphetamine abuse. Protracted withdrawal syndrome might additionally happen with the various symptoms persisting for several months following the ending of usage (Quaak et al. 2021). In this regard, benzodiazepines have been acknowledged as some of the key drugs that induce prolonged withdrawal effects, and its symptoms have been observed to persist for several years following cessation of abuse. Withdrawal from alcohol, benzodiazepine, and barbiturates may be potentially fatal. The abuse of hallucinogens has also been noted to trigger psychotic and delusional phenomena long after one stops using them.

The diagnosis of substance-abuse-related mental disorders is often based on aspects that include social impairment, high risk behaviours, and proof of physical/psychological dependence. Notable symptoms of these mental illnesses include development of tolerance, which leads to one requiring more of the drug or alcohol, increased craving for the substance, and the experience of various withdrawal symptoms following cessation of usage (Vázquez-Abad et al. 2020). Notable kinds of mental illnesses include drug use and alcohol use disorder.

### 11.2.3 Psychosis

Psychosis refers to the abnormal mind condition that leads to challenges in establishing what may be real and what might not be real. The symptoms of psychosis include hallucinations and delusions, as well as incoherent behaviour and speech that are inappropriate in certain circumstances (Gkotsis et al. 2017). The other notable symptoms may include sleeping problems, lack of motivation, social withdrawal, and difficulties in performing everyday activities. Psychosis may have adverse health outcomes for the patient. Moreover, similar to other mental illnesses, psychosis has numerous divergent causes that include mental conditions like bipolar and schizophrenia, sleep deprivation, trauma, certain medications and medical conditions, as well as substances like methamphetamine and cannabis. Post-partum psychosis has also been observed to occur following the birth of a child. In all cases of psychosis, the neurotransmitter dopamine is believed to play vital roles (Potes et al. 2018). Psychosis is considered to be acute in instances where it results in a mental condition and is further regarded as secondary when it is as a result of drug use or a medical condition.

### 11.2.4 Mood Disorders

Mood disorders, commonly referred to as mood affective disorders, refer to a set of mental and behavioural conditions where the disturbance in an individual's mood is the key underlying feature (Maziade 2017). In this regard, mood disorders can be categorized into seven groups: (i) abnormally elevated mood, (ii) mania, (iii) hypomania, (iv) major depression, (v) clinical depression, (vi) unipolar depression, and (vii) bipolar disorder. Numerous types of depressive disorders exist and often feature less austere symptoms like dysthymic disorders alongside cyclothymic disorders. Also, mood disorders may be as a result of substance use or might even occur in response to a specific medical condition.

### 11.2.5 Anxiety Disorders

Anxiety disorders refer to a group of mental disorders marked by a considerable and uncontrollable sense of fear and anxiety, to an extent that an individual's occupational, personal, and social functioning is impaired substantially. Thus, anxiety might result in cognitive and physical symptoms that include irritability, restlessness, difficulties in concentrating, fatigue, chest pains, increase in heart rate, abdominal pains, along with other symptoms that vary according to the person (Horenstein and Heimberg 2020). Several kinds of anxiety disorders exist, including specific phobias, selective mutism, separation anxiety disorder, general anxiety disorder, panic disorders, agoraphobia, and social anxiety disorders. The diagnosis of individual disorders is mainly carried out using certain and special triggering events, timing, and symptoms.

### 11.2.6 Eating Disorders

Eating disorders are mental disorders that have been defined through abnormal eating behaviours that negatively impact on an individual's mental and physical health. Notable kinds of eating disorders include anorexia nervosa, which is marked by an individual's fear of gaining weight, overexercising, and limiting food as a means of managing the fear; binge eating disorder in which the affected person eats increased amounts of food within a short duration; pica, which is marked by the affected person consuming non-food items; bulimia nervosa, which is marked by the affected person eating increased amounts of food and then attempting to purge it; rumination syndrome, marked by the affected person regurgitating minimally or undigested food; as well as the restrictive and avoidant food intake disorders that entail the affected individual having selective or reduced food consumption owing to certain psychological reasons (Rowe 2017). People with eating disorders are also prone to suffer from other conditions that include depression, anxiety disorders, and substance abuse disorders. Though the causes of eating disorders remain unclear, it is believed that environmental and biological disorders play key roles, even as cultural idealization of certain body shapes and sizes are believed to also contribute to certain eating disorders. Further, persons who might have experienced sexual abuse are increasingly prone to develop eating disorders, while disorders such as rumination and pica occur in individuals with intellectual disabilities. Other notable mental illness categories include neurodevelopmental disorders like ADHD; obsessive-compulsive disorders, which often trap individuals in endless behavioural and thought cycles; and trauma and stress-related disorders that often affect individuals who experience scary, dangerous, and shocking events (Vázquez-Abad et al. 2020).

## 11.3 PREVALENCE OF MENTAL HEALTH PROBLEMS DURING THE COVID-19 PANDEMIC

Globally, the COVID-19 pandemic has resulted in major psychological and mental health problems. Despite the burdens being reported among healthcare workers and in the general population, little remains known with regard to the mental health conditions and challenges among patients who have recovered from COVID-19 and related factors. One of the recent studies regarding the mental health and psychological evaluation of 89 COVID-19 patients indicated that 35% presented milder symptoms while 13% suffered from moderate to severe symptoms (Khademi et al. 2021). Other recent research focusing on COVID-19 patients discharged from hospitals indicated that 10.4% of them were acknowledged to have mild to severe anxiety symptoms, while 19% were suffering from considerable symptoms of clinical depression. Moreover, post-traumatic stress disorder (PTSD) resulting from COVID-19 has been diagnosed in 12.4% of COVID-19 patients. As such, in reaction to the pandemic, psychological and mental challenges have become important issues. To tackle these challenges, several measures that include telemedicine guidelines, reinforced mental health guidelines, and mental health helplines have been enforced by numerous nations across the globe (Boldrini et al. 2021). The recent studies focusing on the mental and psychological impacts have mostly concentrated on healthcare workers and the general population, who portrayed anxiety with regard to infection risks, leading to psychological distress (Thapa et al. 2020). However, to this day, no research has reported the prevalence of mental illness that includes anxiety, PTSD symptoms, and depression in COVID-19 patients who have recovered. Furthermore, a dependable approximation of the mental illness prevalence is required for the management of such patients.

## 11.4 POST-COVID-19 NEUROPSYCHIATRIC ABNORMALITIES AND THEIR CLINICAL MANIFESTATIONS

From the beginning of the pandemic in March 2020, increased concerns have been expressed with regard to the survivors being at higher risk of neurological disorders. The concern, originally founded on studies of other coronaviruses, was immediately followed by several case series, emergent proof of the involvement of COVID-19 in the central nervous system (CNS), and the recognition of mechanisms through which this would take place (Fiorillo and Gorwood 2020). Comparable concerns have emerged in relation to COVID-19 psychiatric sequelae, with available evidence indicating that survivors are at high risk of anxiety and mood disorders in the three months following infection. Nevertheless, there is a need for large-scale, long-term, and robust data to aptly identify and quantify COVID-19 consequences on mental health.

In this regard, it has been disclosed that approximately 30% of hospitalized COVID-19 patients have both delayed and acute neuropsychiatric manifestations. Moreover, even patients with asymptomatic and milder disease presentations normally exhibit various mood disorders linked to neurocognitive impairment, sleep-wake rhythm disruption, traumatic memories, delirium, and fatigue. Normally, the post-COVID-19 psychiatric pathology commences with apathy, a decrement in desire for social interaction, acute fatigue, sleep disturbances, and impaired concentration, whose persistence often results in overt depression. Symptoms that include sleep alterations, anhedonia, fatigue, alterations in eating behaviours, and loss of social relationship interests have been noted in overt clinical depression and the neuropsychiatric consequences of systematic infection, even as pessimism, worthlessness, and hopelessness are representative of aspects that are typical of major depression (Daly et al. 2022). Such symptoms are widespread among patients who needed intensive care services following the severe effects of the COVID-19 virus.

## 11.5 DEEP LEARNING

Deep learning (DL) refers to a machine learning subset that is basically a neural network with three layers or more. Such neural networks make attempts towards simulating human brain behaviour, although far from matching its aptitude, and enabling it to effectively learn by drawing from a larger pool of data (Shrestha and Mahmood 2019). Even though a neural network comprising a single layer is capable of making approximate forecasts, additional concealed layers might assist in optimizing and refining for precision. In this regard, DL in its simplest form is perceived as a means of automating the predictive analytics. Despite the conventional machine learning algorithms being linear, in DL the algorithms have been stacked in a certain order of abstraction and in increasing intricacy.

Further, DL drives several different types of artificial intelligence services and applications known to enhance automation, carrying out physical and analytical tasks devoid of human intervention. As a technology, DL underlies daily services and products, including credit card fraud detection, voice-enabled television remote and digital assistants, along with emergent technologies that include self-driving automobiles (Wang et al. 2019). DL also remains a vital aspect of data science that includes predictive modelling and statistics. It is also immensely advantageous to data scientists tasked with the collection, analysis, and interpretation of immense quantities of data, as DL makes the process easy and fast.

## 11.6 APPLICATIONS OF DEEP LEARNING IN THE CLASSIFICATION OF PSYCHIATRIC DISORDERS

Over time, DL algorithms have realized significant success with regard to data analysis tasks, attributable to their aptitude to disclose intricate data patterns. Further, with the advancement of novel sensors, processing hardware, and data storage, DL algorithms have begun dominating different fields, including the field of neuropsychiatry (Vieira et al. 2017). Several kinds of DL algorithms exist for divergent types of data ranging from survey data to the imaging scans derived from functional magnetic resonance. Owing to the observed limitations with regard to the diagnosis and estimation prognosis, as well as the treatment response in relation to neuropsychiatric disorders, DL has become an increasingly promising approach. Thus, DL has been used extensively in neuroimaging data with the objective of identifying patients with neurological and psychiatric disorders.

Normally, the neuropsychiatric disorder diagnosis is conducted using behavioural criteria that have made the diagnosis increasingly challenging. In this regard, the main objective of biomarkers like neuroimaging is required, and upon being coupled with DL, may aid in diagnostic decisions and increase its dependability (Oh et al. 2020). Hence, the vital divergence between DL and machine learning methods entails the observation that DL allows learning permits the learning of optimal feature representations based on the raw data, thereby eliminating the requirement for classical machine learning methods (Craik et al. 2019). The outcomes include increasingly objective and non-biased DL processes. Reviews conducted in 2017 indicated that DL techniques were effective when applied in the neuroimaging and categorization of Alzheimer's disease, ADHD, and in the prediction of disease conversions.

Accordingly, DL has indicated conclusive initial results with regard to the categorization of psychiatric disorders. However, much research has focused on the diagnosis of ADHD and dementia, possibly as a result of increased access to a larger number of publicly accessible datasets on neuroimaging. Based on such datasets and mental illnesses, a balance precision level that is above 90% has been realized, even as a limited number of the studies have examined the aptitude to offer predictions regarding disease trajectories, including the alteration from mild cognitive impairment to Alzheimer's disease that is vital to the detection of that mental illness at the initial stage and to the prevention of its progression (Vázquez-Abad et al. 2020). Studies are accumulating that have utilized DL and neuroimaging to categorize other mental illnesses that include autism, schizophrenia, depression, Parkinson's disease, epilepsy, and substance abuse disorders.

### 11.6.1 Schizophrenia

Schizophrenia is a severe mental disorder with no known aetiology and several divergent symptoms, including disorganized behaviour and speech, and visual and auditory hallucinations. Schizophrenia might also result in cognitive impairment in patients during the illness. Given the lack of specific symptoms and clinical tests for the condition, early interventions and diagnosis of the condition is difficult. Regarding its prevalence, schizophrenia occurs globally and affects approximately 1% of the global population, which is nearly 111.5 per 10,000 individuals (Srinivasagopalan et al. 2019). In the United States, the condition affects nearly 2.6 million individuals over 18 years. Moreover, regarding DL's role in schizophrenia, it can be noted that even though there are distinct structural abnormalities in patients suffering from the illness, detection of it using MRI is a challenge. However, trained DL algorithms have been used in diagnosing schizophrenia through the application of MRI datasets. Recent studies have indicated that DL algorithms presented better performance in detection and diagnosis as it enabled the identification of pertinent structural aspects from the MRI data drawn from the structural brain. Thus, DL algorithms had an acceptable categorization performance in distinct patient groups at the disease's initial stages. DL has, therefore, been used in the delineation of schizophrenia's structural attributes and in offering supplementary diagnostic data in clinical contexts.

### 11.6.2 ADHD

ADHD refers to the neurodevelopmental disorder typified by impulsivity, hyper-activity, and age-inappropriate inattention. The severity of ADHD is mainly evaluated as mild, moderate, and severe, depending on the number of symptoms and their severity based on DSM-5 criteria. ADHD has an approximated global prevalence rate of 5% of the population. Owing to its pathological mechanism's complexities, diagnostic methods have not been developed to this day. As such, imaging parameters have been used in the diagnosis, as they offer an important objective adjunct to the clinical psychiatric assessment.

DL plays an important role in the diagnosis of ADHD, especially in children. For instance, aptly and fully connected deep neural networks have been used in functional connectivity for the identification of children suffering from ADHD. The use of DL networks in diagnosing has been observed to have an accuracy rate of 90%, with ADHD discrimination among patients happening in the brain's cerebellum and frontal areas (Durstewitz et al. 2019). Despite the existence of subtle abnormalities among patients, DL has been used in the extraction of important information from the images of the brain to categorize it and distinguish the disease's subtypes.

### 11.6.3 Autism Spectrum Disorder (ASD)

ASD refers to the development disabilities that are caused by divergences within the brain. ASD severity is rated as mild, moderate, and severe, and is dependent on the level of support required. Still, in relation to the prevalence rate, the World Health Organization estimates that out of every 160 children, 1 is suffering from ASD globally (Heinsfeld et al. 2018). With regard to the role of DL to ASD, it can be noted that it is an increasingly promising tool for studying patterns across larger and more heterogeneous datasets. Thus, DL makes use of data that include personal attributes, social responsiveness scores, and intelligence quotients in the diagnosis of ASD, where the DL algorithms classify brain image data more, compared to some of the existing methods. The DL algorithms make use of intricate data while also depending on minimal intervention from humans for drawing pertinent aspects through the use of learning methods that are unsupervised. The classification of clinical populations through the use of DL and the unsupervised methods enables exploratory searching for neural patterns related to ASD that are less reliant on the generation of hypotheses for feature selection.

## 11.7 RECENT ADVANCES OF DEEP LEARNING IN PSYCHIATRIC DISORDERS

DL is a machine learning subset that has been extensively applied in the fields of academia and breaking benchmark records in the fields of language processing and visual recognition. Divergent from the traditional machine learning algorithm, DL has the ability to learn important features and representations directly from the raw data using nonlinear hierarchical transformations (Chen et al. 2020). Owing to the ability to detect complex and abstract patterns, DL is increasingly being used in neuroimaging research on psychiatric disorders that are marked by diffuse and subtle alterations. Recent reviews of advances in DL have disclosed three distinct advancements that are currently being used in the neuroimaging of various psychiatric and mental health disorders.

Firstly, the development of an autoencoder is considered a major advancement in the field of DL and machine learning. Owing to the intrinsic high dimensional nature of brain image data, a feature simplification approach is necessary prior to model training, which is the important function of the autoencoder. The autoencoder refers to a certain deep neural network comprising two key components, including the encoder that learns to produce low-dimensional original input representation, and the encoder that learns to utilize the low-dimensional representations in the reconstruction of data in close proximity to the original input. The training process entails the extraction of important features. Through the loss function variations, the autoencoder variants may be acquired through the alteration of loss functions, typically denoising autoencoders and sparse autoencoders.

The other key advancement in DL entails the development of the deep belief networks, which are among the models that have successfully resolved optimization challenges in relation to deep neural networks (Zhang et al. 2021). The shallower neural networks, often referred to as the Restricted Boltzmann Machine (RBM), are the deep belief network (DBN) building blocks. An RBM comprises a concealed layer and visible layer, with apt connections between the different layers but none between the layers' nodes. Further, the concealed layer is trained to enable it to capture stochastic representations found in the visible layer. The concatenation of different RBMs occur to enable the development of a DBN, in which the previous RBM's concealed layer becomes the subsequent RBM's visible layer, while the previous RBM's output is the next RBM's input. The successful completion of the layer trainings results in the fine-tuning of the model through back propagation training.

Lastly, the other advancement in DL concerns the development and use of convolutional neural networks. The initial deep neural networks are not effective at tackling vision and image related tasks, given that spatial data is likely to get lost as a result of the image being stretched into vectors, even as several parameters are challenging and inefficient to train (Gehrmann et al. 2018). The convolutional neural networks are inspired by the human visual nervous system, and have been suggested as appropriate for various vison-linked learning tasks. Thus, in the convolutional layer, the different convolutional kernels function like visual neurons and sequentially slide across the images in response to their restricted areas. Several convolution kernels are used concurrently to see the distinct kinds of information related to the image.

## 11.8 PRECISION THERAPEUTICS BY MACHINE LEARNING

The intricacies related to social and environmental dynamics have made it challenging to identify optimal behaviours within real world contexts. In such instances, decision-making entails the use of diverse parts of the brain alongside circuits exacerbated in several psychiatric and neurological disorders (Komatsu et al. 2021). Comprehending the decision-making process is important in the development of apt machine learning tools needed for precision psychiatry. Flaws in the decision-making process have been noted in some of the key psychiatric disorders, and have resulted in poor real-life mental health outcomes. For instance, flaws in decision-making with regard to psychiatric disorders are due to abnormalities in the basic neuropsychological procedures, including reward processing, attention impairment, working memory, and associative learning (Mahmud et al. 2018). Flaws in the decision-making process have also been noted to contributed to various abnormal behaviours that include medication non-adherence, failure to exercise, and poor dieting, which might, in turn, lead to worsening of symptoms, reduction in life contentment levels, impaired daily functioning, and rehospitalization and relapse, among others.

To eliminate the flaws in decision-making, particularly with regard to the prediction, diagnosis, and treatment of mental disorders, machine learning has become increasingly handy. For instance, machine learning methods offer a tool set developed to enable the achievement of precise clinical predictions at a personal level. The predictive models are theoretically located between the genetic susceptibility and an individual's clinical symptoms along with his or her behavioural displays. The use of different endophenotypes presents translational potential in the refinement of clinical management through timely diagnosis, illness stratification, better selection of treatments and medications, and psychiatric care prognosis (Naylor 2018). Still, the various machine learning models have been observed to have a long-lasting concentration on predictions as a statistical quality metric, and have the ability to predict outcomes based on single observations, including the neural, genetic, and behavioural assessment of the person. Furthermore, recent machine learning methodologies have disclosed significant correlations between the functional striatal abnormalities and the severity spectrum across various psychiatric conditions, with dysfunction being more severe in schizophrenia, indistinguishable in ADHD, obsessive-compulsive disorders, and depression, and mild in bipolar disorder.

## 11.9 DEEP LEARNING IN MENTAL HEALTH OUTCOME RESEARCH

As one of the recent artificial intelligence technologies, DL has shown superior performance in several real world usages that include healthcare. DL approaches are aimed at developing mechanisms capable of mapping the input raw aspects directly into outputs using multiple-layer network structures capable of capturing the data's hidden patterns (Miotto et al. 2018). Moreover, as a recent advancement in machine learning and artificial intelligence, the DL that transforms data using layers of computational processing units that are nonlinear offer novel paradigms to efficiently acquire important knowledge from intricate data. In recent times, DL algorithms have indicated superior performance in several data-rich app scenarios that include mental healthcare. In one recent study, the emergent application areas of DL methods in psychiatry focused on subject behaviour and brain dynamics, as well as the embedding of interpretable computational models within statistical settings. (Purushotham et al. 2018). The study's objective was aimed at offering a scope evaluation of extant research, utilizing DL techniques in analysing divergent kinds of data linked to different mental health conditions.

While artificial intelligence becomes increasingly applied in psychiatric research, DL as a facet of artificial intelligence is sparking more interest. DL entails the development of models and algorithms capable of automatically capturing concealed data patterns followed by the development of end-to-end techniques for directly mapping the input data to the outcomes (Shatte et al. 2019). The neural networks and data models are created to enable the analysis of the sequential data, genetic and clinical data, and images. In one piece of recent research, 57 journal-published research articles describing studies founded on DL techniques were analysed (de Bardeci et al. 2021). The researchers disclosed that numerous studies utilized DL in the study of neuroimages that were drawn from functional and structural MRI data. The studies analysed generated data that helped in advancing the comprehension of brain activities related to depression and schizophrenia. Other studies reviewed concentrated on the application of DL for the analysis of the raw electroencephalogram (EEG) signal data. The researchers disclosed that temporal and spectral information pertaining to EEG were vital for effectual depression prediction (Sui et al. 2020). The researchers disclosed that DL had the ability to enhance the predictability of antidepressant and suicide responses. DL was also observed to facilitate genetic data evaluation, and this was attributed to the huge amount of data volumes drawn from the human genome work that is currently accessible. Other notable studies evaluated electronic health records with the objective of studying the different kinds of mental health disorders. The novel DL models were observed to enable the scientists to evaluate the visual and vocal expressions as a mean of estimating mental stress and forecasting various mental health matters (Menke 2018) Further, the social media data analysis that uses DL has concentrated mainly on the detection of stress, thereby identifying depression, and aptly approximating the suicide risks.

## 11.10 LIMITATIONS AND CHALLENGES OF DEEP LEARNING

The notable limitations and challenges of DL concerns the smaller sample size alongside the risk of overfitting. Thus, the various DL models have several millions of weights that have to be learned in the course of the training stage and, therefore, require increased quantities of samples to enable the learning of intricate patterns in comparison to the conventional machine learning techniques. However, it still remains inconclusive as to whether the number of samples are meaningful for DL in relation to neuroimaging researches, and this can be attributed to a restricted number of studies presently available. In instances where a deep network has been trained on a limited number of samples, particularly high dimensional image data, it is feasible that the model (trained) will work excellently on the training set but also perform poorly during the test set, a challenge referred to as overfitting (Stead 2018).

Consequently, the other limitation and challenge of DL concerns the dearth of data acquisition standardization and the uneven quality of data. A larger proportion of existent studies have utilized datasets that are publicly available, including ADHD-200 and ADIBE. Despite the datasets being comparatively larger, the data remain heterogeneous given that they are drawn from different sites that have dissimilar field strengths, imaging sequences, and coil configurations. It has also been shown that the machine learning models' performance can be impacted by different imaging parameters. Furthermore, the widely used echo planar imaging (EPI) sequences that are widely employed in functional MRI and diffusion are increasingly sensitive to inhomogeneity in addition to being increasingly vulnerable to signal loss and image distortion at the air and tissue junctions, including the temporal and frontal lobes, which form the main areas of the brain where psychiatric studies tend to concentrate (Ewbank et al. 2020). Despite the proposal of several correction techniques within the medical imaging and MR physics fields, the requirement for extra scans and intricate calculations have hindered the wider application of such corrective methodologies in clinical studies.

## 11.11 CONCLUSION

The increased prevalence of psychiatric disorders and the requirement for effectual mental health treatment and care, coupled with the advancements in artificial intelligence, has resulted in increased exploration of the field of machine learning, and particularly DL. Most studies have focused on how

DL can be used in the diagnosis, detection, treatment, and prediction of mental disorders. As noted in this chapter, DL has the potential to provide novel routes for human behaviour learning patterns; the detection of the symptoms of mental disorders alongside the risk factors; the prediction of illness progression, as well as the optimization and customization of treatments. Regardless of the several opportunities for DL application in the field of mental health, it is an emergent research field, and the creation of effectual DL-enabled and practice implementable apps is faced with several intricate challenges. Still, given that the DL field in relation to mental health is currently in the infant stages, caution is recommended in presenting DL development to avert premature assertions on the probable significance and impacts of the novel models. The recommendation is vital if one considers the intricacy and challenges faced in the generation of robust and clinically dependable DL outputs. To this end, a larger proportion of the existing models have been infrequently tested in clinical contexts, which leaves a gap in the evaluation of their practicalities and efficiency with regard to the enhancement of mental health treatments and outcomes. Nevertheless, the future holds more promises as an increased amount of work is currently being done to tackle various open issues and ascertain that the science moves forward.

## 11.12 SUMMARY

In summary, mental illness has been defined by the World Health Organization as an array of mental health disorders and conditions affecting an individual's thinking, behaviour, emotions, mood, and physical health. Mental illnesses are linked to distress and challenge functionality within work, family, and social contexts. Mental illnesses have been categorized using two systems, namely the ICD-10 and DSM-5. The systems list mental disorder categories that are distinct and they converge their distinctive codes for the comparability of the manuals, despite the existence of considerable differences. Among the notable categories of mental illnesses are included cognitive disorders, which refer to a class of mental illnesses primarily affecting the cognitive aptitudes that include memory, learning, problem solving, and perception. Substance-abuse-related disorders refer to the addictive problems affecting persons who are highly predisposed to develop such mental disorders. Substance abuse induces symptomatology that resembles mental illness, and is noticeable during intoxication and withdrawal. The other class of mental illnesses is psychosis, which refers to the abnormal mind condition that leads to challenges in establishing what may be real and what might not be real. Psychosis is mainly marked by symptoms like hallucinations, delusions, and incoherent behaviour. Further, mood disorders are another category of mental illnesses and entail a set of mental and behavioural conditions marked by a disturbance in mood. Other notable categories of mental disorders include anxiety and eating disorders.

To effectively diagnose, treat, and manage mental disorders, DL has been developed and widely used. DL implies a machine learning subset that is basically a neural network with three layers or more, which make attempts at simulating human brain behaviour, although far from matching its aptitude, enabling it to effectively learn by drawing from a larger pool of data. The advancement of novel sensors, processing hardware and data storage, has enabled the usage of DL algorithms in neuropsychiatry. Therefore, DL has been used extensively in the neuroimaging data with the objective of identifying patients with neurological and psychiatric disorders. For instance, DL has been used in the delineation of schizophrenia's structural attributes and offering supplementary diagnostic data in clinical contexts. DL has also been used in the diagnosis of ADHD in children, especially in the identification of children suffering from it. Consequently, in ASD, DL has been used as a tool for studying patterns across larger and heterogeneous datasets in ASD studies.

Several advancements have been made with regard to DL algorithms and their usage. Among the recent advancements include the development of an autoencoder, which refers to a deep neural network with two components, the encoder producing low-dimensional original input representation, and an encoder that utilizes low-dimensional representations in the reconstruction of data in close proximity to the original input. The other advancement in DL entails the deep belief networks.

These are among the models that have successfully resolved optimization challenges in relation to deep neural networks.

Nevertheless, regardless of the increased usage in the diagnosis, treatment, and management of mental disorders, DL has certain limitations, including the risks of smaller sample size and overfitting. Thus, DL models comprise millions of weights to be learned during the training stage, which requires increased quantities of samples for the learning of intricate patterns. The other limitation of DL concerns the lack of data acquisition standardization and the uneven quality of data.

## ACKNOWLEDGEMENT

We would like to thank the Institute of Medical Science, BHU for their infrastructural and technical support.

## REFERENCES

Al-Rousan, Tala, Linda Rubenstein, Bruce Sieleni, Harbans Deol, and Robert B. Wallace. "Inside the nation's largest mental health institution: A prevalence study in a state prison system." *BMC Public Health* 17, no. 1 (2017): 1–9.

Bernardini, Francesco, Luigi Attademo, Sean D. Cleary, Charles Luther, Ruth S. Shim, Roberto Quartesan, and Michael T. Compton. "Risk prediction models in psychiatry: toward a new frontier for the prevention of mental illnesses." *The Journal of Clinical Psychiatry* 78, no. 5 (2017): 18451.

Boldrini, Maura, Peter D. Canoll, and Robyn S. Klein. "How COVID-19 affects the brain." *JAMA Psychiatry* 78, no. 6 (2021): 682–683.

Bzdok, Danilo, and Andreas Meyer-Lindenberg. "Machine learning for precision psychiatry: opportunities and challenges." *Biological Psychiatry: Cognitive Neuroscience and Neuroimaging* 3, no. 3 (2018): 223–230.

Chen, Lu, Chunchao Xia, and Huaiqiang Sun. "Recent advances of deep learning in psychiatric disorders." *Precision Clinical Medicine* 3, no. 3 (2020): 202–213.

Craik, Alexander, Yongtian He, and Jose L. Contreras-Vidal. "Deep learning for electroencephalogram (EEG) classification tasks: a review." *Journal of Neural Engineering* 16, no. 3 (2019): 031001.

Daly, Michael, Angelina R. Sutin, and Eric Robinson. "Longitudinal changes in mental health and the COVID-19 pandemic: Evidence from the UK Household Longitudinal Study." *Psychological Medicine* 52, no. 13 (2022): 2549–2558.

de Bardeci, M., Ip, C. T., and Olbrich, S. "Deep learning applied to electroencephalogram data in mental disorders: a systematic review." *Biological Psychology* 108117 (2021).

Durstewitz, Daniel, Georgia Koppe, and Andreas Meyer-Lindenberg. "Deep neural networks in psychiatry." *Molecular Psychiatry* 24, no. 11 (2019): 1583–1598.

Ekhtiari, Hamed, Mehran Zare-Bidoky, and Antonio Verdejo-Garcia. "Neurocognitive disorders in substance use disorders." In *Textbook of Addiction Treatment*, pp. 1159–1176. Springer, Cham, 2021.

Ewbank, Michael P., Ronan Cummins, Valentin Tablan, Sarah Bateup, Ana Catarino, Alan J. Martin, and Andrew D. Blackwell. "Quantifying the association between psychotherapy content and clinical outcomes using deep learning." *JAMA Psychiatry* 77, no. 1 (2020): 35–43.

Fiorillo, Andrea, and Philip Gorwood. "The consequences of the COVID-19 pandemic on mental health and implications for clinical practice." *European Psychiatry* 63, no. 1 (2020).

Gehrmann, Sebastian, Franck Dernoncourt, Yeran Li, Eric T. Carlson, Joy T. Wu, Jonathan Welt, John Foote Jr et al. "Comparing deep learning and concept extraction based methods for patient phenotyping from clinical narratives." *PloS one* 13, no. 2 (2018): e0192360.

Gkotsis, George, Anika Oellrich, Sumithra Velupillai, Maria Liakata, Tim J.P. Hubbard, Richard J.B. Dobson, and Rina Dutta. "Corrigendum: Characterisation of mental health conditions in social media using Informed Deep Learning." *Scientific Reports* 7 (2017).

Graham, Sarah, Colin Depp, Ellen E. Lee, Camille Nebeker, Xin Tu, Ho-Cheol Kim, and Dilip V. Jeste. "Artificial intelligence for mental health and mental illnesses: an overview." *Current Psychiatry Reports* 21, no. 11 (2019): 1–18.

Heinsfeld, Anibal Sólon, Alexandre Rosa Franco, R. Cameron Craddock, Augusto Buchweitz, and Felipe Meneguzzi. "Identification of autism spectrum disorder using deep learning and the ABIDE dataset." *NeuroImage: Clinical* 17 (2018): 16–23.

Horenstein, Arielle, and Richard G. Heimberg. "Anxiety disorders and healthcare utilization: A systematic review." *Clinical Psychology Review* 81 (2020): 101894.
Insel, Thomas R. "Digital phenotyping: a global tool for psychiatry." *World Psychiatry* 17, no. 3 (2018): 276.
Khademi, Mojgan, Roya Vaziri-Harami, and Jamal Shams. "Prevalence of mental health problems and its associated factors among recovered COVID-19 patients during the pandemic: a single-center study." *Frontiers in Psychiatry* 12 (2021): 602244.
Komatsu, Hidetoshi, Emi Watanabe, and Mamoru Fukuchi. "Psychiatric neural networks and precision therapeutics by machine learning." *Biomedicines* 9, no. 4 (2021): 403.
Mahmud, Mufti, Mohammed Shamim Kaiser, Amir Hussain, and Stefano Vassanelli. "Applications of deep learning and reinforcement learning to biological data." *IEEE Transactions on Neural Networks and Learning Systems* 29, no. 6 (2018): 2063–2079.
Martland, Rebecca, Valeria Mondelli, Fiona Gaughran, and Brendon Stubbs. "Can high intensity interval training improve health outcomes among people with mental illness? A systematic review and preliminary meta-analysis of intervention studies across a range of mental illnesses." *Journal of Affective Disorders* 263 (2020): 629–660.
Maziade, Michel. "At risk for serious mental illness–screening children of patients with mood disorders or schizophrenia." *The New England Journal of Medicine* 376, no. 10 (2017): 910–912.
Menke, Andreas. "Precision pharmacotherapy: psychiatry's future direction in preventing, diagnosing, and treating mental disorders." *Pharmacogenomics and Personalized Medicine* 11 (2018): 211.
Miotto, Riccardo, Fei Wang, Shuang Wang, Xiaoqian Jiang, and Joel T. Dudley. "Deep learning for healthcare: review, opportunities and challenges." *Briefings in Bioinformatics* 19, no. 6 (2018): 1236–1246.
Naylor, C. David. "On the prospects for a (deep) learning health care system." *JAMA* 320, no. 11 (2018): 1099–1100.
Oh, Shu Lih, Yuki Hagiwara, U. Raghavendra, Rajamanickam Yuvaraj, N. Arunkumar, M. Murugappan, and U. Rajendra Acharya. "A deep learning approach for Parkinson's disease diagnosis from EEG signals." *Neural Computing and Applications* 32, no. 15 (2020): 10927–10933.
Potes, Angela, Gabriel Souza, Katerina Nikolitch, Romeo Penheiro, Yara Moussa, Eric Jarvis, Karl Looper, and Soham Rej. "Mindfulness in severe and persistent mental illness: A systematic review." *International Journal of Psychiatry in Clinical Practice* 22, no. 4 (2018): 253–261.
Purushotham, Sanjay, Chuizheng Meng, Zhengping Che, and Yan Liu. "Benchmarking deep learning models on large healthcare datasets." *Journal of Biomedical Informatics* 83 (2018): 112–134.
Quaak, Mirjam, Laurens van de Mortel, Rajat Mani Thomas, and Guido van Wingen. "Deep learning applications for the classification of psychiatric disorders using neuroimaging data: systematic review and meta-analysis." *NeuroImage: Clinical* 30 (2021): 102584.
Rowe, Elizabeth. "Early detection of eating disorders in general practice." *Australian Family Physician* 46, no. 11 (2017): 833–838.
Sagar, Rajesh, Rakhi Dandona, Gopalkrishna Gururaj, R.S. Dhaliwal, Aditya Singh, Alize Ferrari, Tarun Dua, et al. "India state-level disease burden initiative mental disorders collaborators. The burden of mental disorders across the states of India: the Global burden of disease study 1990-2017." *Lancet Psychiatry* 7, no. 2 (2020): 148–161. doi: 10.1016/S2215-0366(19)30475-4
Shatte, A. B., D. M. Hutchinson, and S. J. Teague. Machine learning in mental health: a scoping review of methods and applications. *Psychological Medicine* 49 (2019): 1426–1448.
Shrestha, Ajay, and Ausif Mahmood. "Review of deep learning algorithms and architectures." *IEEE Access* 7 (2019): 53040–53065.
Singh, Gagandeep, Meenakshi Sharma, G. Anil Kumar, N. Girish Rao, Kameshwar Prasad, Prashant Mathur, Jeyaraj D. Pandian et al. "The burden of neurological disorders across the states of India: the Global Burden of Disease Study 1990–2019." *The Lancet Global Health* 9, no. 8 (2021): e1129–e1144.
Srinivasagopalan, Srivathsan, Justin Barry, Varadraj Gurupur, and Sharma Thankachan. "A deep learning approach for diagnosing schizophrenic patients." *Journal of Experimental & Theoretical Artificial Intelligence* 31, no. 6 (2019): 803–816.
Stead, William W. "Clinical implications and challenges of artificial intelligence and deep learning." *JAMA* 320, no. 11 (2018): 1107–1108.
Su, Chang, Zhenxing Xu, Jyotishman Pathak, and Fei Wang. "Deep learning in mental health outcome research: a scoping review." *Translational Psychiatry* 10, no. 1 (2020): 1–26.
Sui, Jing, Rongtao Jiang, Juan Bustillo, and Vince Calhoun. "Neuroimaging-based Individualized Prediction of Cognition and Behavior for Mental Disorders and Health: Methods and Promises." *Biological Psychiatry* 88, no. 11 (2020): 818–828.

Thapa, Suraj B., Anustha Mainali, Simone E. Schwank, and Ganesh Acharya. "Maternal mental health in the time of the COVID-19 pandemic." *Acta obstetricia et gynecologica Scandinavica* 99, no. 7 (2020): 817–818.

Trofimova, Irina, and William Sulis. "There is more to mental illness than negative affect: comprehensive temperament profiles in depression and generalized anxiety." *BMC Psychiatry* 18, no. 1 (2018): 1–17.

Vázquez-Abad, Felisa J., Silvano Bernabel, Daniel Dufresne, Rishi Sood, Thomas Ward, and Daniel Amen. "Deep learning for mental illness detection using brain SPECT imaging." In *International Conference on Medical Imaging and Computer-Aided Diagnosis*, pp. 17–26. Springer, Singapore, 2020.

Vieira, Sandra, Walter H.L. Pinaya, and Andrea Mechelli. "Using deep learning to investigate the neuroimaging correlates of psychiatric and neurological disorders: Methods and applications." *Neuroscience & Biobehavioral Reviews* 74 (2017): 58–75.

Wang, Shidan, Donghan M. Yang, Ruichen Rong, Xiaowei Zhan, and Guanghua Xiao. "Pathology image analysis using segmentation deep learning algorithms." *The American Journal of Pathology* 189, no. 9 (2019): 1686–1698.

Yochim, Brian P., and Benjamin T. Mast. "Psychological assessment of neurocognitive disorders." In *Handbook of the psychology of aging*, pp. 251–262. Academic Press, 2021.

Zhang, Xiang, Lina Yao, Xianzhi Wang, Jessica Monaghan, David Mcalpine, and Yu Zhang. "A survey on deep learning-based non-invasive brain signals: recent advances and new frontiers." *Journal of Neural Engineering* 18, no. 3 (2021): 031002.

# Index

Pages in *italics* refer to figures.


**A**

ACE, 38–39, 49
AD, 13, 60, 64, 68
ADEM, 13–15, 26–27
ADHD, 15–16, 174, 177, 179–183
ADL, 45, 49
advantages, 37–40, 45–46
ALS, 58, 61–62
analyte, 113
antenna, 150–151, 153–157
antibody, 116
anxiety, 174, 176–177, 183
AR, 48–49
artefacts, 59, 65–67
artificial intelligence, 112
ASD, 60, 180, 183

**B**

battery, 40–43
biosensors, 113–118, 138–139, 141, 155–156
Bipolar Junction Transistors (BJTs), 78
body sensor networks, 93
bradykinesia, 106
brainstem, 4

**C**

CAD, 56, 60
calibration, 117
cardiovascular disease, 138–140
cerebral cortex, 2
cerebrum, 2
charged-coupled device, 159
cognition, 175
cognitive disorders, 10, 36
cognitive impairment, 10, 21–25
common collector (CC), 80
convolutional neural network (CNN), 102
Covid-19, 177–178

**D**

DALY, 56
deep belief network, 180, 183
deep learning, 174, 178, 180–182
dementia, 16, 19–20, 25
dendrite, 1–2
diagnosis, 10–13, 16, 20–25, 27
digit verbal span task, 159
disadvantages, 37–40, 46
DLB, 11–13
DSM-5, 10, 175, 179, 183
DTI, 64–65

**E**

eating disorder, 176–177, 183
ECG, *see* electrocardiograms
EEG, *see* electroencephalography/electroencephalograms
electrocardiograms (ECGs), 56–58, 63, 65–68, 96
electroencephalography/electroencephalograms (EEG), 56, 58–59, 64–68, 96, 139, 159
electromyography (EMG), 61–62, 66–68, 96
EMG, *see* electromyography
epidemiology, 11, 13, 19, 21, 24, 26
epilepsy, 21–22, 56, 60, 63–65
evaluation, 36–38, 40, 42–43, 46

**F**

Field Effect Transistor (FET), 75, 84
Fin Field Effect Transistor (FinFET), 90
focal seizure, 94
frontal lobe, 2
FTD, 19–20

**G**

GPCOG, 39, 49

**H**

Healthcare Wearable Devices (HWDs), 67–68, 140–143, 145
Hilbert–Huang transform (HHT), 99
HRV, 62–63, 68
HWDs, *see* Healthcare Wearable Devices
hypothalamus, 3

**I**

implantable pulse generator (IPG), 75
Internet of Things (IoT), 67, 121, 138–140, 145–146, 154–157
IoT, *see* Internet of Things

**K**

k-nearest neighbors (kNN), 165

**L**

LBD, 10–13

**M**

MAR, 48
MCI, *see* mild cognitive impairment
MEG, 63–65, 68
memory, 37, 40–45, 47, 49
mental health, 174–175, 177, 180–184
mental illness, 174–177, 179, 183
Metal Oxide Semiconductor Field Effect Transistor (MOSFET), 86
mild cognitive impairment (MCI), 41, 161
mini-mental state examination (MMSE), 36–41, 44–46, 49, 162
mobile cloud computing (MCC), 93
MoCA, 40
mood disorders, 176–178, 183
MR, 36, 48–49
MRI, 36
muscular dystrophy, 62

**N**

NCDs, *see* neurocognitive disorders
neurocognitive disorders (NCDs), 36–40, 43–49, 175
neurological diseases, 56, 59, 63–64
neuron, *1*
neuropsychiatric, 177–178

**O**

occipital lobe, 3
one-class classification (OCC), 166
optical spectroscopy, 158

**P**

parietal lobe, 2
pathogenesis, 11, 13, 16, 21
pathway, 23–24, 26
PCA, 23
PD, 23–25, 57, 59, 61, 63
PET, *see* positron emission tomography
photoplethysmography, 95
point-of-care, 119
positron emission tomography (PET), 64, 158
post-Covid 19, 177–178
prion disease, 10, 23
psychosis, 20, 26, 175–176, 183
pulse width modulation, 80

**R**

real-time monitoring, 121
restricted boltzmann machine, 180

**S**

schizophrenia, 174–176, 179, 181–183
SCI, 62
substance-abuse-related disorders, 175, 183
supervised machine learning, 114
symptoms, 10–12, 14–24, 26–27

**T**

TBI, 65
test, 39–47, 49
therapy, 46–49
transducer, 112
tremors, 106
triaxial accelerometer (ACM), 96

**V**

VR, 43–49

**W**

wearable biosensor, 138–139, 156
wearable sensors, 139, 156

www.ingramcontent.com/pod-product-compliance
Ingram Content Group UK Ltd.
Pitfield, Milton Keynes, MK11 3LW, UK
UKHW050058200926
475702UK00019B/2905
* 9 7 8 1 0 3 2 1 5 6 8 7 3 *